ADVANCES IN

Anesthesia

Editor-in-Chief
Thomas M. McLoughlin, MD

ELSEVIER
An Imprint of Elsevier, Inc.
PHILADELPHIA LONDON TORONTO MONTREAL SYDNEY TOKYO

ADVANCES IN
Anesthesia

VOLUMES 1 THROUGH 28 (OUT OF PRINT)

VOLUME 29

VOLUME 30

VOLUME 31

VP Global Medical Reference: Mary E. Gatsch
Editor: Jennifer Flynn-Briggs

Editorial Office:
Elsevier
1600 John F. Kennedy Blvd,
Suite 1800
Philadelphia, PA 19103-2899

International Standard Serial Number: 0737-6146
International Standard Book Number-13: 978-0-323-26459-4

ADVANCES IN
Anesthesia

Editors

THOMAS M. MCLOUGHLIN

FRANCIS V. SALINAS

LAURENCE TORSHER

Editor-in-Chief

THOMAS M. MCLOUGHLIN, MD, Chair, Department of Anesthesiology, Lehigh Valley Health Network, Allentown, PA; and Professor of Surgery, Division of Surgical Anesthesiology, University of South Florida College of Medicine, Tampa, Florida

Associate Editors

FRANCIS V. SALINAS, MD, Deputy Chief of Anesthesia; Section Head of Orthopedic Anesthesia; and Coordinator of Ultrasound-Guided Regional Anesthesia Education, Virginia Mason Medical Center Department of Anesthesiology, Seattle, Washington

LAURENCE TORSHER, MD Assistant Professor of Anesthesiology, Mayo Clinic, Rochester, Minnesota

CONTRIBUTORS

BASEM ABDELMALAK, MD, Associate Professor of Anesthesiology, Department of General Anesthesiology, Cleveland Clinic Lerner College of Medicine of Case Western Reserve University; Director, Anesthesia for Bronchoscopic Surgery, Departments of General Anesthesiology and Outcomes Research, Anesthesiology Institute, Cleveland Clinic, Cleveland, Ohio

SHEILA RYAN BARNETT, MD, Associate Professor Anesthesiology, Beth Israel Deaconess of Medical Center, Harvard Medical School, Boston, Massachusetts

J. KYLE BOHMAN, MD, Instructor, Division of Critical Care Medicine, Department of Anesthesiology, Mayo Clinic, Rochester, Minnesota

DANIEL R. BROWN, MD, PhD, FCCM, Division of Anesthesiology Critical Care, Department of Anesthesiology, Mayo Clinic, Rochester, Minnesota

KI JINN CHIN, MBBS, MMed, FANZCA, FRCPC, Associate Professor, Department of Anesthesia, Toronto Western Hospital, University of Toronto, Toronto, Ontario, Canada

TIMOTHY B. CURRY, MD, PhD, Departments of Anesthesiology and Physiology and Biomedical Engineering, Mayo Clinic, Rochester, Minnesota

R. ELIOT FAGLEY, MD, Anesthesiologist and Intensivist, Virginia Mason Medical Center, Seattle, Washington

THOMAS R. GILDEA, MD, MS, Head, Section of Bronchoscopy, Staff, Department of Pulmonary, Allergy and Critical Care Medicine, Transplant Center, Respiratory Institute, Cleveland Clinic, Cleveland, Ohio

ASHANPREET S. GREWAL, MD, Assistant Professor, Division of Cardiothoracic Anesthesia, Department of Anesthesiology, University of Maryland School of Medicine, Baltimore, Maryland

ALINA M. GRIGORE, MD, MHS, Associate Professor and Director, Division of Cardiothoracic Anesthesia, Department of Anesthesiology, University of Maryland School of Medicine, Baltimore, Maryland

BRIAN M. ILFELD, MD, MS (Clinical Investigation), Professor of Anesthesiology, In Residence, Division of Regional Anesthesia and Acute Pain Medicine, Department of Anesthesiology, University of California San Diego, California

JAMES EDWARD JOHNSON, MBBS, FANZCA, Clinical Fellow (Regional Anesthesia), Department of Anesthesia, Toronto Western Hospital, University of Toronto, Toronto, Ontario, Canada

DARYL J. KOR, MD, Associate Professor, Division of Critical Care Medicine, Department of Anesthesiology, Mayo Clinic, Rochester, Minnesota

ROHINI KOTHA, MD, PGY-4 Resident, Department of Anesthesiology, University of Pittsburgh School of Medicine, Pittsburgh, Pennsylvania

WALTER MAURER, MD, Section Head, Ambulatory Anesthesia; Staff, Department of General Anesthesia, Cleveland Clinic, Cleveland, Ohio

GREGORY A. NUTTALL, MD, Department of Anesthesiology, Mayo Clinic College of Medicine, Rochester, Minnesota

WILLIAM C. OLIVER Jr, MD, Department of Anesthesiology, Mayo Clinic College of Medicine, Rochester, Minnesota

STEVEN L. OREBAUGH, MD, Professor, Department of Anesthesiology, UPMC Southside/Mercy Anesthesia, University of Pittsburgh School of Medicine, Pittsburgh, Pennsylvania

ANAHI PERLAS, MD, FRCPC, Associate Professor, Department of Anesthesia, Toronto Western Hospital, University of Toronto, Toronto, Ontario, Canada

ALBERT PIERCE, MD, Associate Professor, Head of Trauma and Acute Care Anesthesia, Department of Anesthesiology, University of Alabama at Birmingham, Birmingham, Alabama

JEAN-FRANCOIS PITTET, MD, David Chestnut Professor of Anesthesiology, Vice Chair and Director, Critical Care Division, Department of Anesthesiology, University of Alabama at Birmingham, Birmingham, Alabama

CHARANJIT S. RIHAL, MD, Department of Cardiovascular Disease, Mayo Clinic College of Medicine, Rochester, Minnesota

PHILIP E.F. ROMAN, MD, MPH, Assistant Professor, Division of Cardiothoracic Anesthesia, Department of Anesthesiology, University of Maryland School of Medicine, Baltimore, Maryland

SONALI SETHI, MD, Staff, Department of Pulmonary, Allergy and Critical Care Medicine, Respiratory Institute, Cleveland Clinic, Cleveland, Ohio

BRADLEY S. TAYLOR, MD, MPH, Associate Professor and Director of Coronary Revascularization, Division of Cardiac Surgery, Department of Surgery, University of Maryland School of Medicine, Baltimore, Maryland

JOHN E. TETZLAFF, MD, Professor of Anesthesiology; Staff, Department of General Anesthesia, Cleveland Clinic Lerner College of Medicine of Case Western Reserve University, Cleveland Clinic, Cleveland, Ohio

JOHN VARGO, MD, MPH, Associate Professor of Medicine; Chair, Department of Gastroenterology and Hepatology, Cleveland Clinic Lerner College of Medicine of Case Western Reserve University, Cleveland Clinic, Cleveland, Ohio

ADVANCES IN
Anesthesia

CONTENTS

VOLUME 32 • 2014

Advances in Anesthesia 32 (2014) xix

ADVANCES IN ANESTHESIA

Preface

Dear Readers and Colleagues,

Welcome to the 2014 edition and the 32nd year of *Advances in Anesthesia*. It is our honor to do our best to continue the tradition of this publication in our specialty, as established under the previous editorial guidance of such leaders in our field as Drs Robert Stoelting, Carol Lake, Paul Barash, and Joel Johnson.

We are guided by several priorities in working with our authors to deliver the content of this issue, and each issue, to you. First, we strive to provide balanced content across topics of the general and subspecialty practices of anesthesiology and perioperative medicine and do not assemble issues with dedicated focus to particular patient groups or surgical practices. Second, we aim to include articles that are relevant to practicing anesthesiologists; we endeavor to avoid topics of strictly academic or research interest. Third, we seek to keep the articles timely with respect to new topics or subjects in which the practice of anesthesia is seeing significant change. While not every issue can be identified to have content in every anesthesiology subspecialty, it is our editorial goal to achieve this balance over time and as we perceive important clinical developments and progress.

The editors collaborate to identify areas of recent or evolving investigational or clinical care developments in anesthesiology and perioperative medicine and then work with authors who have the expertise and ability to communicate the context and current or emerging importance of these topics to our readers. As editors, we have different and complementary geographic locations and clinical interests, but a shared mission to bring timely and valuable information to you each year. Please accept our personal invitation and hope that you will reach out to one of us with your ideas for improvement of *Advances in Anesthesia*, for either future content or contributors that would benefit our readership.

Sincerely,

Thomas M. McLoughlin Jr, MD
E-mail address: thomas.mcloughlin@lvhn.org

Francis Salinas, MD
E-mail address: francis.salinas@virginiamason.org

Laurence Torsher, MD
E-mail address: torsher.laurence@mayo.edu

0737-6146/14/$ – see front matter
http://dx.doi.org/10.1016/j.aan.2014.10.001

Advances in Anesthesia 32 (2014) 1–21

ADVANCES IN ANESTHESIA

Practical Understanding of Hemostasis and Approach to the Bleeding Patient in the Operating Room

Albert Pierce, MD[a], Jean-Francois Pittet, MD[b,*]

[a]Department of Anesthesiology, University of Alabama at Birmingham, 804 Jefferson Tower, 619 South 19th Street, Birmingham, AL 35249-6810, USA; [b]Critical Care Division, Department of Anesthesiology, University of Alabama at Birmingham, 804 Jefferson Tower, 619 South 19th Street, JT926, Birmingham, AL 35249-6810, USA

Keywords

• Bleeding • Coagulation • Coagulopathy • Trauma • Inflammation • Massive hemorrhage • Viscoelastic • Damage control resuscitation

Key points

- Coagulation and inflammation are 2 major biologic response systems following tissue trauma.
- A complex interaction between these 2 systems after severe injury may result in coagulopathy and an increased likelihood of poor outcomes.
- Improved understanding of the bleeding seen in severe trauma settings has informed our treatment of poorly controlled bleeding in the operating room.
- Massive hemorrhage is a serious and rapidly changing situation associated with significant increase in mortality rates.
- Identification of high-risk patients and procedures allows preprocedure consideration and preparation promoting good outcomes.

INTRODUCTION

Coagulation and inflammation are biologic damage-response systems activated and amplified after tissue injury. Although they were once thought to be separate and distinct processes, we now know that they are intrinsically linked and interactive systems [1].

The authors do not have any relationship with a commercial company that has a direct financial interest in the subject matter or materials discussed in the article or with a company making a competing product.
Funding Support: National Institutes of Health RO1 GM086416 (J.F. Pittet).

*Corresponding author. *E-mail address:* pittetj@uab.edu

0737-6146/14/$ – see front matter
http://dx.doi.org/10.1016/j.aan.2014.08.009

Bleeding, thrombosis, and maladaptive inflammatory responses are major causes of perioperative morbidity and mortality for trauma and "nontrauma" patients [2–4]. Thus, coagulation and inflammation warrant serious consideration by all who care for surgical patients. New information regarding care of the bleeding trauma patient have led us to revisit our core concepts of caring for other patients with massive bleeding as well.

In this article, we briefly review the different models of coagulation, discuss management of the acute coagulopathy associated with severe trauma, and relate that to the care of other bleeding patients.

CLASSICAL COAGULATION CASCADE

Observation leading to discovery

Astute physicians, noting unusual bleeding tendencies in their patients, in collaboration with brilliant scientists deduced the proteolytic activation of zymogens in plasma leading to fibrin formation. This "waterfall/cascade" described more than 50 years ago, has been the basis for testing and monitoring anticoagulant effects of various medications for decades (Fig. 1) [5].

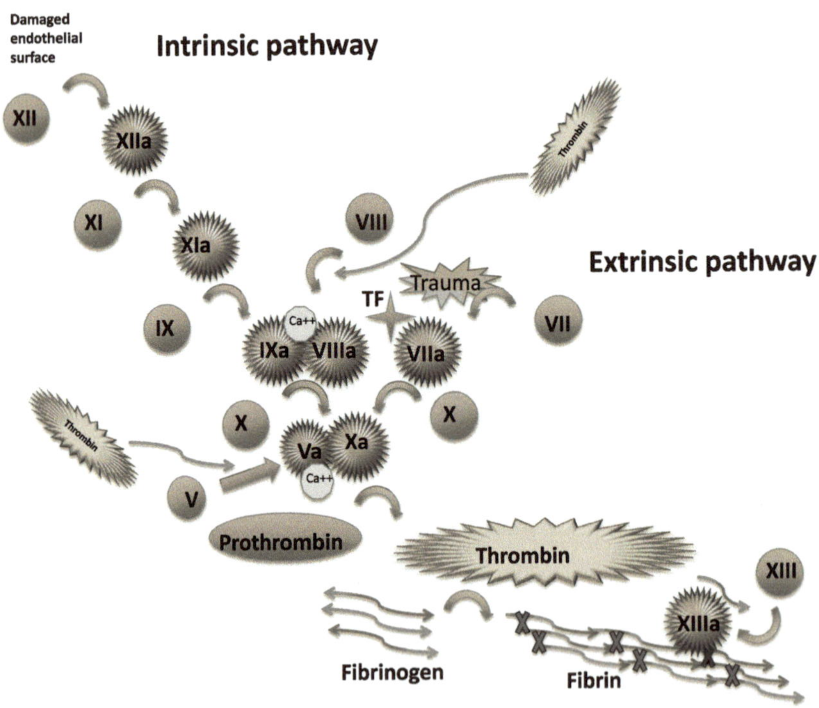

Fig. 1. Waterfall cascade, the classical description of coagulation. Roman numerals indicate the numbered coagulation factors. When followed by an "a," they represent their active forms. Ca++, calcium; TF, tissue factor.

BEYOND THE "WATERFALL/CASCADE"

Although the intrinsic and extrinsic pathways seem somewhat complex, they were never thought to be the full explanation of human hemostasis. This classical model addresses plasma and the factors within it. It does not include considerations of the dynamic cellular processes that are now known to play major roles in procoagulant and anticoagulant physiology. The newer "cellular model" takes some of these into consideration. Thrombus formation within this model is typically divided into 3 overlapping phases: initiation, amplification, and propagation (Fig. 2).

Regulation

In its normal state, blood within the circulatory system remains in a liquid state, freely flowing throughout the body. Excessive and uninhibited procoagulant and inflammatory processes with concomitant lack of tissue perfusion lead to multiorgan failure (MOF) and death. Thrombosis and inflammation must be localized to the site of injury, thus the processes are regulated in several ways. Localization occurs primarily by endothelial processes, flow dilution of factors, and active fibrinolysis. Inhibitory processes within the coagulation system play major roles in regulation of thrombosis (Table 1) [6].

Endothelial roles in regulation

The endothelium has been found to be intrinsically involved in regulation of coagulation in many ways. The endothelium first comes into

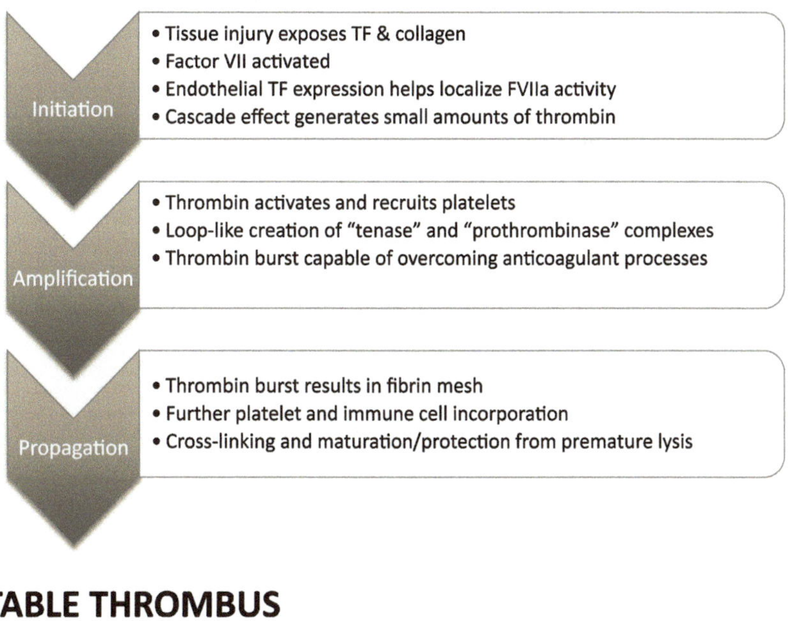

Fig. 2. Cellular model of coagulation. This represents the 3 stages leading to thrombus formation within the cellular model of coagulation, including the contribution of platelets.

Table 1
Effects of the main natural anticoagulant proteins on the coagulation cascade

Anticoagulant protein	Inhibits
Antithrombin	Thrombin, FIXa, Xa, FXIa, FXIIa
Thrombomodulin	Fva, FVIIIa
Protein C	FV, FVIII
Protein S	FV, FVIII
Tissue factor pathway inhibitor	TF:FVIIa, FXa
Intact endothelial glycocalyx	Endothelial platelet bonding

The anticoagulant proteins listed on the left inhibit the corresponding items listed on the right.

play with vasoconstriction as an initial defense against blood loss. Endothelium is known to express antithrombin, thrombomodulin, tissue factor pathway inhibitor, and tissue factor (TF), among other roles (Box 1) [7,8].

Box 1: Examples of endothelial interactions with coagulation

Platelet Interactions
- Activation
- Adhesion
- Von Willebrand factor production
- ADAMTS-13 cleavage of ultralarge von Willebrand factor
- Ectonucleotidase expression
- Release of nitric oxide
- Prostacyclin production

Waterfall Cascade Interactions
- Tissue factor pathway inhibitor release
- Endothelial protein C receptor expression
- Protein C activation via expression of thrombomodulin
- Antithrombin III binding
- Gas6 production and release

Fibrinolysis
- Tissue plasminogen activator (tPA) production
- Urokinase type-plasminogen activator receptor expression
- Plasminogen activator inhibitor-1 induction

The endothelium interacts within the coagulation system via platelets, factors, and fibrinolysis. This is a partial list of these interactions only and is not, by any means, considered exhaustive.

Abbreviations: ADAMTS-13, a disintegrin and metalloproteinase with a thrombospondin type 1 motif member 13; Gas6, growth arrest specific 6 protein.

Importance of the endothelial glycocalyx

The endothelial glycocalyx is now known to be extremely important in both localizing thrombosis and preventing inappropriate thrombosis, in preventing tissue edema, and in modulating immune activation. If this luminal anticoagulant covering is damaged, endothelial activation of coagulation and inflammation occur. This is considered one of the important mechanisms of MOF from trauma at distant sites [9–11].

Continued evolution of our understanding

We are continuing to develop our understanding of many aspects of plasma, vascular, and extravascular processes important in coagulation. TF expression and its regulation, flow dynamics, shear stress–related conformational changes, turbulence, and spatial and temporal considerations and other more basic processes continue to be elucidated. One recent example is the role of the growth arrest specific-6 (Gas6) protein in expression of TF by endothelial cells. The vitamin K–dependent protein Gas6 binds to endothelial *T*yro, *A*xyl, *M*er (TAM) receptors, inducing vascular tissue factor expression. This tissue factor then binds factor VIIa, initiating coagulation [12,13].

TRAUMA/INFLAMMATION/COAGULOPATHY

It follows that tissue damage sufficient to require hemostasis would have subsequent healing promoted by protection from bacterial invasion, clearance of cellular debris, and other inflammatory responses. Therefore, it is not surprising that coagulation and inflammation are linked (Box 2) [1]. Many components of one system affect processes within the other and they also share many regulatory processes.

Immune response to injury

The inflammatory response is absolutely necessary for healing and recuperation after injury, but if not appropriately balanced and controlled, may lead to life-threatening complications of its own. Excessive and prolonged proinflammatory response after trauma has been associated with MOF and death [14,15].

The neutrophils and macrophages of the innate immune system carry most of the responsibility for tissue defense and clearance of cellular debris after traumatic tissue injury. Excessive response, however, leads to the systemic inflammatory response syndrome (SIRS) and sepsis in a manner surprisingly similar to other causes [4,16–18]. Xiao and colleagues [4] demonstrated the remarkably uniform nature of inflammatory responses to bacterial pathogens, burns, and trauma at a transcriptomic and genomic level. They also showed that proinflammatory and anti-inflammatory processes both begin immediately after tissue injury.

Coagulopathy from excessive, dysregulated inflammatory response is well documented in SIRS and sepsis. More recently, its importance in trauma-induced coagulopathy (TIC) has become increasingly evident [19]. Additional support for this concept came recently from a secondary analysis of the Inflammation and the Host Response to Injury Large Scale Collaborative Program (Glue Grant; https://www.gluegrant.org/). Neal and colleagues [20] revealed

Box 2: Interactions between coagulation and inflammation

Anti-inflammatory roles of anticoagulants

Antithrombin:

- Via induction of endothelial prostacyclin release
  - Blocks neutrophil/endothelial tethering
  - Decreases endothelial cytokine production
- Blocks neutrophil, monocyte, and lymphocyte endothelial interactions
- P-selectin downregulation

Protein C:

- Via PAR-1, blocks nuclear factor-κB translocation
- Vascular permeability barrier preservation
- Downregulates inflammatory response

Protein S:

- Facilitates apoptotic cell phagocytosis
- Downregulates intracellular inflammatory pathways via acting as a ligand for innate immune cell tyrosyl, axyl, mer (TAM) receptors

Inflammatory activation of coagulation

Cytokines induce tissue factor expression

Inflammation down regulates the Protein-C system

Inflammation inhibits fibrinolysis

Inflammatory platelet activation

Coagulation activation of inflammation

Platelet activation of monocytes

uPA/uPAR macrophage activation

Fibrin, thrombin, FXa, and FXa complexes activate monocytes, macrophages, mast cells, and endothelium

Coagulation and inflammation are inextricably linked biologic defense mechanisms. Multiple interrelated processes exist that aid in defense and healing. Extreme activation of these processes may also be considered maladaptive at times, as is the case with activated protein-C–related trauma-induced coagulopathy.

Abbreviations: PAR-1, protease activated receptor-1; uPA, urokinase-type plasminogen activator; uPAR, uPA receptor.

an association between prehospital nonsteroidal anti-inflammatory use and a significant reduction in TIC.

A mechanism of tissue injury–induced inflammation

Tissue injury causes the release of intracellular components into the circulation at concentrations much higher than is seen with programmed cell death. Much like the pathogen-associated molecular patterns that cause inflammatory response to bacterial invasion, intracellular debris may serve as damage-associated molecular patterns (DAMPs), or "alarmins" [21]. Mitochondrial DNA, with significant bacterial similarity, is one such DAMP [22].

Pattern recognition receptors, such as Toll-like receptors and the receptor for advanced glycation end products, recognize these DAMPs and initiate cytokine production and inflammatory response. Of note, additional evidence of the interdependence of coagulation and inflammation is seen in the fact that DAMPs cause direct activation of coagulation [23].

Severity of tissue injury is associated with proportional increases in proinflammatory markers, including cytokine interleukin (IL)-6. Increased IL-6 levels from surgery or trauma are also associated with activation of coagulation, endocrine response, and postsurgical complications [24–31].

Importance of trauma-induced coagulopathy

Coagulopathy has long been recognized as a lethal component of trauma. When combined with acidemia and hypothermia, it forms the "lethal triad." Our understanding of the coagulopathy associated with trauma has progressed over the years. The dilution of factors and platelets secondary to resuscitation and hypothermia that was recognized years ago is still considered an important factor. In fact, it should be considered in any "massive resuscitation."

However, research into TIC revealed a severe coagulopathy (demonstrable before resuscitation) that had not been previously clinically appreciated. TIC is now known to be a consequence of severe tissue injury and shock-induced hypoperfusion with other contributing factors (Box 3) [32,33]. To have a significant impact on this problem, early identification of patients at risk and prompt treatment is extremely important.

Box 3: Contributors to trauma-induced coagulopathy (TIC)

TIC Contributors

- Severe tissue injury
- Shock-induced tissue hypoperfusion
- Excessive and prolonged inflammatory response
- Systemic endothelial degradation
  - Auto-heparinization
  - Weible-Palade body degranulation and tPA-associated hyperfibrinolysis
- Platelet dysfunction
- Maladaptive protein C response
- Fibrinogen depletion

TIC, an acute coagulopathy seen immediately after severe trauma, is a multifactorial disorder.

MANAGEMENT GOALS

Newer models of treatment for trauma resuscitation

For decades, crystalloid-based resuscitation of the severely injured patient was standard, but this practice is increasingly being reevaluated and modified. Large-volume crystalloid resuscitation leads to tissue edema, thus worsening tissue oxygenation and perfusion. This worsens a pathologic cycle of hypoperfusion, tissue injury, and inflammatory complications (Fig. 3).

Our current practice of goal-directed resuscitation aims to break this cycle by using a technique that has been referred to as "damage-control resuscitation" (DCR) (Box 4). DCR describes an approach to resuscitation that may be broken down into 2 major components: hypotensive and hemostatic resuscitation. It is usually combined with damage-control surgery in an attempt to improve the survival of severely traumatized patients.

Time is of the essence when treating a bleeding patient, and temporary control via direct pressure or tourniquet is very important. The very best resuscitation with fractionated blood components still falls short of providing the function of native blood with its own inflammatory mediators, antigens, and coagulation components. Herein lies the importance of direct control of bleeding via surgical and topical therapies aided by DCR techniques, including hypotensive resuscitation: it helps maintain the patients' intrinsic blood volume.

Identification of the need for massive transfusion

Certain clinical indicators and laboratory values have been demonstrated in trauma patients to be associated with a need for massive transfusion (MT).

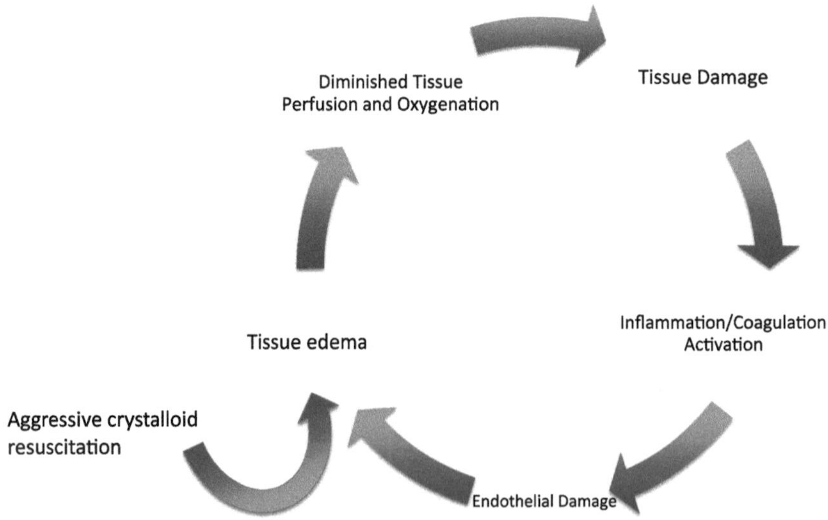

Fig. 3. The pathologic cycle of hypoperfusion, tissue injury, and inflammatory complications. Tissue edema is worsened by aggressive crystalloid-based resuscitation, thus propagating this cycle.

Box 4: Damage control resuscitation

Goals of Trauma Resuscitation addressed by Damage Control Resuscitation

- Identify patients at risk for "massive transfusion"
- Prompt initiation of appropriate hemostatic resuscitation
- Prevent bleeding induced by excessive blood pressure
- Balance intentional hypotension with critical organ perfusion
- Improve tissue perfusion
- Minimize crystalloid resuscitation
- Minimize hemodilution of factors
- Treat/prevent hypothermia
- Correct acidemia

Trauma resuscitation must be goal directed and prompt to attain the best potential outcome.

These have been assimilated into scoring systems that may be used as triggers for initiating a massive transfusion protocol (MTP). If a patient meets the appropriate criteria, the MTP should be initiated immediately to avoid lost opportunity for corrections [32]. There are common factors associated with a need for MT and a simple clinical scoring system is available that aids in identifying trauma patients at high risk for MT (Tables 2 and 3) [32,34].

Two models of resuscitation

There are 2 competing models that aim to best implement the concepts of DCR. A protocol-driven model that uses a ratio (eg, 1:1:1 = red blood cells (RBCs):fresh frozen plasma (FFP):platelets) of available blood components versus a point-of-care (POC) coagulation-testing model that uses rapid coagulation testing and specific therapy (including concentrated factors) for abnormalities that are discovered. There are specific rationales and concerns associated with each of these approaches (Table 4).

Table 2
Major indicators of need for massive transfusion in trauma

Clinical indicators	Laboratory indicators
Injury severity score >15	Base deficit <−6
Systolic pressure <90 mm Hg	International normalized ratio >1.2
Temperature <35.5°C	Hemoglobin <11 g/dL
Heart rate >120 beats per minute	pH <7.25
Positive FAST examination	
GCS <9	

These (and other) indicators have been utilized in different scoring systems to help predict the need for massive transfusion in trauma.

Abbreviations: FAST, Focused Assessment with Sonography in Trauma; GCS, Glascow Coma Scale.

Table 3
A simple system to help predict massive transfusion needs in trauma

Assessment of blood consumption (ABC) score	
Penetrating mechanism	1
Arrival systolic blood pressure $\leq$90 mm Hg	1
Arrival heart rate $\geq$120/min	1
FAST examination positive	1

The ABC score uses readily available clinical indicators to help predict the need for massive transfusion in trauma.
Abbreviation: FAST, Focused Assessment with Sonography in Trauma.
Sum $\geq$2 correctly classified 85% of massive transfusion patients.

Point-of-care coagulation testing

In a situation of rapid exsanguination, the patient's clinical status continues to change very rapidly and it takes far too long to receive the results from traditional coagulation testing to provide direction for current treatment [35]. In this situation, the patient's clinical status continues to change very rapidly. Within the hour or more that it takes for the information to return, the patient has continued to bleed and may have received several procoagulant therapies.

Traditional coagulation testing is also considered unreliable in characterizing TIC. Prothrombin time (PT), international normalized ratio (INR), and activated partial thromboplastin times (aPTT) all use plasma samples devoid of blood's cellular components that play major roles in vivo. These tests also do not consider clot stability, fibrin functionality, or fibrinolysis [36].

Table 4
The 2 major models of trauma resuscitation

Model	Rationale	Concern	Location
Ratio-driven protocol	• Improved early survival in MT patients • Early intervention decreases overall transfusion requirements • Rapid POC testing and concentrated products largely unavailable	• Morbidity and mortality associated with nonspecific transfusion rationale • Waste of preprepared blood products • Cost of blood products	United States
POC testing protocol	• Indiscriminant use of blood products is harmful • Rapid POC testing allows specificity of therapy, including blood products	• Potential for delay in therapy and lost opportunity • FFP contains some beneficial components not commercially available • Cost of therapies	Europe

These models were developed based on prior experiences and considerations within 2 different health care systems. Availability of testing and products is dissimilar as well.
Abbreviations: FFP, fresh frozen plasma; MT, massive transfusion; POC, point of care.

The recently published Society of Thoracic Surgeons Blood Conservation Guideline Task Force recommendations (2007) and the update (2011) include POC coagulation testing in their recommendations [37]. Also, POC testing is featured prominently in the European guidelines regarding "Management of bleeding and coagulopathy following major trauma" updated in December 2013 [38].

Rapid viscoelastic and platelet function testing is increasingly proving beneficial in this area. Thromboelastography (TEG; Haemonetics, Braintree, Massachusetts; Tem Innovations GmbH, Munich, Germany) and rotational thromboelastometry (ROTEM; Pentapharm, Germany) both use whole blood samples to help rapidly evaluate coagulation processes including blood cellular contributions and fibrinolysis.

HOW VISCOELASTIC TESTS HELP

Normal thromboelastography/rotational thromboelastometry

One of the strengths of TEG/ROTEM lies in the strong negative predictive power [39]. In other words, if the TEG/ROTEM is normal, observed clinical bleeding is almost certainly not due to coagulopathy, and is more likely due to uncontrolled surgical bleeding or "suture" deficiency (Fig. 4A). The source should be discovered and controlled if discreet. Topical prothrombotic agents should be strongly considered. Interventional radiological procedures may be necessary and should be considered as well.

Abnormal thromboelastography/rotational thromboelastometry

Different components of the TEG/ROTEM reveal different defects in hemostasis. Inadequate factor, fibrinogen, and platelet function all show different TEG/ROTEM abnormalities, as does hyperfibrinolysis. Abnormal results in

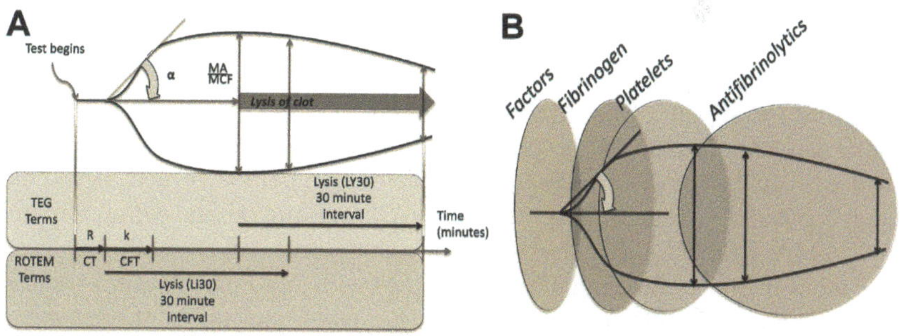

Fig. 4. (*A*) Normal-appearing TEG/ROTEM graph and parameters. The appearance of TEG and ROTEM graphs are quite similar, yet with different nomenclature and lysis interval timing. CFT, clot formation time; CT, clotting time; k, kinetics; Li30, lysis index 30 minutes after CT; LY30, lysis 30 minutes after MA; MA, maximum amplitude; MCF, maximum clot firmness; R, reaction time; α, alpha angle. (*B*) Treatments based on areas of abnormal values. Abnormal results in different areas of the graph help direct therapy by revealing the problematic area within the coagulation system. As shown, there is overlap in the therapies indicated by certain abnormal results.

the TEG/ROTEM help direct therapy by indicating the source of the coagulation dysfunction [39].

Prolonged coagulation initiation (R/CT), decreased kinetics of formation (k/CFT), inability to attain an adequate maximum strength (MA/MCF), and excessive fibrinolysis (LY30/Li30) each has a specific associated therapy (see Fig. 4B).

Just as traditional coagulation testing does not reveal the entire in vivo clotting process, viscoelastic testing is limited as well. Unfortunately, it does not reflect vascular (eg, glycocalyx, endothelium, vessel wall) or extravascular contributions to clotting. Also, the activators used in the testing process cause generation of thrombin. As such, TEG/ROTEM may not identify problems associated with platelet dysfunction secondary to antiplatelet therapies (eg, aspirin, clopidogrel) or associated with trauma [40,41]. Specific platelet function testing is usually performed by other methods, as discussed in the following section.

Platelet testing

Turbidimetric platelet aggregometry is the trusted "gold standard" assay for platelet function; however, some drawbacks, including long "turn-around" time, render it rather useless in the treatment of acute massive bleeding. Newer tests, including viscoelastic platelet mapping, impedance aggregometry (IA), and platelet function analysis, offer rapid POC assessment of platelet function.

Platelet mapping

TEG PlateletMapping (Haemonetics, Braintree, Massachusetts) assay allows the evaluation of platelet function as it relates to antiplatelet therapy. It reports the percentage of inhibition or aggregation compared with the patient's uninhibited maximum response. PlateletMapping shows promise; however, this function is not a simple test, not a standard TEG test, and is currently unavailable on ROTEM. Also, TEG platelet mapping uses 3 channels, thus requiring 2 machines.

Impedance aggregometry

IA testing (Multiplate, Roche, Switzerland) offers rapid POC platelet function testing. Impedance increases as platelets aggregate on the electrodes in the sample. IA is capable of determining platelet functional defects related to vascular injury (collagen) and antiplatelet therapy (ADP) among others, within minutes.

Using IA, Kutcher and colleagues [41] recently revealed clinically significant defects in platelet functionality associated with trauma. Trauma-induced platelet dysfunction was present despite adequate quantitative platelet values (and other traditional coagulation tests) and was found predictive of both early and late mortality.

IA and ROTEM are components of the POC testing guided approach to TIC, as both tests offer results within a few minutes and evaluate different aspects of coagulopathy. IA is currently used for clinical testing in Europe but is currently unavailable in the United States, except for use in research. A somewhat limited version has recently received approval by the Food and Drug Administration for clinical use and may be available by the end of 2014 [42].

Fibrinolysis testing

Traditional testing for fibrinolysis includes quantification of the cross-linked fibrin-degradation product D-dimer and the euglobulin clot lysis time (ECLT). D-dimer testing results are typically available in 1 to 2 hours. Elevated D-dimer is nonspecific, as it may be associated with many different entities, including venous thromboembolism, syncope, heart failure, trauma, and cancer [43]. The ECLT is labor intensive and takes 3 to 6 hours to complete, and in many laboratories is thus routinely processed once each morning. TEG/ROTEM accurately reveals significant hyperfibrinolysis within 30 minutes from clot initiation (ROTEM) or from maximum amplitude (TEG).

Role of traditional coagulation tests

Care should be exercised when interpreting any laboratory data, including viscoelastic tests, thus additional testing is warranted to provide confirmatory and complementary data. Traditional screening tests, such as aPTT and PT/INR, along with quantitative fibrinogen and platelet values, help to ensure correct interpretation and performance of advanced tests.

A COMBINED APPROACH TO RESUSCITATION

In resuscitation from acute massive hemorrhage, a combination of the 2 models (protocol-driven and POC-testing–driven) may provide improved results. This combined model may address limitations in each individually (Fig. 5). The

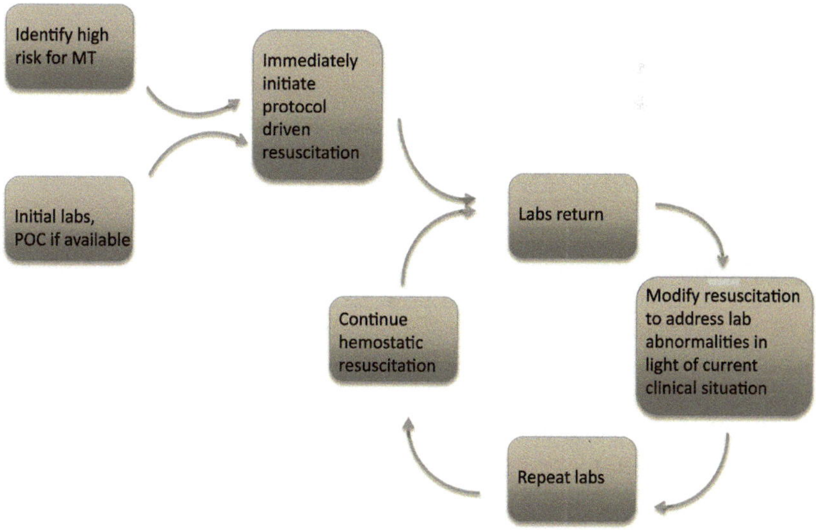

Fig. 5. A combined resuscitation approach. Combining the 2 models of massive transfusion, a reasonable and effective strategy such as this may best address concerns raised by both. labs, laboratory tests.

recently updated European guidelines that promote POC coagulation testing also support this combined approach. It states:

> Recommendation 26. We recommend the initial administration of plasma (fresh frozen plasma (FFP) or pathogen-inactivated plasma) (Grade 1B) or fibrinogen (Grade 1C) in patients with massive bleeding.
>
> If further plasma is administered, we suggest an optimal plasma: RBC ratio of at least 1:2 (Grade 2C).
>
> We recommend that plasma transfusion be avoided in patients without substantial bleeding (Grade 1B) [38].

In this manner, early identification of a serious clinical problem, immediate institution of therapy, monitoring of coagulation changes, and rapid adjustment of treatment is possible. Benefits to the patient would include treatment of the major components of the lethal triad, prevention of an escalating problem of inflammation with minimization of total blood product utilization and their inherent risks.

DAMAGE-CONTROL RESUSCITATION IN NONTRAUMA PATIENTS

Surgical hemorrhage as trauma-induced bleeding

As previously noted, tissue injury when combined with hemorrhagic shock initiates a massive inflammatory response capable of proceeding to TIC, SIRS, MOF, and death. Tissue injury of sufficient magnitude, regardless of its source, including surgery, along with hemorrhagic shock, is sufficient to enact this scenario.

Massive hemorrhage is a major cause of death after severe trauma. It is also associated with significantly increased mortality from surgery [44,45]. When bleeding continues or is acutely intense enough to warrant consideration of treatment with blood components or procoagulants, rapid assessment of coagulation is warranted. Often, blood products are used despite a lack of understanding of the benefits, risks, options, and costs involved [46].

Coagulopathy

Although most intraoperative hemorrhage is associated with surgical technique or "suture deficiency" requiring direct control, coagulopathy resulting in additional microvascular bleeding may develop and contribute to the clinical challenge [44]. TIC develops in association with a maladaptive protein-C response, massive inflammatory response to DAMPs, and tissue hypoperfusion; in analogous fashion, coagulopathy from "surgical trauma" may develop. As evaluated by TEG results, early administration of FFP and platelets, along with RBCs has been shown to maintain coagulation capacity in a variety of massively bleeding patients [47].

Predicting hemorrhage

In the operating room, the likelihood of massive hemorrhage is associated with the type or complexity of the procedure. Cardiac, major vascular, trauma, major orthopedic, organ transplantation, and complex oncological procedures are all likely candidates for increased risks of operative bleeding. Patients with a higher likelihood of perioperative hemorrhage include those with incompetent coagulation systems (intrinsic or iatrogenic), and comorbidities characterized by diminished physiologic states (eg, malnutrition, chronic steroid use, advanced age, American Society of Anesthesiologists (ASA) III-IV, hepatic or renal insufficiency) [37,48].

Blood conservation

In 2007, the Society of Thoracic Surgeons Blood Conservation Guideline Task Force made recommendations regarding blood conservation for cardiac surgery. A planned revision, incorporating newer information, was published in 2011. These guidelines contain considerations appropriate for other procedures associated with bleeding risk as well (Box 5) [49].

Coagulation testing for perioperative massive hemorrhage

Advanced POC testing, including viscoelastic and rapid platelet function tests, would be best suited to provide results rapidly enough to help evaluate coagulopathy in massive hemorrhage. In a prospective, randomized study, Weber and colleagues [50] evaluated POC testing (ROTEM and IA) in patients clinically considered to be coagulopathic after complex cardiac surgery. They performed a planned interim analysis and terminated their study early because of a significantly decreased erythrocyte transfusion rate in the POC cohort. Several secondary outcome parameters, including decreased FFP and platelet transfusion rates, length of ICU stay, and 6-month mortality rates, were also found to be lower in the POC group.

Trigger of massive transfusion protocol

As discussed before, in trauma, certain clinical indicators and laboratory values have been developed into triggers for initiating an MTP. This is not the case for operative procedures. Resuscitation often proceeds as indicated by estimated blood loss and hemodynamic instability. Uncontrolled bleeding resulting in hypotension should be considered a trigger, as well. As we understand the mechanisms of TIC more fully, we realize that emphasis should be placed on maintenance of coagulation capacity in massive hemorrhage as well as in TIC.

APPLICATION OF DAMAGE-CONTROL RESUSCITATION METHODS TO NONTRAUMA PATIENTS

Massive hemorrhage, regardless of the cause, must be treated rapidly with the same basic goals of trauma resuscitation.

- *Rapid surgical control of bleeding* cannot be overemphasized, and its absence cannot be overcome with medical treatment.
- Identify patients requiring "massive transfusion" as early as possible.
  Inability to directly control the source of bleeding due to a cryptic source, anatomic challenge, and so forth, leading to hemorrhagic shock is similar to the sequence in the development of TIC. Clear and direct communication between the surgical and anesthesia teams is paramount. Early

Box 5: Modified Society of Thoracic Surgeons recommendations

- Creation of multidisciplinary blood management teams is considered important in prevention and treatment of massive bleeding.
- Identification of patients at high risk of requiring blood transfusions
  - Advanced age
  - Low preoperative red cell volume
  - Antiplatelet/antithrombotic drugs preoperatively
  - Complex procedures
  - Emergency operations
  - Comorbidities
- Preoperative risk-reduction strategies
  - Correction of anemia before surgery
  - Use of antifibrinolytic drugs
  - Selective use of alternative procedures with lower bleeding risk
  - Appropriate modification of antiplatelet/anticoagulant therapy
    - Discontinuation/bridging based on most recent guidelines
  - Prothrombin complex concentrates (PCC) reversal of warfarin for emergency surgery
  - Platelet function testing for those on antiplatelet therapies
- Intraoperative
  - Cell salvage
  - Factor replacement when rapid point-of-care (POC) testing shows specific source(s)
    - Fractionated products if available
    - Plasma acceptable when safer fractionated products are unavailable
  - Factor replacement when rapid POC testing unavailable
    - Plasma acceptable when used as part of a massive transfusion algorithm
  - Topical hemostatic agents
    - Compression devices
    - Sealants after cell salvage
    - Antifibrinolytics poured into the wound after cell salvage
- Postoperatively
  - Continued monitoring of bleeding and coagulation status
  - Treatment as indicated

The 2011 Society of Thoracic Surgeons blood conservation guidelines have been condensed and modified for broader application.

recognition of poorly controlled bleeding allows rapid conversion to more appropriate resuscitation methods.

- Promptly initiate an appropriate hemostatic resuscitation (MTP).
  Baseline laboratory evaluation and if available POC testing should be initiated. Early considerations include
  - Adequate intravenous access for resuscitation is critical.
  - Arterial pressure monitoring is helpful but should not delay therapy. Waveform analysis and changes associated with therapy provide rapid information regarding contractility and volume status, and blood sampling for serial laboratory tests is simplified.
  - Tranexamic acid has proven beneficial in trauma and other settings [51].
  - Desmopressin (DDAVP) induces endothelial release of factor VIII and von Willebrand factor, and improves primary hemostasis in settings of von Willebrand disease, antiplatelet therapy, acidemia, and hypothermia [38].
  - Excessive crystalloid-based resuscitation is detrimental.
  - Early administration of available replacement therapy is indicated. FFP, fractionated products, fibrinogen concentrates, cryoprecipitate, platelets, and so forth should be instituted as indicated to maintain coagulation function. In this specific subset of patients, much greater use of blood products and other procoagulants is seen when therapy is delayed, and thus early intervention helps decrease utilization of these resources.
- Improve/maintain tissue perfusion.
  - Adequate tissue perfusion promotes correction of acidemia.
  - Base excess and lactate levels at baseline and sequentially, helps monitor adequacy of perfusion.
  - Maintenance of the microcirculation with appropriate resuscitation and support of cardiac output when needed, helps prevent global inflammatory activation, hopefully decreasing the likelihood of progression to MOF and worse.
  - Norepinephrine may be used as bridging therapy, but continued use of vasoconstricting medications may be counterproductive in leading to worsening global tissue perfusion, thus promoting acidemia. However, if volume resuscitation alone fails to attain adequate blood pressure because of other factors, norepinephrine infusion may indeed need to be continued.
- Permissive hypotension is considered beneficial in uncontrolled bleeding.
  - Prevention of the excess bleeding associated with increased blood pressure must be balanced with the need for critical organ perfusion. In a non-vasoconstricted patient, tissue perfusion is typically adequate with minimal adverse effect. Regional perfusion to critical organs in the setting of comorbidities is a concern, however. Specific limitations to the degree of hypotension that should be permitted exist in the setting of traumatic brain injury: recommendations for no less than a systolic blood pressure of 90 mm Hg (American Association of Neurologic Surgeons) [52] and a mean arterial pressure of 80 mm Hg (European guidelines) [38] have been established.

NOTE: Intentional hypotension should be discontinued after surgical control of bleeding is attained so as to improve tissue perfusion. There is also concern that in an artificially hypotensive state, vascular bleeding can be masked. For this reason, blood pressure should be allowed to rise to the levels expected postoperatively, before wound closure. This allows visual confirmation of hemostasis and may prevent some immediate postoperative "rebleeding" and emergent reentry.

- Minimize crystalloid resuscitation
  Restricting crystalloid administration minimizes hemodilution of coagulation factors, decreases tissue edema, and avoids excessive chloride load.
- Treat/prevent hypothermia
  All resuscitation fluids should be warmed where appropriate and active warming devices should be used.
- Correct electrolyte abnormalities
  In the setting of massive resuscitation, electrolyte abnormalities are common. Administration of citrate-containing blood products, along with consumption of calcium during clotting processes, often leads to decreased ionized calcium levels that should be monitored and replaced.

SUMMARY

Coagulation and inflammation are 2 major biologic response systems following tissue trauma. A complex interaction between these 2 systems after severe injury may result in coagulopathy and an increased likelihood of poor outcomes. Improved understanding of the bleeding seen in severe trauma settings has informed our treatment of poorly controlled bleeding in the operating room. Massive hemorrhage is a serious and rapidly changing situation associated with significant increase in mortality rates. We recommend that a multidisciplinary blood-management team establish rapid response systems and algorithms to facilitate the clinical response to massive hemorrhage.

Identification of high-risk patients and procedures allows preprocedure consideration and preparation promoting good outcomes. Once high risk is identified, concepts of blood product conservation should be used before, during, and after the procedure. Rapid, acute hemorrhage is not immediately reflected in decreased hemoglobin/hematocrit nor is acute coagulopathy able to be characterized by standard coagulation tests. Appropriate therapy must be rapidly instituted to avoid a "bloody vicious cycle" of bleeding and coagulopathy. In the setting of massive hemorrhage where coagulopathy may be contributory, damage control resuscitation concepts should be used. POC testing is capable of guiding therapy in this dynamic situation, and we recommend blending protocol-driven and testing-driven approaches to the bleeding patient. New information and capabilities arise continuously; therefore, we must continue to stay abreast of current recommendations and developments.

References

[1] Petaja J. Inflammation and coagulation. An overview. Thromb Res 2011;127(Suppl 2):S34–7.
[2] Adams GL, Manson RJ, Turner I, et al. The balance of thrombosis and hemorrhage in surgery. Hematol Oncol Clin North Am 2007;21(1):13–24.

[3] Desai KH, Tan CS, Leek JT, et al. Dissecting inflammatory complications in critically injured patients by within-patient gene expression changes: a longitudinal clinical genomics study. PLoS Med 2011;8(9):e1001093.
[4] Xiao W, Mindrinos MN, Seok J, et al. A genomic storm in critically injured humans. J Exp Med 2011;208(13):2581–90.
[5] Davie EW. A brief historical review of the waterfall/cascade of blood coagulation. J Biol Chem 2003;278(51):50819–32.
[6] Adams RL, Bird RJ. Review article: coagulation cascade and therapeutics update: relevance to nephrology. Part 1: overview of coagulation, thrombophilias and history of anticoagulants. Nephrology (Carlton) 2009;14(5):462–70.
[7] van Hinsbergh VW. Endothelium–role in regulation of coagulation and inflammation. Semin Immunopathol 2012;34(1):93–106.
[8] Rivera J, Lozano ML, Navarro-Nunez L, et al. Platelet receptors and signaling in the dynamics of thrombus formation. Haematologica 2009;94(5):700–11.
[9] Mulivor AW, Lipowsky HH. Inflammation- and ischemia-induced shedding of venular glycocalyx. Am J Physiol Heart Circ Physiol 2004;286(5):H1672–80.
[10] Chappell D, Westphal M, Jacob M. The impact of the glycocalyx on microcirculatory oxygen distribution in critical illness. Curr Opin Anaesthesiol 2009;22(2): 155–62.
[11] Torres LN, Sondeen JL, Ji L, et al. Evaluation of resuscitation fluids on endothelial glycocalyx, venular blood flow, and coagulation function after hemorrhagic shock in rats. J Trauma Acute Care Surg 2013;75(5):759–66.
[12] Foley JH, Conway EM. Gas6 gains entry into the coagulation cascade. Blood 2013;121(4):570–1.
[13] Robins RS, Lemarie CA, Laurance S, et al. Vascular Gas6 contributes to thrombogenesis and promotes tissue factor up-regulation after vessel injury in mice. Blood 2013;121(4): 692–9.
[14] Gentile LF, Cuenca AG, Efron PA, et al. Persistent inflammation and immunosuppression: a common syndrome and new horizon for surgical intensive care. J Trauma Acute Care Surg 2012;72(6):1491–501.
[15] Gando S, Kameue T, Matsuda N, et al. Combined activation of coagulation and inflammation has an important role in multiple organ dysfunction and poor outcome after severe trauma. Thromb Haemost 2002;88(6):943–9.
[16] Chow CC, Clermont G, Kumar R, et al. The acute inflammatory response in diverse shock states. Shock 2005;24(1):74–84.
[17] Lenz A, Franklin GA, Cheadle WG. Systemic inflammation after trauma. Injury 2007;38(12):1336–45.
[18] Tsukamoto T, Chanthaphavong RS, Pape HC. Current theories on the pathophysiology of multiple organ failure after trauma. Injury 2010;41(1):21–6.
[19] Pierce A, Pittet JF. Inflammatory response to trauma: implications for coagulation and resuscitation. Curr Opin Anaesthesiol 2014;27(2):246–52.
[20] Neal MD, Brown JB, Moore EE, et al. Prehospital use of nonsteroidal anti-inflammatory drugs (NSAIDs) is associated with a reduced incidence of trauma-induced coagulopathy. Ann Surg 2014;260(2):378–82.
[21] Matzinger P. The danger model: a renewed sense of self. Science 2002;296(5566): 301–5.
[22] Zhang Q, Raoof M, Chen Y, et al. Circulating mitochondrial DAMPs cause inflammatory responses to injury. Nature 2010;464(7285):104–7.
[23] Esmon CT, Xu J, Lupu F. Innate immunity and coagulation. J Thromb Haemost 2011;9(Suppl 1):182–8.
[24] Pullicino EA, Carli F, Poole S, et al. The relationship between the circulating concentrations of interleukin 6 (IL-6), tumor necrosis factor (TNF) and the acute phase response to elective surgery and accidental injury. Lymphokine Res 1990;9(2):231–8.

[25] Yilmaz S, Arioz DT, Altindis M, et al. Short period of preconditioning protects by decreasing the TNF-alpha and IL-6 values before laparoscopic surgery (a rat experiment). Med Sci Monit 2010;16(2):BR75–9.
[26] Hisano S, Sakamoto K, Ishiko T, et al. IL-6 and soluble IL-6 receptor levels change differently after surgery both in the blood and in the operative field. Cytokine 1997;9(6):447–52.
[27] Uchida I, Ueo H, Takamatsu T, et al. An increase in circulating IL-6 levels correlates to endocrine response to abdominal surgery: preliminary report. Nihon Geka Gakkai Zasshi 1991;92(12):1726 [in Japanese].
[28] Sanders J, Hawe E, Brull DJ, et al. Higher IL-6 levels but not IL6 -174G>C or -572G>C genotype are associated with post-operative complication following coronary artery bypass graft (CABG) surgery. Atherosclerosis 2009;204(1):196–201.
[29] Sedlar M, Kudrnova Z, Erhart D, et al. Older age and type of surgery predict the early inflammatory response to hip trauma mediated by interleukin-6 (IL-6). Arch Gerontol Geriatr 2010;51(1):e1–6.
[30] Tschoeke SK, Hellmuth M, Hostmann A, et al. The early second hit in trauma management augments the proinflammatory immune response to multiple injuries. J Trauma 2007;62(6):1396–403 [discussion: 1403–4].
[31] Jiang J, Tian K, Chen H, et al. Kinetics of plasma cytokines and its clinical significance in patients with severe trauma. Chin Med J (Engl) 1997;110(12):923–6.
[32] Maegele M, Spinella PC, Schochl H. The acute coagulopathy of trauma: mechanisms and tools for risk stratification. Shock 2012;38(5):450–8.
[33] Chambers LA, Chow SJ, Shaffer LE. Frequency and characteristics of coagulopathy in trauma patients treated with a low- or high-plasma-content massive transfusion protocol. Am J Clin Pathol 2011;136(3):364–70.
[34] Nunez TC, Voskresensky IV, Dossett LA, et al. Early prediction of massive transfusion in trauma: simple as ABC (assessment of blood consumption)? J Trauma 2009;66(2): 346–52.
[35] Davenport R, Manson J, De'Ath H, et al. Functional definition and characterization of acute traumatic coagulopathy. Crit Care Med 2011;39(12):2652–8.
[36] Schochl H, Maegele M, Solomon C, et al. Early and individualized goal-directed therapy for trauma-induced coagulopathy. Scand J Trauma Resusc Emerg Med 2012;20:15.
[37] Society of Thoracic Surgeons Blood Conservation Guideline Task Force, et al. Perioperative blood transfusion and blood conservation in cardiac surgery: the Society of Thoracic Surgeons and the Society of Cardiovascular Anesthesiologists clinical practice guideline. Ann Thorac Surg 2007;83(5 Suppl):S27–86.
[38] Spahn DR, Bouillon B, Cerny V, et al. Management of bleeding and coagulopathy following major trauma: an updated European guideline. Crit Care 2013;17(2):R76.
[39] Ganter MT, Hofer CK. Coagulation monitoring: current techniques and clinical use of viscoelastic point-of-care coagulation devices. Anesth Analg 2008;106(5): 1366–75.
[40] McMichael MA, Smith SA. Viscoelastic coagulation testing: technology, applications, and limitations. Vet Clin Pathol 2011;40(2):140–53.
[41] Kutcher ME, Redick BJ, McCreery RC, et al. Characterization of platelet dysfunction after trauma. J Trauma Acute Care Surg 2012;73(1):13–9.
[42] FDA medical devices online database. 2014. Available at: http://www.accessdata.fda.gov/cdrh_docs/reviews/k103555.pdf. FDA online medical device database. Accessed May 15th, 2014.
[43] Lippi G, Bonfanti L, Saccenti C, et al. Causes of elevated D-dimer in patients admitted to a large urban emergency department. Eur J Intern Med 2014;25(1):45–8.
[44] Marietta M, Facchini L, Pedrazzi P, et al. Pathophysiology of bleeding in surgery. Transplant Proc 2006;38(3):812–4.
[45] Marietta M, Pedrazzi P, Girardis M, et al. Massive bleeding: are we doing our best? Transfus Apher Sci 2011;45(3):287–90.

[46] Shander A. Financial and clinical outcomes associated with surgical bleeding complications. Surgery 2007;142(4 Suppl):S20–5.
[47] Johansson PI, Bochsen L, Stensballe J, et al. Transfusion packages for massively bleeding patients: the effect on clot formation and stability as evaluated by Thrombelastograph (TEG). Transfus Apher Sci 2008;39(1):3–8.
[48] Odumala AO, Ayekoloye CI, Packer G. Predictors of excessive blood loss during operative treatment of hip fractures. J R Coll Surg Edinb 2002;47(3):552–6.
[49] Society of Thoracic Surgeons Blood Conservation Guideline Task Force, et al. 2011 update to the Society of Thoracic Surgeons and the Society of Cardiovascular Anesthesiologists blood conservation clinical practice guidelines. Ann Thorac Surg 2011;91(3): 944–82.
[50] Weber CF, Gorlinger K, Meininger D, et al. Point-of-care testing: a prospective, randomized clinical trial of efficacy in coagulopathic cardiac surgery patients. Anesthesiology 2012;117(3):531–47.
[51] Ker K, Edwards P, Perel P, et al. Effect of tranexamic acid on surgical bleeding: systematic review and cumulative meta-analysis. BMJ 2012;344:e3054.
[52] Brain Trauma F, American Association of Neurological S, Congress of Neurological S, et al. Guidelines for the management of severe traumatic brain injury. I. Blood pressure and oxygenation. J Neurotrauma 2007;24(Suppl 1):S7–13.

Advances in Anesthesia 32 (2014) 23–36

ADVANCES IN ANESTHESIA

Update on Perioperative Myocardial Injury and Infarction

Definitions, Diagnosis, Biomarkers, Implications, and Approach to Care in the Perioperative Period

Gregory A. Nuttall, MD[a,*], William C. Oliver Jr, MD[a], Charanjit S. Rihal, MD[b]

[a]Department of Anesthesiology, Mayo Clinic College of Medicine, 200 First Street Southwest, Rochester, MN 55905, USA; [b]Department of Cardiovascular Disease, Mayo Clinic College of Medicine, 200 First Street Southwest, Rochester, MN 55905, USA

Keywords

• Myocardial infarction • ST-elevation myocardial infarction • Troponin • Natriuretic peptide • Myocardial injury after noncardiac surgery • MINS

Key points

- Elevations of biomarkers of myocardial infarction are more common and clinically important than once thought.
- Elevated biomarkers are associated with an increased risk of death following noncardiac surgery.
- The concept of myocardial injury after noncardiac surgery should be embraced, and studies should be performed to determine which therapies are most effective in preventing perioperative death.

INTRODUCTION

Most noncardiac surgery is undertaken to extend or improve the quality of a patient's life. There is a growing awareness that perioperative myocardial infarction (MI) is more common than initially appreciated and is associated with significant patient mortality. A recent analysis of data from the PeriOperative Ischemia Evaluation (POISE) trial indicates that perioperative MI is the most common cardiovascular complication following noncardiac surgery [1]. This study found that of the 8351 patients who were enrolled and were 45 years

*Corresponding author. *E-mail address*: nuttall.gregory@mayo.edu

0737-6146/14/$ – see front matter
http://dx.doi.org/10.1016/j.aan.2014.08.007

or older with cardiac risk factors, 415 patients (5.0%) who were diagnosed as having an MI. Most of the MIs occurred within 48 hours of surgery (74.1%). Of greater importance, the 30-day mortality rate was 11.6% among those who had an MI versus 2.2% for those who did not ($P<.001$). Of note, most of the MI patients were asymptomatic (65.3%) and the mortality was similar between those with (9.7%) and without (12.5%) ischemic symptoms.

DEFINITIONS

There are many pathologic factors and clinical scenarios that can result in myocardial injury. The detection of myocardial cell death resulting from prolonged ischemia is central to the diagnosis of acute MI. The time from onset of myocardial ischemia to heart-cell death can take anywhere between 20 minutes and more than 4 hours, depending on the cell's oxygen and nutrient demand and the cell's resistance to ischemia from ischemic preconditioning. In 2007 an international task force created a "universal definition of MI" [2], containing 5 sets of diagnostic criteria and 5 types of MI. The 5 types of MI are:

- Type 1, which is a spontaneous MI related to ischemia attributable to a primary coronary event such as plaque rupture, erosion, fissuring, or dissection. Type 1 MIs were further divided into unstable angina, Non–ST-elevation MI (NSTEMI), and ST-elevation MI (STEMI).
- Type 2 MIs are MIs resulting from ischemia induced by either increased myocardial demand or decreased coronary supply, such as arrhythmias, anemia, systemic hypotension or hypertension, coronary artery spasm, or embolism.
- Type 3 MIs are those that lead to sudden unexpected cardiac death.
- Type 4 MIs are associated with percutaneous coronary intervention (PCI) or coronary stent thrombosis.
- Type 5 MIs are associated with coronary artery bypass grafting (CABG) in the operating room and intensive care unit (ICU).

Types 1 and type 2 MI are most commonly encountered. Only for type 1 MI are there detailed, evidence-based management guidelines, which stress the time-critical nature of successful medical and/or percutaneous intervention [3,4].

DIAGNOSIS

The most recent universal definition describes MI as an increased plasma cardiac troponin concentration greater than 99% of the normal reference population range along with one of the following: (1) ST-segment, T-wave changes, new left bundle branch block, or pathologic Q-waves on electrocardiogram (ECG); (2) symptoms of cardiac ischemia; (3) new cardiac wall motion abnormalities or loss of viable myocardium on imaging; or (4) detection of intracoronary thrombus [5]. Many common abnormalities other than MI can result in an elevation of biomarkers of myocardial necrosis.

Symptoms of MI are rare or masked in the operating room and ICU, thus making the detection of inducible angina, especially unstable angina, very difficult. The physiologic changes that could result from an MI in the operating room and ICU are common and nonspecific, such as ST changes, new-onset atrial fibrillation, or worsening ratio of partial pressure of arterial oxygen/fraction of inspired oxygen. The 12-lead changes of the ECG of a new-onset MI may be caused by other pathologic factors or be absent [2], and ischemic ECG changes are not always present in patients who have elevated troponin levels [6]. Only 14% (95% confidence interval [CI] 3%–28%) of surgical patients who suffer an MI present with chest pain [7]. In a study of 415 noncardiac surgery patients who had a perioperative MI, 65.3% did not have ischemic symptoms [1]. Detecting new cardiac wall-motion abnormalities or the loss of viable myocardium or intracoronary thrombus on imaging requires specialized equipment and expertise that may not be rapidly available.

BIOMARKERS

Biomarkers now play a pivotal role in the diagnosis and management of acute coronary syndromes. Until 20 years ago biomarkers only retrospectively detected cardiac necrosis. These tests utilized lactate dehydrogenase (LDH) and creatine kinase (CK), and their isoenzymes. The average peak times after infarction were 6 hours for CK-MB, 18 hours for CK, and 48 hours for LDH. The CK-MB assay supported by clinical history, physical examination, and ECG findings represented the gold standard for detection of myocardial injury.

Troponin has become the biomarker of choice for the detection of myocardial injury. The troponin complex is composed of troponins I, T, and C. The troponin complex is located on the actin filament along with tropomyosin [8]. The troponin complex consists of regulatory proteins that control the calcium-mediated interaction of actin and myosin [9]. The cardiac-specific isoforms of troponin are known as cTnI and cTnT. Troponin C exists in skeletal muscle and thus is not cardiac specific. The early release of troponin from an MI is thought to arise from what has been termed the cytosolic pool. Subsequent release of troponin is prolonged from the degradation of actin and myosin in the area of damage.

There are variations in the sensitivity and specificity of the various cTnI and cTnT immunoassays [10,11]. This variation is due to lack of standardization, modified cTnI and cTnT in the plasma, and variations in antibody cross-reactivities to the various detectable forms of cTnI that follow its degradation. Point-of-care tests are thought to have lower sensitivity than laboratory-based tests [12]. Because all cTnI and cTnT assays are unique, a value from one assay cannot be extrapolated to another. Therefore, the 99th percent value needs be known for the assay being used, along with the level of 10% coefficient of variance for each individual test and hospital. Troponins can be elevated by a variety of other conditions, such as moderate to severe pulmonary embolism with right heart overload, heart failure, myocarditis, cardiac contusion, cardiotoxic agents, stress (Takotsubo) cardiomyopathy, sepsis, renal failure, severe neurologic diseases, hemorrhage infiltrative diseases, rhabdomyolysis with cardiac involvement, severe anemia, and even running a marathon.

Other biomarkers are also being used. Brain natriuretic protein (BNP), atrial natriuretic protein (ANP), and amino-terminal pro–B-type natriuretic peptide (NT-proBNP) are the most characterized natriuretic peptides [13]. ANP is secreted mostly by the cardiac atria, and BNP is secreted primarily by the cardiac ventricles. The most important stimulus for secretion of these peptides is stretching of myocardial fibers caused by volume overload or myocardial ischemia. These peptides have diuretic, natriuretic, and vasorelaxant properties. There is evidence that measuring BNP before major vascular surgery and cTnI after surgery provides additional prognostic information for major adverse cardiac events (MACE) and mortality [14]. A recent meta-analysis of 18 studies demonstrated that patients undergoing noncardiac surgery with elevated postoperative BNP were at increased risk for mortality, MI, and cardiac failure at 30 days and beyond 180 days after surgery [15]. Other biochemical markers of MI are under development [8].

Recent studies suggest that perioperative elevated plasma troponin is common and strongly associated with mortality for both cardiac surgery [16] and noncardiac surgery [17], and any acute severe illness [18–20]. Biomarkers also improve the risk stratification for surgery. Choi and colleagues [21] demonstrated that the addition of a preoperative NT-proBNP to the Revised Cardiac Risk Index (RCRI) significantly improved the RCRI's ability to predict MACE. A meta-analysis of preoperative natriuretic proteins (NPs) showed they could significantly alter RCRIs in vascular surgical patients [22]. Another meta-analysis of patients undergoing intermediate and major noncardiac surgery showed improved accuracy of RCRI with preoperative NP values [23]. In both of these studies there was an increased risk for MACE with each incremental increase in NP.

RISK FACTORS

The American College of Cardiology and American Heart Association (ACC/AHA) 2007 perioperative guidelines specify 4 active cardiac conditions that require evaluation and treatment before noncardiac surgery [24]. Unstable coronary syndromes such as unstable or severe angina or recent MI, within 30 days, are the first condition. Recent unstable coronary syndromes are hypercoagulable states. Noncardiac surgery is also associated with a hypercoagulable state, which can aggravate the existing hypercoagulable state and result in myocardial ischemia. The incidence of perioperative MI or death has been shown to as high as 28% in patients with unstable angina undergoing noncardiac surgery [25]. Decompensated heart failure is the second condition. New York Heart Association functional class IV or worsening or new-onset heart failure are included in this group. The third condition is the presence of significant arrhythmias, including heart block, symptomatic ventricular arrhythmias, or bradycardia. The fourth condition is severe aortic stenosis or severe symptomatic mitral stenosis [26].

The RCRI devised by Lee and colleagues [27] continues to be the best paradigm for stratifying cardiac risk before noncardiac surgery. There are 6 independent predictors of cardiac complications in this validated index:

- High-risk surgery (intraperitoneal, intrathoracic, or suprainguinal vascular procedures)
- Known ischemic heart disease
- History of congestive heart failure
- History of cerebrovascular disease
- Insulin-dependent diabetes mellitus
- Preoperative creatine greater than 2.0 mg/dL

The greater the number of predictors a patient has, the greater the risk of perioperative complications with noncardiac surgery. Recently, another cardiac risk calculator has been developed [28]. Although not as well validated as the RCRI, this calculator may be more accurate. The cardiac risk calculator includes the patient's functional capacity, which appears to be an important determinant of patient risk. A study by Reilly and colleagues [29] showed that patients who were undergoing major noncardiac surgery and who reported poor exercise capacity, including inability to walk 4 blocks or climb 2 flights of stairs, had much worse perioperative complications than those who had good exercise capacity.

There are surgery-specific cardiac risk predictors before noncardiac surgery, especially in those patients with more than 2 clinical factors on the RCRI [30]. Vascular surgery and emergency surgery are considered the highest-risk procedures, with cardiac morbidity rates of greater than 5%. Vascular surgery includes aortic and other major vascular surgery along with peripheral vascular surgery. The risk of endovascular aortic surgery is not well defined, but is generally thought to be intermediate-risk surgery [31]. Intermediate-risk surgery is thought to have a cardiac morbidity risk of 1% to 5%, and would include head and neck surgery, carotid endarterectomy, and orthopedic and prostate surgery. Unlike the RCRI, intraperitoneal or intrathoracic surgery in this definition is considered intermediate risk. Low-risk surgery is thought to have a cardiac risk of less than 1%, and would include endoscopic and superficial surgery, breast surgery, ambulatory surgery, and cataract surgery.

APPROACH TO CARE

The accurate identification of those patients who are at higher risk of perioperative MI and increased mortality has multiple advantages. The physician and the patient have a better understanding of the risk versus benefit of the expected surgical procedure. Together they may decide to modify the surgical procedure (eg, performing an endovascular abdominal aortic replacement rather than an open procedure), or may decide to decline or defer the procedure. Preoperative identification of high-risk patients enables physicians to direct their efforts toward those patients most likely to benefit from additional interventions. In addition, postoperative management, monitoring, and therapies can be individualized in accordance with the patient's risk of perioperative MI [32].

One option would be to perform coronary artery revascularization via either PCI or CABG before noncardiac surgery. PCI requires anticoagulation with clopidogrel and/or aspirin following the procedure. Surgery induces a procoagulant state, which puts the patient at risk for stent thrombosis and MI. It is the recommendation of the ACC/AHA that noncardiac surgery be delayed for 2 weeks following coronary balloon angioplasty and 30 to 45 days following placement of a bare-metal stent [30]. Noncardiac surgery should be delayed at least 1 year following the placement of a coronary drug-eluting stent.

A major question concerns whether antiplatelet therapy be continued throughout surgery. A study of 647 consecutive vascular surgery patients showed no difference in bleeding and blood transfusion between patients taking clopidogrel and those not taking it [33]. A retrospective study of drug-eluting stents and noncardiac surgery did show increased bleeding in patients who continued clopidogrel though surgery [34]. A large study of noncardiac surgical patients who were randomized to either aspirin or placebo found that 351 of 4998 patients (7.0%) had composite MI or death at 30 days in the aspirin group, compared with 355 of 5012 patients (7.1%) in the placebo group (hazard ratio [HR] in the aspirin group, 0.99; 95% CI, 0.86–1.15; $P =$ .92) [35]. Major bleeding was more common in the aspirin group (330 patients, 4.6%) than in the placebo group (188 patients, 3.8%; hazard ratio 1.23; 95% CI, 1.01–1.49; $P =$ .04). A smaller study of 291 patients, called the STATAGEM trial, randomized patients to either aspirin or placebo for noncardiac surgery [36]. No difference was found between the aspirin group and placebo group regarding the incidence thrombotic or bleeding outcomes. A study of 4149 vascular surgery patients found that patients taking aspirin, β-blockers, and statins had a 3-fold lower incidence of MI (2.5% vs 7.8%; odds ratio [OR] 0.31; 95% CI, 0.15–0.61, $P =$ .001) compared with those patients not taking these drugs [37]. After adjusting for propensity to use various therapies, aspirin (HR 0.35; 95% CI, 0.24–0.53, $P <$.0001), β-blockers (HR 0.65; 95% CI, 0.43–1, $P =$ .05), and statins (HR 0.36; 95% CI, 0.25–0.53, $P <$.0001) remained associated with improved 12-month survival. Aspirin use did not predict severe/moderate bleeding. A report by Schouten and colleagues [38] of prospectively collected Dutch registry data found that stopping antiplatelet therapy with noncardiac surgery and a recent PCI increased risk MACE to 30.7%, compared with 0% in those patients who continued antiplatelet therapy in their surgery. The relative risk of bleeding, especially into an enclosed space such as the brain, spinal cord, or eye, compared with the risk of perioperative MI needs to be determined. If the patient has a recent PCI and is at high risk for MI, it may be beneficial to continue antiplatelet therapy throughout the surgery or delay the surgery until there is time for the stent to endothelialize.

The first randomized trial comparing CABG with PCI before major elective vascular surgery was the Coronary Artery Revascularization Prophylaxis (CARP) study [39]. This trial randomized 510 patients and found that revascularization failed to affect any outcome measure, including mortality and MI, with 6 years' follow-up. The study population all had single-, double-, or triple-vessel coronary artery disease. A reanalysis of the CARP data according to type of revascularization procedure, CABG or PCI, showed that patients undergoing CABG had lower rates of death, MI, and need for additional revascularization procedures following surgery in comparison with PCI [40]. Further analyses of the CARP data show that patients with left main disease did have improvement in survival with perioperative coronary revascularization. The DECREASE-V pilot study was a small study of 101 patients with extensive coronary ischemia randomized to prophylactic revascularization (PCI with bare-metal stent, or drug-eluting stent, or CABG) or best medical management before major vascular surgery. No short-term or long-term benefits of prophylactic revascularization were found [41]. One reason why prophylactic revascularization is not beneficial is timing. A retrospective cohort trial showed similar rates of adverse cardiac outcomes in patients who had their PCI performed less than 90 days before noncardiac surgery and in matched nonrevascularized controls [42]. If PCI was performed greater than 90 days before noncardiac surgery, the PCI patients had a lower risk of adverse outcomes in comparison with matched controls.

For many years β-blockers were considered the best drugs to protect patients with or without known coronary artery disease from perioperative MACE. In 2007 the perioperative guidelines of the ACC/AHA advocated the continuation of β-blocker therapy in patients who are already taking these agents [30]. For those patients not already taking β-blockers, they recommended initiating β-blocker therapy for those patients who have ischemia on preoperative testing and are undergoing vascular surgery. A large meta-analysis of all prospective randomized trials of perioperative β-blocker therapy showed no statistically significant protection from β-blockers. This finding resulted in the PeriOperative Ischemic Evaluation (POISE) trial [43], the largest randomized placebo-controlled trial of β-blocker therapy to date, with 8351 patients with or at risk of coronary atherosclerotic disease and undergoing noncardiac surgery. The β-blocker group received extended-release metoprolol succinate, 100 mg 2 to 4 hours before surgery, continued for 30 days postoperatively. There was less MACE in the metoprolol group, 244 patients (5.8%), versus 290 patients (6.9%) in the placebo group (HR 0.84; 95% CI, 0.7–0.99; $P = .0399$). There were fewer MIs in the metoprolol group than in the placebo group: 176 (4.2%) versus 239 (5.7%). Unfortunately, there was greater mortality in metoprolol group (129; 3.1%) than in the placebo group (97; 2.3%). There also was a greater number of cerebrovascular accidents in the metoprolol group (41 patients; 1.0%) than in the placebo group (19 patients; 0.5%). A meta-analysis following POISE has confirmed the cardioprotective effects of β-blockers but also the significant risk associated with β-blocker therapy before noncardiac surgery [44]. Time of β-blocker use may an important factor. A very large database trial found that compared with patients having a duration of β-blockade greater than 31 days, patients who had a duration of β-blockade of 1 to 7 days had a greater 30-day mortality (OR 1.49; 95% CI, 1.03–2.16; $P = .03$) [45]. Curiously the choice of β-blocker may be a factor in the results. Wallace and colleagues [46] has shown in 3789 patients with continuing β-blocker treatment that atenolol was associated with better protection for 30-day and 1-year mortality than metoprolol. Guidelines for the perioperative use of β-blockers were published in 2009 [47], recommending continuing long-term treatment with β-blockers, avoidance of high-dose β-blockade, and consideration of introducing β-blocker treatment in patients with known coronary artery disease, reversible ischemia on stress testing, and at risk of coronary artery disease undergoing high-risk surgery, especially vascular surgery.

Does cardiac stress testing improve outcomes? It is recommended that the need for stress testing should depend on cardiac and surgical risk factors [48]. The European Society of Cardiology guidelines for preoperative cardiac risk assessment and perioperative management recommend additional cardiac testing in patients with 3 or more clinical risk factors on the RCRI and undergoing high-risk surgery [49].

Statin therapy should not be stopped for surgery. A meta-analysis of 12 retrospective and 3 prospective trials with a total of 223,010 patients showed that preoperative statin therapy was associated with 38% reduction in the risk of mortality after cardiac surgery (1.9% vs 3.1%; $P = .0001$) and a 59% reduction in the risk of mortality after vascular surgery (1.7% vs 6.1%; $P = .0001$) [50]. Schouten and colleagues [51] reported that statin discontinuation was associated with an increased risk of troponin release (HR 4.6; 95% CI, 2.2–9.6) and combined MI and death (HR 7.5; 95% CI, 2.8–20.1) Similar results were reported by Welten and colleagues [52].

Clonidine is an α2-adrenergic agonist used to treat hypertension and other conditions. Should patients be on clonidine before noncardiac surgery? In a large, prospective randomized trial, POISE-2, patients were randomized to either low-dose clonidine or placebo [53]. Clonidine use was not associated with a reduction in composite death and MI at 30 days (HR 1.08; 95% CI, 0.93–1.30; $P = .29$). More patients in the clonidine group had clinically important hypotension (47.6%) than in the placebo group (37.1%) (HR 1.32; 95% CI, 1.24–1.40; $P < .0001$). There also was a higher rate of nonfatal cardiac arrest in the clonidine group (0.3%) compared with the placebo group (0.1%) (HR 3.20; 95% CI, 1.17–8.73; $P = .29$).

Anemia is a theoretic risk for perioperative MI. Anemia reduces oxygen delivery and increases oxygen demand for the heart. A retrospective study by Beattie and colleagues [54] showed that as nadir hemoglobin decreased, the risk of MACE increased. In these anemic patients, MACE was much worse in β-blocked patients than in those who were not β-blocked. Anemia is associated with the need for red blood cell transfusions. A meta-analysis by Biccard and Rodseth [55] identified independent intraoperative predictors of adverse cardiac events. The need for intraoperative blood transfusion (OR 2.3; 95% CI, 1.4–3.3), vascular surgery (OR 2.3; 55% CI, 1.2–3.4), and emergent or urgent surgery (OR 2.3; 95% CI, 1.1–3.5) were the only independent intraoperative risk predictors of adverse cardiac events. Other hemodynamic risk factors they identified were hypotension, tachycardia, or hypothermia in the recovery room, and ischemic preconditioning.

Theoretically regional anesthesia is better than general anesthesia at blunting the stress response and inflammatory reaction to surgery. Neuraxial block causes sensory block, resulting in reduced opioid requirements and improved pain outcomes after surgery. Neuraxial block can also block the sympathetic system; however, the sympathetic blockade may result in hypotension. A meta-analysis of 17 studies demonstrated that postoperative epidurals resulted in a reduction in perioperative MIs compared with no epidural [56]. A recent analysis of data from the POISE trial found that neuraxial block was associated with an increased risk of death and perioperative MI (7.3% vs 5.7%; OR 1.24; 95% CI, 1.02–1.49) [57]. The mechanism of this association with increased adverse events is not known.

IMPLICATIONS

What should be done if a patient has elevated biomarkers following surgery but is totally asymptomatic? This situation represents a true clinical dilemma. First, a comprehensive search for a cardiac explanation should be conducted. This search includes ECG and, in most cases, echocardiography. Essentially any cardiac abnormality or underlying condition, including common ones such as left ventricular hypertrophy, can result in some myocyte necrosis following anesthesia and noncardiac surgery. An attempt should be made to categorize postoperative MI as type 1 (a primary acute coronary problem) or type 2 (demand ischemia). As noted earlier, the postoperative state is proinflammatory and procoagulant, and is associated with plaque erosion and rupture. If a primary type 1 MI is suspected, urgent catheterization with coronary angiography is indicated as soon as is safe from a surgical standpoint. Minimum antiplatelet and antithrombin requirements include aspirin, 81 to 162 mg and unfractionated heparin, 50 U/kg. Often it is safe to proceed on the day of surgery, although this is variable. PCI can be performed, but the risk of stent thrombosis is likely higher than usual. If safe, the addition of clopidogrel should be considered. On the other hand, a type 2 MI is suspected if there are no acute ECG changes in the face of known heart disease (eg, prior known coronary occlusions, old MI, left ventricular hypertrophy, severe valve disease). Prior angiograms, if any, should be reviewed carefully, and echocardiography performed to evaluate left ventricular function and to exclude less common causes of postoperative troponin elevation such as Takotsubo cardiomyopathy (apical balloon syndrome). If left ventricular function is normal or unchanged, the patient can be treated medically and followed. Medical treatment can include addition of β-blocker and/or statin therapy. Subsequently, noninvasive and/or invasive cardiac evaluation can be performed if indicated for standard clinical indications.

In noncardiac surgical patients, an elevated troponin independently predicts both short-term and long-term mortality [58,59]. Moreover, the greater the increase in troponin, the greater the risk of 30-day mortality with or without symptoms [17,60]. There is also evidence that elevated biomarkers may predict noncardiac-related death [61]. A new perioperative clinical entity called myocardial injury after noncardiac surgery (MINS) has been proposed [6]. MINS is a major cause of 30-day mortality. In the VISON trial, the risk for MINS was 34.0% (95% CI, 26.6–41.5), comparable with the risk of sepsis and infection, which was 30.5% (95% CI, 23.7–37.2) [62]. To date there are no prospective randomized trials on the management of MINS, but there is evidence for improvement in care. The POISE trial demonstrated that statin and aspirin therapy were associated with cardiovascular protection [1]. There is therefore an opportunity to optimize patients' medical management if the patients are not already on aspirin and statin therapy. Prior studies indicate that a large number of patients with elevated troponins are not on these medications [1,63]. The European Society of Cardiology has put forward guidelines for preoperative cardiac risk assessment and perioperative management [49]. Application of these guidelines resulted in a reduction in postoperative MI in

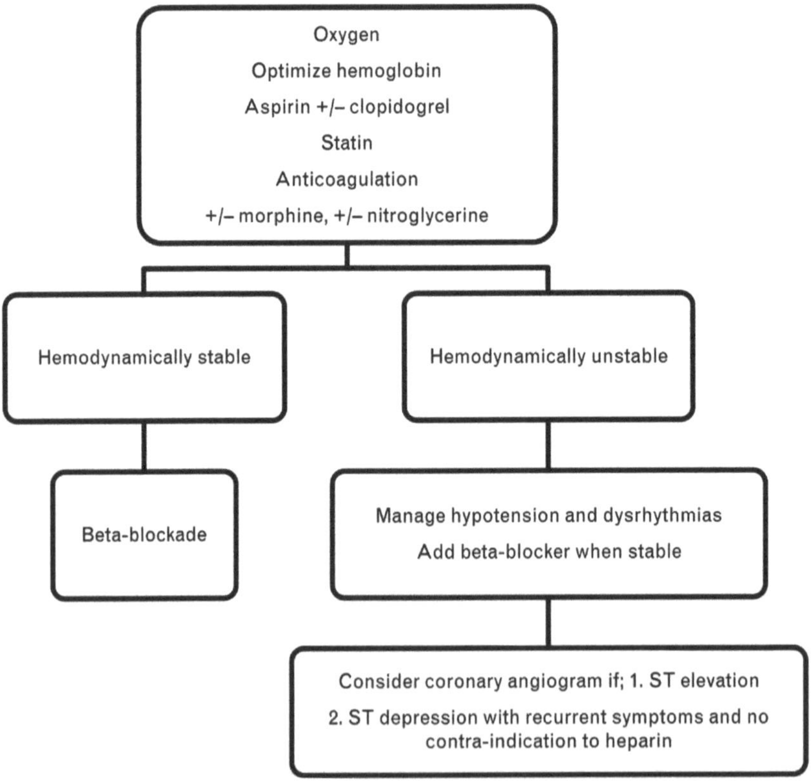

Fig. 1. Proposed algorithm for the management of patients with myocardial injury after noncardiac surgery. (*From* Biccard B. Detection and management of perioperative myocardial ischemia. Curr Opin Anaesthesiol 2014;27(3):342; with permission.)

orthopedic surgical patients [64]. It appears there is a 24-hour period before maximal increase in troponins, and the median time after peak troponin to death from MINS is 9 to 12 days [60,62,65]. Therefore, there is time for medical therapy. A management algorithm for MINS has been proposed (Fig. 1) [6].

SUMMARY

Elevations of biomarkers of MI are more common and clinically important than once thought. Elevated biomarkers are associated with an increased risk of death following noncardiac surgery. The concept of MINS should be embraced, and studies performed to determine which therapies are most effective in preventing perioperative death.

References

[1] Devereaux PJ, Xavier D, Pogue J, et al. Characteristics and short-term prognosis of perioperative myocardial infarction in patients undergoing noncardiac surgery: a cohort study. Ann Intern Med 2011;154:523–8.
[2] Thygesen K, Alpert JS, White HD, et al. Universal definition of myocardial infarction. Circulation 2007;116:2634–53.
[3] Hamm CW, Bassand JP, Agewall S, et al. ESC Guidelines for the management of acute coronary syndromes in patients presenting without persistent ST-segment elevation: The Task Force for the management of acute coronary syndromes (ACS) in patients presenting without persistent ST-segment elevation of the European Society of Cardiology (ESC). Eur Heart J 2011;32:2999–3054.
[4] Jneid H, Anderson JL, Wright RS, et al. 2012 ACCF/AHA focused update of the guideline for the management of patients with unstable angina/Non-ST-elevation myocardial infarction (updating the 2007 guideline and replacing the 2011 focused update): a report of the American College of Cardiology Foundation/American Heart Association Task Force on practice guidelines. Circulation 2012;126:875–910.
[5] Thygesen K, Alpert JS, Jaffe AS, et al. Third universal definition of myocardial infarction. Circulation 2012;126:2020–35.
[6] Biccard BM. Detection and management of perioperative myocardial ischemia. Curr Opin Anaesthesiol 2014;27:336–43.
[7] Devereaux PJ, Goldman L, Yusuf S, et al. Surveillance and prevention of major perioperative ischemic cardiac events in patients undergoing noncardiac surgery: a review. CMAJ 2005;173:779–88.
[8] Ramasamy I. Biochemical markers in acute coronary syndrome. Clin Chim Acta 2011;412:1279–96.
[9] Adams JE 3rd, Abendschein DR, Jaffe AS. Biochemical markers of myocardial injury. Is MB creatine kinase the choice for the 1990s? Circulation 1993;88:750–63.
[10] Panteghini M, Pagani F, Yeo KT, et al. Evaluation of imprecision for cardiac troponin assays at low-range concentrations. Clin Chem 2004;50:327–32.
[11] Apple FS, Quist HE, Doyle PJ, et al. Plasma 99th percentile reference limits for cardiac troponin and creatine kinase MB mass for use with European Society of Cardiology/American College of Cardiology consensus recommendations. Clin Chem 2003;49:1331–6.
[12] Thygesen K, Alpert JS, White HD. Universal definition of myocardial infarction. Eur Heart J 2007;28:2525–38.
[13] Battistoni A, Rubattu S, Volpe M. Circulating biomarkers with preventive, diagnostic and prognostic implications in cardiovascular diseases. Int J Cardiol 2012;157:160–8.
[14] Bolliger D, Seeberger MD, Lurati Buse GA, et al. A preliminary report on the prognostic significance of preoperative brain natriuretic peptide and postoperative cardiac troponin in patients undergoing major vascular surgery. Anesth Analg 2009;108:1069–75.

[15] Rodseth RN, Biccard BM, Chu R, et al. Postoperative B-type natriuretic peptide for prediction of major cardiac events in patients undergoing noncardiac surgery: systematic review and individual patient meta-analysis. Anesthesiology 2013;119:270–83.
[16] Domanski MJ, Mahaffey K, Hasselblad V, et al. Association of myocardial enzyme elevation and survival following coronary artery bypass graft surgery. JAMA 2011;305: 585–91.
[17] Devereaux PJ, Chan MT, Alonso-Coello P, et al. Association between postoperative troponin levels and 30-day mortality among patients undergoing noncardiac surgery. JAMA 2012;307:2295–304.
[18] Lim W, Cook DJ, Griffith LE, et al. Elevated cardiac troponin levels in critically ill patients: prevalence, incidence, and outcomes. Am J Crit Care 2006;15:280–8.
[19] Kelley WE, Januzzi JL, Christenson RH. Increases of cardiac troponin in conditions other than acute coronary syndrome and heart failure. Clin Chem 2009;55:2098–112.
[20] Reynolds T, Cecconi M, Collinson P, et al. Raised serum cardiac troponin I concentrations predict hospital mortality in intensive care unit patients. Br J Anaesth 2012;109:219–24.
[21] Choi JH, Cho DK, Song YB, et al. Preoperative NT-proBNP and CRP predict perioperative major cardiovascular events in non-cardiac surgery. Heart 2010;96:56–62.
[22] Rodseth RN, Lurati Buse GA, Bolliger D, et al. The predictive ability of pre-operative B-type natriuretic peptide in vascular patients for major adverse cardiac events: an individual patient data meta-analysis. J Am Coll Cardiol 2011;58:522–9.
[23] Rodseth RN, Biccard BM, Le Manach Y, et al. The prognostic value of pre-operative and post-operative B-type natriuretic peptides in patients undergoing noncardiac surgery: B-type natriuretic peptide and N-terminal fragment of pro-B-type natriuretic peptide: a systematic review and individual patient data meta-analysis. J Am Coll Cardiol 2014;63: 170–80.
[24] Fleisher LA, Beckman JA, Brown KA, et al. ACC/AHA 2007 Guidelines on Perioperative Cardiovascular Evaluation and Care for Noncardiac Surgery: Executive Summary: A Report of the American College of Cardiology/American Heart Association Task Force on Practice Guidelines (Writing Committee to Revise the 2002 Guidelines on Perioperative Cardiovascular Evaluation for Noncardiac Surgery): Developed in Collaboration With the American Society of Echocardiography, American Society of Nuclear Cardiology, Heart Rhythm Society, Society of Cardiovascular Anesthesiologists, Society for Cardiovascular Angiography and Interventions, Society for Vascular Medicine and Biology, and Society for Vascular Surgery. Circulation 2007;116:1971–96.
[25] Shah KB, Kleinman BS, Rao TL, et al. Angina and other risk factors in patients with cardiac diseases undergoing noncardiac operations. Anesth Analg 1990;70:240–7.
[26] Tashiro T, Pislaru SV, Blustin JM, et al. Perioperative risk of major non-cardiac surgery in patients with severe aortic stenosis: a reappraisal in contemporary practice. Eur Heart J 2014; http://dx.doi.org/10.1093/eurheartj/ehu044.
[27] Lee TH, Marcantonio ER, Mangione CM, et al. Derivation and prospective validation of a simple index for prediction of cardiac risk of major noncardiac surgery. Circulation 1999;100:1043–9.
[28] Gupta PK, Gupta H, Sundaram A, et al. Development and validation of a risk calculator for prediction of cardiac risk after surgery. Circulation 2011;124:381–7.
[29] Reilly DF, McNeely MJ, Doerner D, et al. Self-reported exercise tolerance and the risk of serious perioperative complications. Arch Intern Med 1999;159:2185–92.
[30] Fleisher LA, Beckman JA, Brown KA, et al. ACC/AHA 2007 guidelines on perioperative cardiovascular evaluation and care for noncardiac surgery: a report of the American College of Cardiology/American Heart Association Task Force on Practice Guidelines (Writing Committee to Revise the 2002 Guidelines on Perioperative Cardiovascular Evaluation for Noncardiac Surgery) developed in collaboration with the American Society of Echocardiography, American Society of Nuclear Cardiology, Heart Rhythm Society, Society of Cardiovascular Anesthesiologists, Society for Cardiovascular Angiography and

Interventions, Society for Vascular Medicine and Biology, and Society for Vascular Surgery. J Am Coll Cardiol 2007;50:e159–241.
[31] Paravastu SC, Jayarajasingam R, Cottam R, et al. Endovascular repair of abdominal aortic aneurysm. Cochrane Database Syst Rev 2014;(1):CD004178.
[32] Biccard BM, Devereaux PJ, Rodseth RN. Cardiac biomarkers in the prediction of risk in the non-cardiac surgery setting. Anaesthesia 2014;69:484–93.
[33] Saadeh C, Sfeir J. Discontinuation of preoperative clopidogrel is unnecessary in peripheral arterial surgery. J Vasc Surg 2013;58:1586–92.
[34] Rabbitts JA, Nuttall GA, Brown MJ, et al. Cardiac risk of noncardiac surgery after percutaneous coronary intervention with drug-eluting stents. Anesthesiology 2008;109: 596–604.
[35] Devereaux PJ, Mrkobrada M, Sessler DI, et al. Aspirin in patients undergoing noncardiac surgery. N Engl J Med 2014;370:1494–503.
[36] Mantz J, Samama CM, Tubach F, et al. Impact of preoperative maintenance or interruption of aspirin on thrombotic and bleeding events after elective non-cardiac surgery: the multicentre, randomized, blinded, placebo-controlled, STRATAGEM trial. Br J Anaesth 2011;107:899–910.
[37] Lau WC, Froehlich JB, Jewell ES, et al. Impact of adding aspirin to β-blocker and statin in high-risk patients undergoing major vascular surgery. Ann Vasc Surg 2013;27:537–45.
[38] Schouten O, van Domburg RT, Bax JJ, et al. Noncardiac surgery after coronary stenting: early surgery and interruption of antiplatelet therapy are associated with an increase in major adverse cardiac events. J Am Coll Cardiol 2007;49:122–4.
[39] McFalls E, Ward H, Moritz T, et al. Coronary-artery revascularization before elective major vascular surgery. N Engl J Med 2004;351:2795–804.
[40] Ward HB, Kelly RF, Thottapurathu L, et al. Coronary artery bypass grafting is superior to percutaneous coronary intervention in prevention of perioperative myocardial infarctions during subsequent vascular surgery. Ann Thorac Surg 2006;82:795–800.
[41] Schouten O, van Kuijk JP, Flu WJ, et al. Long-term outcome of prophylactic coronary revascularization in cardiac high-risk patients undergoing major vascular surgery (from the randomized DECREASE-V Pilot Study). Am J Cardiol 2009;103:897–901.
[42] Posner K, Van Norman G, Chan V. Adverse cardiac outcomes after noncardiac surgery in patients with prior percutaneous transluminal coronary angioplasty. Anesth Analg 1999;89:553–60.
[43] Devereaux PJ, Yang H, Yusuf S, et al. Effects of extended-release metoprolol succinate in patients undergoing non-cardiac surgery (POISE trial): a randomised controlled trial. Lancet 2008;371:1839–47.
[44] Bangalore S, Wetterslev J, Pranesh S, et al. Perioperative β blockers in patients having noncardiac surgery: a meta-analysis. Lancet 2008;372:1962–76.
[45] Wijeysundera DN, Beattie WS, Wijeysundera HC, et al. Duration of preoperative β-blockade and outcomes after major elective noncardiac surgery. Can J Cardiol 2014;30:217–23.
[46] Wallace AW, Au S, Cason BA. Perioperative β-blockade: atenolol is associated with reduced mortality when compared to metoprolol. Anesthesiology 2011;114:824–36.
[47] Fleischmann KE, Beckman JA, Buller CE, et al. 2009 ACCF/AHA focused update on perioperative β blockade: a report of the American college of cardiology foundation/American heart association task force on practice guidelines. Circulation 2009;120: 2123–51.
[48] Hoeks SE, Poldermans D. European Society of Cardiology 2009 guidelines for preoperative cardiac risk assessment and perioperative cardiac management in noncardiac surgery: key messages for clinical practice. Pol Arch Med Wewn 2010;120:294–9.
[49] Schouten O, Sillesen H, Poldermans D. New guidelines from the European Society of Cardiology for perioperative cardiac care: a summary of implications for elective vascular surgery patients. Eur J Vasc Endovasc Surg 2010;39:1–4.

[50] Hindler K, Shaw AD, Samuels J, et al. Improved postoperative outcomes associated with preoperative statin therapy. Anesthesiology 2006;105:1260–72.
[51] Schouten O, Hoeks SE, Welten GM, et al. Effect of statin withdrawal on frequency of cardiac events after vascular surgery. Am J Cardiol 2007;100:316–20.
[52] Welten GM, Chonchol M, Hoeks SE, et al. Statin therapy is associated with improved outcomes in vascular surgery patients with renal impairment. Am Heart J 2007;154:954–61.
[53] Devereaux PJ, Sessler DI, Leslie K, et al. Clonidine in patients undergoing noncardiac surgery. N Engl J Med 2014;370:1504–13.
[54] Beattie WS, Wijeysundera DN, Karkouti K, et al. Acute surgical anemia influences the cardioprotective effects of β-blockade: a single-center, propensity-matched cohort study. Anesthesiology 2010;112:25–33.
[55] Biccard BM, Rodseth RN. What evidence is there for intraoperative predictors of perioperative cardiac outcomes? A systematic review. Perioper Med (Lond) 2013;2:14.
[56] Beattie WS, Badner NH, Choi P. Epidural analgesia reduces postoperative myocardial infarction: a meta-analysis. Anesth Analg 2001;93:853–8.
[57] Leslie K, Myles P, Devereaux P, et al. Neuraxial block, death and serious cardiovascular morbidity in the POISE trial. Br J Anaesth 2013;111:382–90.
[58] Nagele P, Brown F, Gage BF, et al. High-sensitivity cardiac troponin T in prediction and diagnosis of myocardial infarction and long-term mortality after noncardiac surgery. Am Heart J 2013;166:325–32.e1.
[59] Levy M, Heels-Ansdell D, Hiralal R, et al. Prognostic value of troponin and creatine kinase muscle and brain isoenzyme measurement after noncardiac surgery: a systematic review and meta-analysis. Anesthesiology 2011;114:796–806.
[60] van Waes JA, Nathoe HM, de Graaff JC, et al. Myocardial injury after noncardiac surgery and its association with short-term mortality. Circulation 2013;127:2264–71.
[61] Oluleye OW, Folsom AR, Nambi V, et al. Troponin T, B-type natriuretic peptide, C-reactive protein, and cause-specific mortality. Ann Epidemiol 2013;23:66–73.
[62] Botto F, Alonso-Coello P, Chan MT, et al. Myocardial injury after noncardiac surgery: a large, international, prospective cohort study establishing diagnostic criteria, characteristics, predictors, and 30-day outcomes. Anesthesiology 2014;120:564–78.
[63] Hietala P, Strandberg M, Strandberg N, et al. Perioperative myocardial infarctions are common and often unrecognized in patients undergoing hip fracture surgery. J Trauma Acute Care Surg 2013;74:1087–91.
[64] Ausset S, Auroy Y, Verret C, et al. Quality of postoperative care after major orthopedic surgery is correlated with both long-term cardiovascular outcome and troponin Ic elevation. Anesthesiology 2010;113:529–40.
[65] Le Manach Y, Perel A, Coriat P, et al. Early and delayed myocardial infarction after abdominal aortic surgery. Anesthesiology 2005;102:885–91.

Advances in Anesthesia 32 (2014) 37–57

ADVANCES IN ANESTHESIA

ELSEVIER
MOSBY

Shoulder Surgery in the Beach Chair Position

Current Anesthetic Concepts and Controversies in Hemodynamic Management and Cerebral Perfusion

Rohini Kotha, MD[a], Steven L. Orebaugh, MD[b,*]

[a]Department of Anesthesiology, University of Pittsburgh School of Medicine, 910 LSK, 3471 Fifth Avenue, Pittsburgh, PA 15213, USA; [b]Department of Anesthesiology, UPMC Southside/Mercy Anesthesia, University of Pittsburgh School of Medicine, 2000 Mary Street, Pittsburgh, PA 15203, USA

Keywords

• Beach chair position • Shoulder surgery • Anesthesia • Hemodynamics
• Cerebral ischemia • Neurologic outcomes

Key points

- Reduced cerebral perfusion seems to occur frequently during shoulder surgery in the beach chair position (BCP), primarily in patients under general anesthesia, with positive pressure ventilation, which may be magnified by deliberate hypotension.
- Interscalene brachial plexus blockade with sedation may protect against cerebral hypoperfusion by allowing preservation of autoregulation, as well as avoiding the diminished cardiac output that occurs with controlled ventilation.
- The overall incidence of severe neurologic injury is quite low, but the occurrence of clinically subtle forms of neurologic dysfunction, such as delirium and postoperative cognitive dysfunction, has not been well delineated.
- Although its importance may be the subject of scientific debate, most clinicians consider that blood pressure measured at the arm level overestimates cerebral pressure in the upright position and so they deliberately correct for this factor in determining perfusion pressures of the brain.
- The lower limit of autoregulation is likely variable between individuals and is altered by pathologic entities, such as chronic hypertension or preexisting cerebrovascular pathologic abnormality.
- Monitors of cerebral perfusion have not been definitively shown to prevent central nervous system injury, but may be useful in vulnerable individuals.

Conflicts: The authors have no conflicts of interest to declare.

*Corresponding author. *E-mail address:* orebaughsl@anes.upmc.edu

0737-6146/14/$ – see front matter
http://dx.doi.org/10.1016/j.aan.2014.08.008

INTRODUCTION

There has been an exponential growth in the volume of shoulder surgery in the last 2 decades. In one study examining the epidemiology of upper extremity ambulatory procedures performed in the United States [1] for the year 2006, the estimates for these common procedures include

- 272,148 rotator cuff repairs (RCRs)
- 257,541 shoulder arthroscopies, excluding RCRs

Colvin and colleagues [2] performed an investigation to determine trends in resource utilization for RCRs, including type and setting of surgical treatment from 1996 to 2006. They reported that overall there was a 141% increase in the number of RCRs performed, from approximately 41 per 100,000 population in 1996 to approximately 98 per 100,000 population in 2006. Open repairs were increased by 21%, whereas arthroscopic repairs increased to a much greater extent, by 530%. The ambulatory surgery setting witnessed much greater growth than inpatient procedures, more than quadrupling during this period (from 22 to 91 per 100,000 capita), whereas inpatient surgical procedures decreased by 63%. In addition, shoulder arthroplasty procedures have increased dramatically as well. Kim and colleagues [3] described a marked increase in total shoulder arthroplasty, by more than 2.5-fold in a 15-year period from 1993 to 2008, with a less significant increase in hemi-arthroplasties.

Many, if not most, of these shoulder procedures are conducted in the upright beach chair position (BCP). In this article, current concepts, controversies, and practicalities of anesthetic practice for shoulder surgery in the seated, or BCP position, are reviewed.

HISTORY/UTILITY OF BEACH CHAIR POSITION

Since its introduction for shoulder arthroscopy by Skyhar and colleagues [4] in 1988, orthopedic surgeons have debated whether the BCP or the lateral decubitus position (LDP) is superior for shoulder surgery. Although other positioning techniques have their proponents, the BCP has spread widely and is now favored by many surgeons because of several apparent benefits [5]:

- Upright anatomic position
- Decreased brachial plexus injury
- Increased operative arm mobility
- Easier examination under anesthesia
- Easier anterior port placement
- Easier conversion to open procedure
- More conducive positioning for a regional anesthetic peripheral nerve block (PNB) technique

MANAGEMENT GOALS FOR ANESTHESIA IN BEACH CHAIR POSITION

General considerations

A thorough preoperative assessment is essential before choosing the anesthetic technique, because there are certain patients with comorbidities and ailments that can make anesthesia in the BCP challenging. These ailments include cerebrovascular disease, orthopedic problems, or body habitus, which may make adoption of the seated position difficult. In addition, surgical factors should also be considered. Minor procedures that are of relatively short duration may be carried out with regional anesthesia and sedation alone, whereas more extensive procedures and/or prolonged surgical duration may require a combination of regional and general anesthesia, because remaining seated and immobile for longer periods may be quite uncomfortable, and longer procedures are more likely to lead to potential airway management issues.

Position-related considerations

There are unique complications associated with the use of the upright BCP. Maintaining a safe position for the head can be challenging, and stretch or pressure on nerves must be conspicuously avoided. Park and Kim [6] reviewed 3 cases of neurapraxia of the cutaneous branches of the cervical plexus after shoulder surgery in the BCP. Involved nerves included the lesser occipital and greater auricular, both of which were thought to have sustained direct compression from the headrest holder. Recommendations were made for consideration of headrest redesign, extra-auricular padding, and frequent head position checks. Hypoglossal nerve palsy had been described as well [7,8]. In these cases, the postulated cause was thought to have been because of a change in posture of the head and neck during the operative procedure, thus leading to an unintended compression of the hypoglossal nerve and a subsequent palsy.

Anesthetic-related considerations

Interscalene nerve block

Possible risks and complications of this peripheral block include brachial plexus neurapraxia/transient neuropathy, inadvertent central neuraxial injection, local anesthetic systemic toxicity (LAST), hypotensive bradycardic episodes (HBE), and unintended blockade of adjacent nerves–phrenic, recurrent laryngeal, sympathetic chain–resulting in undesirable side effects, such as symptomatic hemi-diaphragmatic paralysis, hoarseness, and Horner syndrome, respectively.

Serious complications, including signs of LAST, pneumothorax, arrhythmias, peripheral neurologic complications, and death, have been described [9]. When symptoms of abnormal neurologic function are aggressively sought after interscalene nerve block (ISB) and shoulder surgery, as many as 14% of patients note sensory loss that is apparently unrelated to the surgery, but these symptoms are mostly self-limited and abate over several weeks or months [10,11]. Authors of a recent systematic review [12] concluded that the use of an ISB for shoulder procedures resulted in significant decreases in postoperative pain compared with general anesthesia alone, and in the amount of postoperative supplemental analgesia required in patients undergoing arthroscopic procedures. The overall complication rate attributable to the block in the randomized trials evaluated was negligible. In addition, ISB was found to be more cost-effective compared with general anesthesia alone. In a prospective study of 1319 patients who underwent ultrasound-guided ISB anesthesia for shoulder arthroscopy [13], the block was reportedly successful in 99.6%. A total of 38 major and minor complications occurred, for a rate of 2.88%. Most complications were transient neurologic events: 3 cases of postoperative brachial plexitis, 14 cases of ear numbness (likely due to compression from headrest), 8 cases of digital numbness, and a single case of distal ulnar neuropathy. Three patients had permanent sequelae, including a case of perioperative myocardial infarction, one of transverse myelitis, and a persistent brachial plexopathy in a patient ultimately diagnosed with multiple sclerosis.

Deliberate hypotensive anesthesia

In many orthopedic cases, the use of controlled hypotensive anesthesia can be beneficial by decreasing blood loss, and enhancing surgical exposure, thus limiting surgical time–especially surgeries of the hip and shoulder, where tourniquet use is not possible. However, major concerns have been raised regarding the use of hypotensive anesthesia in patients in the BCP. Pohl and Cullen [14] reported 4 cases of ischemic brain and spinal cord injury after shoulder procedures performed under hypotensive anesthesia. They noted that the BCP provides several unusual risk factors for cerebral hypoperfusion: the decrease in blood pressure associated with general anesthesia and upright posture, the requirement to correct for the effects of gravity on cerebral perfusion pressure (CPP), and vascular compression related to malpositioning of the head and neck. The authors noted that vigilant monitoring of blood pressure, with correction for differences in height between measurement site and circle of Willis and careful maintenance of adequate CPP, are recommended to optimize patient safety. In addition, it is crucial to consider individual patients' susceptibilities to reduced perfusion, especially in the elderly and in those with cardiovascular and cerebrovascular comorbidities.

Irrigation-related considerations

Inadequate preoperative mixing of epinephrine into the irrigating fluid, if used, can result in a rapid administration of a highly concentrated epinephrine solution, which has resulted in life-threatening dysrhythmias, but this can be prevented by thoroughly mixing before spiking the bag [15,16].

Airway compromise

Airway obstruction due to extra-articular spread of arthroscopic irrigation fluid has been reported in a few cases [17–19]. Although rare in the upright position, this potentially fatal complication can be prevented by restricting the duration of the procedure and minimizing the arthroscopy pump pressures and amount of fluid used for joint irrigation. In addition, frequent evaluation of the degree of neck swelling can forewarn the occurrence of severe edema and allow cessation of the procedure and tracheal intubation if necessary [19].

PATHOPHYSIOLOGY OF CEREBRAL BLOOD FLOW IN BEACH CHAIR POSITION

The upright position is the normal position for humans during most of waking life as well as the normal reference position for obtaining outpatient arterial blood pressure measurements. The hydrostatic effect of gravity produces a decrease in systemic arterial pressure on adoption of the upright position due to venous pooling the lower extremities. The volume of blood accumulating in the venous system depends on patient factors, including body mass index, sympathetic tone, intravascular volume status, and preexisting hypertension. As a result, in an awake subject, upright positioning activates the sympathetic nervous system, over a short interval, producing increases in heart rate (15%–30%), systemic vascular resistance (30%–40%), and systemic blood pressure (10%–15%) [20]. In anesthetized patients, however, the response of the autonomic nervous system is blunted by the vasodilating and cardiac depressant effects of intravenous and volatile anesthetics, as well as the effects of positive pressure ventilation, resulting in an attenuated increase in systemic vascular resistance, reduced preload, a decrease in mean arterial pressure (MAP), and a greater reduction in cardiac output compared with the awake state [21], which may be further compounded by surgical requests for controlled hypotension. Together, these effects may result in relative central nervous system (CNS) hypoperfusion, particularly in the watershed regions of perfusion.

Stroke is a potentially devastating consequence of prolonged cerebral hypoperfusion. Perioperative stroke is relatively unusual, but has been well recognized after major cardiac and vascular surgery. Following lower extremity major joint surgery, the incidence of perioperative stroke in the United Kingdom was found to be around 0.03% [22], but the mortality incurred was 29%. Other reports place the incidence at a somewhat higher level, between 0.1% and 0.7% for noncardiac, nonneurologic surgery [23,24].

The most concerning complications reported during shoulder surgery in the BCP follow the use of controlled hypotensive anesthesia, with resultant rare but devastating neurologic complications that have included ischemic brain and spinal cord injury and visual loss in otherwise healthy patients [14,25,26]. These adverse neurologic events are generally attributed to inadequate cerebral perfusion secondary to intraoperative hypotension. In a review of stroke and death related to shoulder surgery in the sitting position, Papadonikolakis and colleagues [27] explored the concept of correct interpretation of patients' blood pressure, noting that, in particular, use of blood pressure determinations on the leg and use of controlled hypotension during anesthesia are major adverse influences, which may predispose to catastrophic complications.

There has long been a common acceptance that there exists a critical CPP below which cerebral blood flow will be compromised (lower limit of cerebral autoregulation), usually in the range of 50 mm Hg. However, there is no rigorous available evidence that supports this pressure recommendation, nor that such a pressure reflects the physiology of any given individual patient, raising the question: "What is the safe lower limit of autoregulation of the brain?" Drummond [28], in an insightful report, noted that this threshold may be as high as 60 to 90 mm Hg in awake normotensive volunteers, and that the results of multiple studies suggest that the lower limit of cerebral autoregulation may be actually be closer to 70 mm Hg, with the significant ranges reported reflecting interindividual variation.

In an interesting study performed on healthy rats under anesthesia, Jones and colleagues [29] observed the autoregulatory curve in a controlled setting to analyze variations from the classic patterns of the response near its lower limit. Intracranial pressure was fixed, and MAP was varied with progressive hemorrhage, while cerebral blood flow (CBF) was measured using laser Doppler flowmetry. Three different patterns of vasoregulatory response to falling perfusion pressures were noted: a "peak" response in 31% of animals, with a greater-than-expected degree of vasodilation and blood flow; a normal response observed in 52% of specimens; and a "none" response in 17%, in which there was a failure of autoregulatory vasodilation, allowing CBF to decrease in a pressure-dependent manner (Fig. 1). However, when these observations were averaged together, the classic, textbook pattern of autoregulation resulted.

Loss of autoregulation similar to the "none" pattern is well described in humans following acute events such as stroke and traumatic brain injury [30,31]. Studies using transcranial Doppler (TCD) to assess dynamic cerebral autoregulation show impairment of this reflex for a variable period after the insult and may affect even uninjured portions of the brain [32]. In these patients, it is not just the lower limit of autoregulation that is altered; rather, it is the actual shape of the curve. In recent studies, evidence has accumulated demonstrating that autoregulation is impaired by a variety of factors, including chronic hypertension, diabetes, smoking, peripheral vascular disease, and hypertension-associated disorders, including obstructive sleep apnea [28,31,33–35]. This impairment results in a change in the shape of the autoregulatory curve

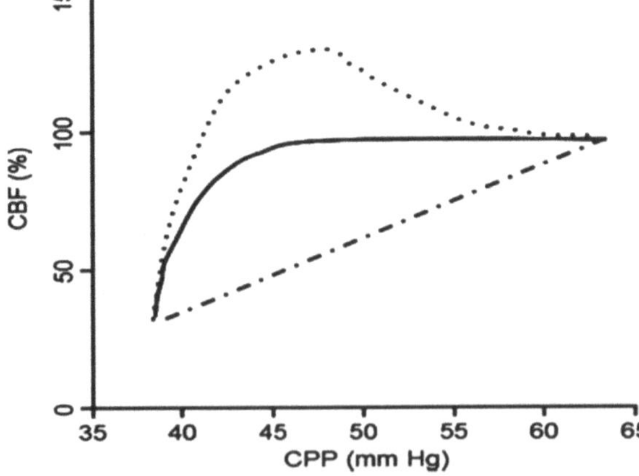

Fig. 1. Physiologic heterogeneity in cerebral autoregulation. Schematic representation of 3 different patterns of CBF following a decrease in CPP (classical [*solid line*], peak [*dotted line*], and none [*dashed line*]) observed in anesthetized rats.

from sigmoidal to more linear [31–33]. Changes related to chronic hypertension include vascular hypertrophy and increased sympathetic activity, both of which may adversely affect the autoregulatory response to changes in perfusion pressure. This failure of autoregulation (a "none" pattern) leads to a situation in which cerebral blood flow becomes dependent on systemic blood pressure (Fig. 2) [34].

Another important feature of the current debate regarding blood pressure management in the head-up position revolves around whether blood pressure should be adjusted to account for the difference in height between the site of measurement (most commonly a noninvasive blood pressure cuff on the nonoperative arm) and the level of the brain. There are currently 2 schools of thought regarding this: the closed/siphon theory and the open/waterfall theory.

The presence or absence of a siphon effect is the key point of differentiation in closed and open systems. The siphon concept or "closed model" is based on the presence of a continuous column of blood between the arterial and venous limbs of the circulation. For the brain, a siphon mechanism would involve a circuit of vessels including the thoracic aorta, the cerebral arteries, and the cerebral veins where they leave the skull, and the superior vena cava draining into to the right atrium. When a siphon is functional, no work is done on blood to increase its gravitational potential energy because the pressure gradients are equal and opposite in direction in the ascending and the descending limbs of the loop [36,37] and hence no "correction factor" is needed; the sitting position results in equivalent decreases in MAP and central venous pressure.

According to the waterfall or "open model," cerebral veins collapse, preventing a siphon effect from operating. Gravitational effects cause blood to drain to the heart on the venous side of the cerebral circuit, veins and venules collapse

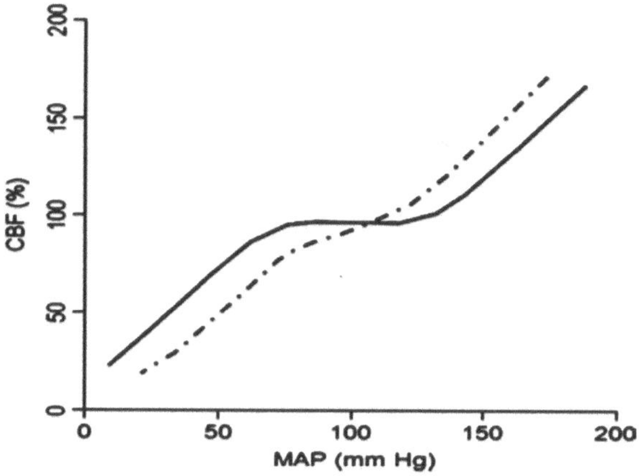

Fig. 2. Pathologic disturbance of autoregulation. Schematic representation of the "classic" autoregulation curve (*solid line*) and the change in patients with chronic hypertension (*dashed line*).

completely, and the heart is responsible for pumping a column of blood toward the brain against a gravity-derived pressure gradient [37]. In this situation, a correction factor is required to account for the weight of this column of blood, in determining the perfusion pressure at the level of the brain (the blood pressure is reduced approximately 2 mm Hg for every 1-inch, or 2.5 cm, of height difference between the site of measurement and the brain).

Of interest, a recent experiment in anesthetized giraffes demonstrated that cerebral blood flow was determined by arterial pressure without contribution from a siphon mechanism. Simultaneous measurements of blood flow and pressure showed that cerebral perfusion of anesthetized upright-positioned giraffes is maintained by the high arterial blood pressure, and that the jugular vein is collapsed in the upright position, favoring the waterfall theory. This waterfall theory implies that the vascular resistance of the jugular vein counterbalances the gravitational pressure profile and, thus, there is no indication of a functional siphon, at least in this long-neck animal model [38]. However, neither the open nor the closed mechanism completely explains the variations in cerebral perfusion with changes of position. Munis [37] noted that several limitations exist with the open model, including the impracticality to explain cerebral perfusion in weightlessness or the upside down position, the lack of a correspondingly high venous pressure at the level of the heart in seated patients, and the occurrence of venous air embolism during positive pressure ventilation.

Multiple other contributing factors that may influence CBF in the upright position have been identified [39,40], including physical and anatomic factors, such as:

- Intraluminal atherosclerosis
- Deviations from classic vessel configurations within the neck, such as a diminutive or nonfunctioning vertebral artery unilaterally
- Changing relationships between the geography of the brain stem and vertebral vessels during head flexion
- External compression of the carotid and vertebral arteries by osteophytes or even normal bony vertebral anatomy.

The influence of posture and anesthesia on total cerebral oxygen delivery is complex and multifactorial; it is affected not only by changes in MAP but also by variations in intracranial pressure, vascular reactivity, moment-to-moment changes in cerebral oxygen extraction, and the dynamics of cerebral venous outflow. On head elevation, a decrease in intracranial pressure and central venous pressure will augment CPP, whereas a reduction in MAP will tend to decrease it. Predicting the balance of these many factors is challenging and may vary from individual to individual.

Several investigators have demonstrated that reduced cerebral perfusion in association with decreased blood pressure is not infrequent during surgery in BCP, as shown in Table 1 [41]. Various modes of assessment of cerebral perfusion have been used. Although some investigators have used near-infrared spectroscopy (NIRS) for determination of cerebral oximetry to examine the

Table 1
Investigations examining the effect of beach chair position on cerebral blood flow and oxygenation

Publication	Study design	Outcome measure	Results
Fischer et al [42], 2009	Case report 63 y/o–ASA 3	$S(ct)O_2$	↓$S(ct)O_2$ correlated with ↓MAP, ↓$etCO_2$
Dippmann et al [43], 2010	Case report 1. 46 y/o–ASA 1 2. 58 y/o–ASA 2	$S(ct)O_2$	↓$S(ct)O_2$ correlated with ↓MAP
McCulloch et al [49], 2010	TCD supine vs 45° BCP (n = 19)	MCAv	SBP_{arm} 142 → 96 mm Hg SBP_{eam} 141 → 76 mm Hg MAP_{eam} 95 → 50 mm Hg (47%↓) MCA_v 46 → 36 cm/s (22%↓)
Lee et al [44], 2011	$S(ct)O_2$ supine vs BCP (n = 27)	S(ct)O2	MAP_{eam} 85 → 75 mm Hg $S(ct)O_2$ 74 → 67%
Jeong et al [46], 2012	$S(ct)O_2$ and $SjvO_2$ supine vs 65°–70° BCP w/P/R vs S/N (n = 56)	$S(ct)O_2$ and $SjvO_2$	MAP_{eam} goal w/in 20% baseline. MAP_{eam} <20% baseline: P/R group, 69%; S/N group, 38% $SjvO_2$ <50%: P/R group, 56%; S/N group, 21% P/R Anesth (OR 4.76) MAP_{eam} <50 mm Hg (OR 3.85) (P = .02) $S(ct)O_2$ >20% ↓ from baseline: P/R group, 28%; S/N group, 25% ($S(ct)O_2$ sensitivity and specificity for detecting $SjvO_2$ <50% was 30.4% and 75.8%)
Gillespie et al [66], 2012	EEG supine vs 60° BCP (n = 52)	EEG	MAP/SBP goal <20% below baseline and SBP >90 mm Hg All patients fell below BP goals 3 patients w/EEG ischemia

Abbreviations: ECG, electroencephalogram; MCAv, middle cerebral artery velocity; $S(ct)O_2$, cerebral oximetry saturation.
Data from Shear T, Murphy G. Impact of the beach chair position on cerebral perfusion: what do we know so far? APSF Newsletter 2013;18–9.

effect of the BCP on oxygen supply to the brain, others have used TCD to determine middle cerebral artery velocity, electroencephalography, and/or jugular venous oxygen saturation ($SjvO_2$). Despite differing methodologies for assessment, all of these studies suggest that considerable reductions in perfusion occur as MAP decreases with anesthesia in the upright position.

CLINICAL OUTCOMES

In 2005, Pohl and Cullen [14] published their startling 4-patient case series describing catastrophic neurologic outcomes after shoulder surgery in the BCP. This case series has prompted several investigators to study how management of intraoperative factors like blood pressure and type of anesthesia may potentially affect outcomes following shoulder surgery in the BCP.

Multiple monitoring modalities have been used to estimate the adequacy of cerebral oxygenation, the most common one being cerebral oximetry. NIRS is a commercially available noninvasive technology that provides continuous monitoring of regional cerebral oxygen saturation (rSO_2).

Beach chair position versus supine

Several case reports have provided evidence that a reduction in MAP may lead to a diminished rSO_2 in the BCP after induction of general anesthesia, to levels that are concerning for cerebral ischemia, although absolute threshold values have not been definitely established [42,43]. In these cases, administration of vasopressor or inotropic agents to restore blood pressure resulted in rapid elevation of cerebral saturation values. Lee and colleagues [44] prospectively investigated 28 patients under general anesthesia and mechanical ventilation in the BCP, with induced hypotension to MAP of 60 to 65 mm Hg, measured with a radial arterial cannula referenced to the level of the external auditory meatus (EAM). Cerebral oxygen saturation was measured by NIRS. Adoption of upright position resulted in a significant decrease in MAP as compared with supine, with a corresponding drop in rSO_2. However, further reductions in blood pressure to the desired levels of hypotension did not result in further decline in cerebral oxygenation. Two patients developed a more severe reduction in cerebral perfusion, with rSO_2 decreasing to less than 80% of baseline; this was readily corrected when blood pressure was increased to higher levels. No adverse neurologic outcomes were noted.

In a prospective study of 20 patients under general anesthesia, receiving usual anesthetic care by providers blinded to values of NIRS-determined rSO_2, Moerman and colleagues [45] reported an 80% incidence of cerebral desaturation events (CDE), defined as a relative decrease in rSO_2 of greater than 20%, when an upright position was adopted for shoulder surgery. Postural decreases in rSO_2 were consistent and related to both blood pressure and end-tidal CO_2. Airway management was not specified. Deliberate hypotension was not used for these cases, and systolic arterial blood pressure (SBP) less than 80 mm Hg (measured with a noninvasive cuff on the nonoperative arm) or heart rate less than 50 beats per minute were treated with vasoconstrictors or chronotropic agents as indicated. However, the significance of the CDEs is not clear, because none of the patients developed gross neurologic abnormalities or cognitive dysfunction postoperatively.

In a randomized trial, Jeong and colleagues [46] studied 56 patients undergoing surgery in the BCP with general anesthesia provided by either propofol/remifentanil (P/R) or sevoflurane/N_2O (S/N). Patients were relaxed with rocuronium and mechanical ventilation was used to maintain end-tidal carbon dioxide (ET CO_2) tension at 35 to 40 mm Hg. The authors demonstrated that jugular venous desaturation ($SjvO_2$ <50%), indicative of cerebral hypoperfusion, occurred in 41% of patients undergoing shoulder surgery in BCP–three in the S/N group and 12 in the P/R group. Of those who developed $SjvO_2$ less than 40%, a value consistent with actual cerebral ischemia, all were in the propofol group. Risk factors for jugular venous desaturation included P/R anesthesia and MAP less than 50 mm Hg. Patients in the P/R group had significantly lower presitting baseline values of $SjvO_2$ and also showed a more profound decrease in MAP compared with those in the S/N group. The use of propofol for maintenance anesthesia likely reduces jugular venous saturation because of decreased cerebral oxygen delivery in the presence of an unfavorable cerebral oxygen balance, because propofol decreases CBF more than $CMRO_2$ and also because of a greater reduction of MAP and CPP. The authors also reported that NIRS-determined $SctO_2$ was not different between groups and correlated only weakly with $SjvO_2$. None of the patients developed neurologic signs or symptoms postoperatively.

Interestingly, in a prospective study of 40 American Society of Anesthesiologists (ASA) I/II patients Jo and colleagues [47] found that not only preload but also measures of preoperative cardiac performance may be important factors in the development of hypotension after repositioning from supine to sitting during general anesthesia. Using a radial artery catheter and a noninvasive hemodynamic assessment system, they demonstrated that the preinduction hemodynamic values of stroke volume index (SVI) and cardiac index (CI), and the postinduction value of stroke volume variation, determined before a positional change, could predict hypotension in the BCP under general anesthesia with mechanical ventilation and sevoflurane for maintenance.

Murphy and colleagues [48] evaluated 124 patients under general anesthesia with sevoflurane and controlled ventilation during shoulder arthroscopy using noninvasive cerebral oximetry. Sixty-one patients had the procedure in the BCP and 63 in the lateral decubitus position (LDP), depending on surgeon preference. Blood pressure measurements were carried out at the level of the upper arm rather than correcting for the level at the brain in the seated position. Despite the use of a protocol designed to optimize CPP, the incidence of CDE (defined as a reduction in rSO_2 of $\geq$20% from baseline or absolute value <55% for >15 seconds) was significantly higher in the BCP: 80.3% versus 0% in LDP. In contrast with results from other studies, the intraoperative values of HR, MAP, SpO_2, and bispectral index (BIS) did not differ between the 2 groups. A significantly higher incidence of postoperative nausea

(50% vs 6.7%, $P = .0001$) and vomiting (27.3% vs 3.3%, $P = .011$) was observed in subjects with intraoperative CDEs compared with subjects with no CDE. Anesthesia management varied considerably in this study, with 71% of patients in LDP receiving regional anesthesia, and only 8% of BCP patients, but variations in nausea and vomiting persisted even after multiple logistic regression analysis was used to factor in the anesthesia type.

In an investigation of 19 patients undergoing shoulder surgery in the BCP under general anesthesia using desflurane for maintenance of anesthesia with positive pressure ventilation, McCulloch [49] measured middle cerebral artery blood velocity (MCAv) using TCD. When hypotension was induced, with a decrease in SBP from 142 mm Hg to 96 mm Hg at the level of the arm (which corresponded to 76 at the EAM), a mean 22% decrease in MCAv was noted compared with the supine-normotensive state. The authors also found that mean apparent zero flow pressure (aZFP)–an index of critical closing pressure–decreased significantly with sitting position and induced hypotension. In addition, they calculated the resistance area product (RAP), an indicator of cerebrovascular resistance, which likewise decreased with adoption of the sitting position and decrease in blood pressure. Although MCAv was diminished in this setting, its decrement was less than the decrease in perfusion pressure, suggesting that autoregulation was at least partially preserved. The authors opined that the decline in aZFP and RAP contributed an equal measure to the decrease in MCAv as components of autoregulation.

In addition to the above compensatory mechanisms, severity and duration of ischemia are critical determinants of tissue damage, and viability-time thresholds must be exceeded to produce irreversible damage to the CNS. In a pig model, low rSO_2 values that persisted for less than 2 hours did not result in neurologic injury [50]. An analysis of NIRS data from 265 coronary artery bypass graft patients revealed a desaturation-time threshold of 50 minutes that was associated with cognitive decline and longer hospital length of stay [51]. Because shoulder surgery is often a relatively short procedure, the duration of most CDEs in many of the above investigations was probably limited, which may explain why no cerebrovascular events (CVEs) leading to gross neurologic injury were identified despite their frequent occurrence.

Type of anesthesia and mode of ventilation

Yadeau and colleagues [52] examined a cohort of 99 patients undergoing ambulatory shoulder arthroscopy in the BCP to examine the effect of deliberate hypotension on cerebral oxygenation with regional anesthesia. Cerebral oximetry was used to assess the adequacy of cerebral oxygenation as a surrogate of cerebral blood flow. The authors noted that the use of regional anesthesia with sedation as the primary anesthetic approach seemed to reduce the risk of CDEs compared with reported rates as high as 80% in patients who underwent surgery in the BCP under general anesthesia [48], although there was no control group receiving general anesthesia. In this study, 99% of patients met the definition for hypotension, but only 10% developed CDEs. With adjustment for baseline factors, CDE was not associated with hypotension, but was associated with risk factors for cerebrovascular disease. The blood pressure in this study was corrected to account for the distance between the heart and the brain (waterfall model) and all patients were breathing spontaneously.

In a recent prospective study, Koh and colleagues [53] evaluated 60 patients who underwent shoulder surgery after self-selection to an either an awake (interscalene block-propofol sedation) group or an asleep (general anesthesia, with controlled ventilation) group. NIRS was used to assess the adequacy of CBF. CDEs occurred in 57% of the asleep group, with nearly 3 episodes per patient, but there were no ischemic occurrences in the awake group. In addition, substantially more interventions were performed for hypotension in the asleep group (Fig. 3). However, MAP was successfully maintained and no significant differences were noted between the awake, asleep, and baseline blood pressure measurements at almost all time points. It was striking that, despite apparently adequate MAP, more than half of the patients in the asleep group (56.7%) demonstrated substantial decreases in rSO_2 (Fig. 4). Although there were no adverse neurologic outcomes reported, the authors concluded that avoidance

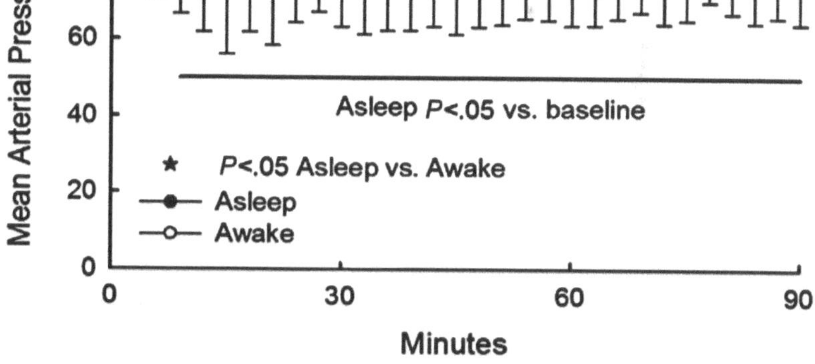

Fig. 3. Mean (standard deviation) arterial pressure (mm Hg) is shown for the general anesthesia (asleep) and interscalene block (awake) groups. The horizontal lines indicate the times whereby blood pressure was statistically different from baseline measures, from 9 to 90 minutes in the asleep group (*solid line*; overall P<.05) and from 39 to 45 minutes in the awake group (*dashed line*; overall P<.05). The only difference between the groups was at 12 minutes (overall P<.05). Note that data were collected throughout the entire procedure, but beyond 90 minutes there were fewer values for meaningful comparisons and trends did not significantly differ. (*From* Koh JL, Levin SD, Chehab EL, et al. Neer award 2012: cerebral oxygenation in the beach chair position: a prospective study on the effect of general anesthesia compared with regional anesthesia and sedation. J Shoulder Elbow Surg 2013;22:1328; with permission.)

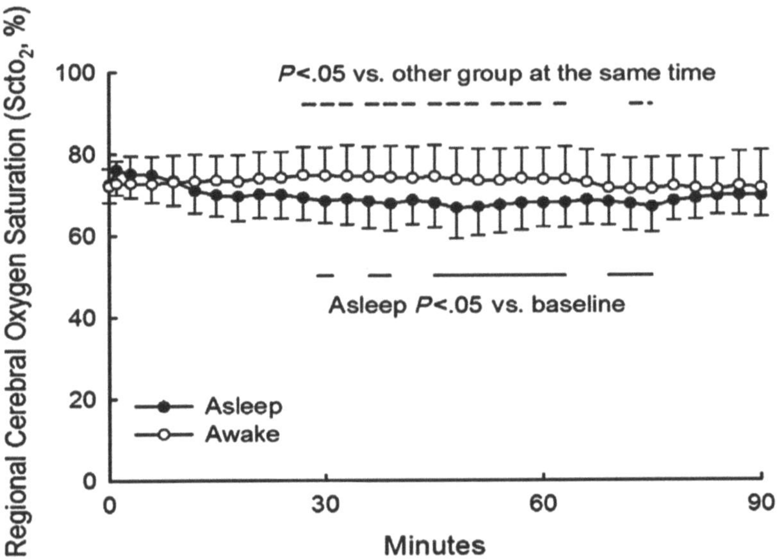

Fig. 4. Mean (standard deviation) regional cerebral oxygen saturation ($SctO_2$, %) for the patients in the general anesthesia (asleep) and interscalene block (awake) groups. A solid horizontal line marks the times when there was a statistically significant difference from baseline in the asleep group. The $SctO_2$ values in the awake patients never differed from their baseline measures. The dashed line marks significant differences between the asleep and awake groups. (*From* Koh JL, Levin SD, Chehab EL, et al. Neer award 2012: cerebral oxygenation in the beach chair position: a prospective study on the effect of general anesthesia compared with regional anesthesia and sedation. J Shoulder Elbow Surg 2013;22:1329; with permission.)

of general anesthesia (GA) for patients in the BCP might potentially reduce the risk of ischemic neurologic injury.

Comparing anesthesia regimens in 90 patients in BCP with controlled hypotension for shoulder surgery, and their impact on cerebral perfusion, hemodynamics, and neurobehavioral/neurologic outcome, Aguirre and colleagues [54] found that patients undergoing regional anesthesia had significantly fewer CDE ($P<.001$), and fewer decreases in rSO_2 values ($P<.001$). In addition, these patients maintained greater hemodynamic stability in the BCP compared with the patients in the general anesthesia group and manifested significantly better neurobehavioral test results the day after surgery.

There are several important, potentially relevant physiologic differences between general anesthesia and regional anesthesia in the BCP. Deleterious hemodynamic effects of the sitting position can be minimized with regional anesthesia, as sedated patients can better compensate for the decrease in venous return from the sitting position by increasing systemic vascular resistance. In addition, negative inotropic effects of anesthetics may be reduced, because overall doses are diminished. Furthermore, spontaneous ventilation helps to maintain venous return. In contrast, positive pressure ventilation that often accompanies GA can cause a decrease in cardiac output and cerebral perfusion secondary to decreased venous return, right ventricular dysfunction, and alteration of left ventricular distensibility.

In an evaluation of the importance of the technique of anesthesia in preserving CBF in upright position, Soeding and colleagues [55] evaluated the effects of general anesthesia versus sedation in 40 spontaneously breathing patients who had undergone interscalene block. General anesthesia consisted of sevoflurane delivered through a laryngeal mask airway and titrated to a bispectral index range of 40 to 60, whereas sedation consisted of a propofol infusion at 10 to 20 mg/h, with intent to preserve patient responsiveness. CBF was estimated using pulsed wave Doppler analysis of internal carotid artery blood flow. Although MAP, measured invasively and referenced to the level of the EAM, decreased to a much greater degree with general anesthesia than with sedation (34 mm Hg vs 4 mm Hg), and in addition, these patients had a markedly higher requirement for vasopressor agents and fluids to maintain the MAP at 70 or greater, there was no change in estimated CBF from the supine to sitting position in either group, and no difference between groups. The authors concluded that this preservation of CBF was evidence of intact autoregulation [55]. These results also suggest that the mode of ventilation may have a more profound effect than some of the other variables evaluated in the studies discussed.

EPIDEMIOLOGIC OUTCOMES

The exact incidence of stroke or significant cerebral or spinal cord injury during shoulder surgery in the BCP remains poorly defined. Friedman and colleagues [56] attempted to quantify the prevalence of intraoperative CVE during shoulder surgery through a survey of 287 members of the American Shoulder and Elbow Surgeons. A total of 93 members (32%) responded. The overall rate of CVE was reported as 8 of 274,225 or approximately 0.003%. All 8 cases occurred in patients who were in the BCP. Details of the anesthetics were not noted.

Yadeau and colleagues [57] reviewed 4169 (3000 retrospective and 1169 prospective) shoulder surgery cases in the sitting position, greater than 97% of which were managed with brachial plexus block, moderate sedation, and spontaneous ventilation. Forty percent of the patients had risk factors for stroke, and 47% experienced hypotension by one of several measures, but no patient had evidence of CNS ischemia or infarction. Notably, all of these were ambulatory surgical procedures, and some of the data was retrospective. More recently, a large retrospective review of 15,014 patients in BCP for shoulder surgery, over an 11-year period, was performed [58]. All patients received ISB and propofol/ketamine sedation. Only one neurologic deficit was reported, secondary to ischemic stroke, which occurred 24 hours after the surgery.

Pin-on et al [59] performed a comprehensive retrospective interrogation of the electronic medical record for 5177 patients who underwent either orthopedic shoulder surgery or neurologic surgery in the sitting position at Mayo

Clinic Rochester between 2002 and 2009, 4227 of which were orthopedic. In all of these cases, patients underwent general anesthesia with controlled ventilation. There were no patients who experienced ischemic brain or spinal cord injury. MAP during the first 2 hours of surgery was reduced significantly from baseline for both neurosurgical and orthopedic patients regardless of the method of BP measurement, and the average reduction in intraoperative SBP ranged from 12% to 19%, depending on the type of surgery and method of BP measurement. Hypertensive patients were found to have a greater magnitude of intraoperative BP reduction compared with normotensive patients regardless of the method of BP measurement.

In another epidemiologic study, a cohort of 1319 ASA 1 or 2 patients undergoing arthroscopic shoulder surgery at an outpatient surgery center [13] was prospectively evaluated. All of the patients had an interscalene block performed using ultrasound guidance, followed by general anesthesia with a laryngeal mask airway. Patients were queried by a physician 24 hours postoperatively regarding their satisfaction with the ISB and screened for a comprehensive registry of minor and major adverse events in the perioperative period. None of these patients suffered an acute, central neurologic injury related to surgery in the BCP. There were 3 admissions for cardiac-related complaints.

Monitoring cerebral perfusion

Cerebral hypoperfusion and ischemia are likely the major contributors to poor neurologic outcome related to the BCP, but the accurate determination of cerebral perfusion during the perioperative period still remains a challenge. Numerous methods and devices have been evaluated, including $SjvO_2$, middle cerebral artery blood flow velocity determined by Doppler, electroencephalogram, and regional cerebral oxygen saturation using near-infrared spectroscopy. As some of these are invasive or logistically challenging and may not be appropriate for ambulatory shoulder surgery in the BCP, most emphasis has been on cerebral oximetry using NIRS.

Cerebral oximetry is a noninvasive optical technology that integrates frontal cortex blood hemoglobin-oxygen saturation, providing real-time assessment of regional cerebral blood flow. Although several studies have shown a correlation between reduced perfusion pressures in the upright position and a decrement in frontal lobe oxygenation, there is little evidence that these episodes are related to postoperative outcomes. In addition, some studies have shown poor agreement between oximetry and other methods of assessment of perfusion, such as jugular venous saturation [46].

Several limitations of this technology should be borne in mind. NIRS monitored cerebral oxygenation values may be confounded by hyperthermia and norepinephrine-determined skin oxygenation [60]. Cerebral oximetry seems to have a high negative predictive value, but the positive predictive value is low, and its overall usefulness in predicting cerebral ischemia is modest [61,62]. In a comparison of cerebral oximetry values to awake testing during carotid endarterectomy, Stilo and colleagues [61] determined a sensitivity of

60% and specificity of only 25% when a drop of 20% in cerebral oximetry was used as an indicator of cerebral ischemia. Davie and Grocott [63] studied 3 brands of currently available NIRS devices and found that external contamination related to induced scalp ischemia significantly influenced regional cerebral oxygenation (rSO_2) readings.

Preventative strategies

In addition to avoidance of severe hypotension (ie, more than 20% less than a patient's baseline blood pressure), provision of a regional anesthetic [52–54,56] and maintenance of spontaneous ventilation [55] are some of the few measures that are thought to decrease the incidence of cerebral hypoperfusion. Measures to reduce venous pooling in the upright position may also be helpful. Kwak and colleagues [64] performed a randomized, controlled trial to evaluate the effect of a sequential compression device (SCD) on hemodynamics in arthroscopic shoulder surgery in the BCP. Patients underwent general anesthesia with sevoflurane and controlled ventilation. The authors noted that hypotension less than 80% of the patient's baseline, or MAP of lower than 60, occurred in 64% of control patients, but only 28% of those with the compression devices. In addition, cardiac output (CO) and stroke volume index (SVI) were maintained at a higher level in this group. These differences were very transient, however, perhaps because of rapid treatment of hypotension with ephedrine under the conditions of the study.

Adjustment of mechanical ventilation to maintain ET CO_2 at 40 to 42 mm Hg compared with 30 to 32 mm Hg significantly improves cerebral oxygenation during shoulder surgery in the BCP [65].

SUMMARY

Reduced cerebral perfusion seems to occur frequently during shoulder surgery in the BCP, primarily in patients under general anesthesia with positive pressure ventilation. General anesthesia effects may be magnified by deliberate hypotension. Interscalene brachial plexus blockade with sedation may protect against cerebral hypoperfusion by allowing preservation of autoregulation, as well as avoiding the diminished cardiac output that occurs with controlled ventilation. The overall incidence of severe neurologic injury is quite low, but the occurrence of clinically subtler forms of neurologic dysfunction, such as delirium and postoperative cognitive dysfunction, has not been well delineated. Although its importance may be the subject of scientific debate, most clinicians consider that blood pressure measured at the arm level overestimates cerebral pressure in the upright position and deliberately correct for this factor in determining perfusion pressures of the brain. The lower limit of autoregulation is likely variable between individuals and is altered by pathologic entities, such as chronic hypertension or preexisting cerebrovascular pathologic abnormality. Therefore, confident prediction of a lowest safe blood pressure in a given individual in the BCP remains difficult. Basing the acceptable blood pressure on the patient's baseline in the sitting position seems most prudent, and safest. Monitors of cerebral perfusion have not been definitively shown to prevent CNS injury, but may be useful in vulnerable individuals.

RECOMMENDATIONS

- Thorough preoperative evaluation to assess for risk factors for inadequate cerebral perfusion in the perioperative period to determine whether or not the patient is a candidate for the BCP.
- Avoid placing the noninvasive blood pressure cuff on the lower extremities.
- Establish an acceptable lower limit of blood pressure based on the individual patient's baseline determined in the sitting position; while this is somewhat arbitrary, most clinicians choose 20% lower than the baseline pressure.
- Reference systolic/mean arterial blood pressures to the level of the midbrain/circle of Willis, taking into account the effect of gravity (2mm Hg decrease in pressure for every 1-inch, or 2.5 cm, difference in height between the site of measurement and the brain).
- Use a regional technique as the primary anesthetic whenever possible.
- Avoid excessive depths of general anesthesia, which may lead to more severe decrements in blood pressure and flow. BIS monitoring may be useful in avoiding excessive depths of general anesthesia.
- Maintain spontaneous ventilation when possible, even if an airway is placed. If positive pressure ventilation is used, minute ventilation should be adjusted to avoid hyperventilation.
- Consider use of HBE prophylaxis when using interscalene nerve block, especially when exogenous epinephrine is used in the injectate.
- Minimize sudden changes in position.
- Provide frequent evaluation for neck swelling/edema, which may lead to airway obstruction in a patients without an endotracheal tube.
- Maintain euvolemia and administer vasopressors or inotropic agents as necessary to maintain MAP above the threshold identified for the individual patient.
- Consider use of sequential compression devices (SCDs).

References

[1] Jain NB, Higgins LD, Losina E, et al. Epidemiology of musculoskeletal upper extremity ambulatory surgery in the United States. BMC Musculoskelet Disord 2014;15:4; http://dx.doi.org/10.1186/1471-2474-15-4.
[2] Colvin AC, Egorova N, Harrison AK, et al. National trends in rotator cuff repair. J Bone Joint Surg Am 2012;94:227–33.
[3] Kim SH, Wise BL, Zhang Y, et al. Increasing incidence of shoulder arthroplasty in the United States. J Bone Joint Surg Am 2011;93:2249–54.
[4] Skyhar MJ, Altchek DW, Warren RF, et al. Shoulder arthroscopy with the patient in the beach-chair position. Arthroscopy 1988;4:256–9.
[5] Peruto CM, Ciccotti MG, Cohen SB. Shoulder arthroscopy positioning: lateral decubitus versus beach chair. Arthroscopy 2009;25:891–6.
[6] Park TS, Kim YS. Neuropraxia of the cutaneous nerve of the cervical plexus after shoulder arthroscopy. Arthroscopy 2005;21:631.
[7] Mullins RC, Drez D Jr, Cooper J. Hypoglossal nerve palsy after arthroscopy of the shoulder and open operation with the patient in the beach-chair position. A case report. J Bone Joint Surg Am 1992;74:137–9.
[8] Rhee YG, Cho NS. Isolated unilateral hypoglossal nerve palsy after shoulder surgery in beach-chair position. J Shoulder Elbow Surg 2008;17:e28–30.

[9] Lenters TR, Davies J, Matsen FA 3rd. The types and severity of complications associated with interscalene brachial plexus block anesthesia: local and national evidence. J Shoulder Elbow Surg 2007;16:379–87.
[10] Borgeat A, Ekatodramis G, Kalberer F, et al. Acute and nonacute complications associated with interscalene block and shoulder surgery: a prospective study. Anesthesiology 2001;95:875–80.
[11] Liu SS, Gordon MA, Shaw PM, et al. A prospective clinical registry of ultrasound-guided regional anesthesia for ambulatory shoulder surgery. Anesth Analg 2010;111:617–23.
[12] Hughes MS, Matava MJ, Wright RW, et al. Interscalene brachial plexus block for arthroscopic shoulder surgery: a systematic review. J Bone Joint Surg Am 2013;95: 1318–24.
[13] Singh A, Kelly C, O'Brien T, et al. Ultrasound-guided interscalene block anesthesia for shoulder arthroscopy: a prospective study of 1319 patients. J Bone Joint Surg Am 2012;94:2040–6.
[14] Pohl A, Cullen DJ. Cerebral ischemia during shoulder surgery in the upright position: a case series. J Clin Anesth 2005;17:463–9.
[15] Rains DD, Rooke GA, Wahl CJ. Pathomechanisms and complications related to patient positioning and anesthesia during shoulder arthroscopy. Arthroscopy 2011;27:532–41.
[16] Cho SH, Yi JW, Kwack YH, et al. Ventricular tachycardia during arthroscopic shoulder surgery: a report of two cases. Arch Orthop Trauma Surg 2010;130:353–6.
[17] Hynson JM, Tung A, Guevara JE, et al. Complete airway obstruction during arthroscopic shoulder surgery. Anesth Analg 1993;76:875–8.
[18] Antonucci S, Orlandi P, Mattei PA, et al. Airway obstruction during arthroscopic shoulder surgery: anesthesia for the patient or for the surgeon? Minerva Anestesiol 2006;72: 995–1000.
[19] Orebaugh SL. Life-threatening airway edema resulting from prolonged shoulder arthroscopy. Anesthesiology 2003;99:1456–8.
[20] Smith JJ, Porth CM, Erickson M. Hemodynamic response to the upright posture. J Clin Pharmacol 1994;34:375–86.
[21] Porter JM, Pidgeon C, Cunningham AJ. The sitting position in neurosurgery: a critical appraisal. Br J Anaesth 1999;82:117–28.
[22] Sanders RD, Jameson SS, James P, et al. Major medical complications and mortality following total hip arthroplasty: is thromboembolism a priority? Anesthesiology 2011;115:A1507.
[23] Mashour GA, Shanks AM, Kheterpal S. Perioperative stroke and associated mortality after noncardiac, nonneurologic surgery. Anesthesiology 2011;114:1289–96.
[24] Bateman BT, Schumacher HC, Wang S, et al. Perioperative acute ischemic stroke in noncardiac and nonvascular surgery. Anesthesiology 2009;110:231–8.
[25] Bhatti MT, Enneking FK. Visual loss and ophthalmoplegia after shoulder surgery. Anesth Analg 2003;96:899–902.
[26] Cullen DJ, Kirby RR. Beach chair position may decrease cerebral perfusion: catastrophic outcomes have occurred. APSF Newsletter 2007;22:25–7.
[27] Papadonikolakis A, Wiesler ER, Olympio MA, et al. Avoiding catastrophic complications of stroke and death related to shoulder surgery in the sitting position. Arthroscopy 2008;24:481–2.
[28] Drummond JC. The lower limit of autoregulation: time to revise our thinking. Anesthesiology 1997;86(6):1431–3.
[29] Jones SC, Radinsky CR, Furlan AJ, et al. Variability in the magnitude of the cerebral blood flow response and the shape of the cerebral blood flow pressure autoregulation curve during hypotension in normal rats [corrected]. Anesthesiology 2002;97:488–96.
[30] Novak V, Chowdhary A, Farrar B, et al. Altered cerebral vasoregulation in hypertension and stroke. Neurology 2003;60:1657–63.

[31] Hu K, Peng CK, Czosnyka M, et al. Nonlinear assessment of cerebral autoregulation from spontaneous blood pressure and cerebral blood flow fluctuations. Cardiovasc Eng 2008;8:60–71.
[32] Aries MJ, Elting JW, De Keyser J, et al. Cerebral autoregulation in stroke: a review of transcranial Doppler studies. Stroke 2010;41:2697–704.
[33] Novak V, Hajjar I. The relationship between blood pressure and cognitive function. Nat Rev Cardiol 2010;7:686–98.
[34] Sanders RD, Degos V, Young WL. Cerebral perfusion under pressure: is the autoregulatory 'plateau' a level playing field for all? Anaesthesia 2011;66:968–72.
[35] Urbano F, Roux F, Schindler J, et al. Impaired cerebral autoregulation in obstructive sleep apnea. J Appl Physiol (1985) 2008;105:1852–7.
[36] Gisolf J. Postural changes in humans: effect of gravity on the circulation. Enschede: Universiteit van Amsterdam; 2005.
[37] Munis J. The problems of posture, pressure, and perfusion. APSF Newsletter 2008;22: 82–3.
[38] Brondum E, Hasenkam JM, Secher NH, et al. Jugular venous pooling during lowering of the dead affects blood pressure of the anesthetized giraffe. Am J Physiol Regul Integr Comp Physiol 2009;297:R1058–65.
[39] Toole JF, Tucker SH. Influence of head position upon cerebral circulation. Studies on blood flow in cadavers. Arch Neurol 1960;2:42–9.
[40] Toole JF. Effects of change of head, limb and body position on cephalic circulation. N Engl J Med 1968;279:307–11.
[41] Shear T, Murphy G. Impact of the beach chair position on cerebral perfusion: what do we know so far? APSF Newsletter 2013;28:18–9.
[42] Fischer GW, Torrillo TM, Weiner MM, et al. The use of cerebral oximetry as a monitor of the adequacy of cerebral perfusion in a patient undergoing shoulder surgery in the beach chair position. Pain Pract 2009;9:304–7.
[43] Dippmann C, Winge S, Nielsen HB. Severe cerebral desaturation during shoulder arthroscopy in the beach-chair position. Arthroscopy 2010;26(Suppl 9):S148–50.
[44] Lee JH, Min KT, Chun YM, et al. Effects of beach-chair position and induced hypotension on cerebral oxygen saturation in patients undergoing arthroscopic shoulder surgery. Arthroscopy 2011;27:889–94.
[45] Moerman AT, De Hert SG, Jacobs TF, et al. Cerebral oxygen desaturation during beach chair position. Eur J Anaesthesiol 2012;29:82–7.
[46] Jeong H, Lee SH, Jang EA, et al. Haemodynamics and cerebral oxygenation during arthroscopic shoulder surgery in beach chair position under general anaesthesia. Acta Anaesthesiol Scand 2012;56:872–9.
[47] Jo YY, Jung WS, Kim HS, et al. Prediction of hypotension in the beach chair position during shoulder arthroscopy using pre-operative hemodynamic variables. J Clin Monit Comput 2014;28:173–8.
[48] Murphy GS, Szokol JW, Marymont JH, et al. Cerebral oxygen desaturation events assessed by near-infrared spectroscopy during shoulder arthroscopy in the beach chair and lateral decubitus positions. Anesth Analg 2010;111:496–505.
[49] McCulloch TJ, Liyanagama K, Petchell J. Relative hypotension in the beach-chair position: effects on middle cerebral artery blood velocity. Anaesth Intensive Care 2010;38: 486–91.
[50] Kurth CD, McCann JC, Wu J, et al. Cerebral oxygen saturation-time threshold for hypoxic-ischemic injury in piglets. Anesth Analg 2009;108:1268–77.
[51] Slater JP, Guarino T, Stack J, et al. Cerebral oxygen desaturation predicts cognitive decline and longer hospital stay after cardiac surgery. Ann Thorac Surg 2009;87:36–44.
[52] Yadeau JT, Liu SS, Bang H, et al. Cerebral oximetry desaturation during shoulder surgery performed in a sitting position under regional anesthesia. Can J Anaesth 2011;58: 986–92.

[53] Koh JL, Levin SD, Chehab EL, et al. Neer Award 2012: cerebral oxygenation in the beach chair position: a prospective study on the effect of general anesthesia compared with regional anesthesia and sedation. J Shoulder Elbow Surg 2013;22:1325–31.
[54] Aguirre J, Borgeat A, Trachsel T, et al. Cerebral oxygenation in patients undergoing shoulder surgery in beach chair position: comparing general to regional anesthesia and the impact on neurobehavioral outcome. Rev Esp Anestesiol Reanim 2014;61:64–72.
[55] Soeding PF, Wang J, Hoy G, et al. The effect of the sitting upright or 'beach chair' position on cerebral blood flow during anaesthesia for shoulder surgery. Anaesth Intensive Care 2011;39:440–8.
[56] Friedman DJ, Parnes NZ, Zimmer Z, et al. Prevalence of cerebrovascular events during shoulder surgery and association with patient position. Orthopedics 2009;32:256–61.
[57] Yadeau JT, Casciano M, Liu SS, et al. Stroke, regional anesthesia in the sitting position, and hypotension: a review of 4169 ambulatory surgery patients. Reg Anesth Pain Med 2011;36:430–5.
[58] Rohrbaugh M, Kentor ML, Orebaugh SL, et al. Outcomes of shoulder surgery in the sitting position with interscalene nerve block: a single-center series. Reg Anesth Pain Med 2013;38:28–33.
[59] Pin-on P, Schroeder D, Munis J. The hemodynamic management of 5177 neurosurgical and orthopedic patients who underwent surgery in the sitting or "beach chair" position without incidence of adverse neurological events. Anesth Analg 2013;116:1317–24.
[60] Sørensen H, Secher NH, Siebenmann C, et al. Cutaneous vasoconstriction affects near-infrared spectroscopy determined cerebral oxygen saturation during administration of norepinephrine. Anesthesiology 2012;117(2):263–70.
[61] Stilo F, Spinelli F, Martelli E, et al. The sensibility and specificity of cerebral oximetry, measured by INVOS - 4100, in patients undergoing carotid endarterectomy compared with awake testing. Minerva Anestesiol 2012;78(10):1126–35.
[62] Samra SK, Dy EA, Welch K, et al. Evaluation of a cerebral oximeter as a monitor of cerebral ischemia during carotid endarterectomy. Anesthesiology 2000;93:964–70.
[63] Davie SN, Grocott HP. Impact of extracranial contamination on regional cerebral oxygen saturation: a comparison of three cerebral oximetry technologies. Anesthesiology 2012;116:834–40.
[64] Kwak HJ, Lee JS, Lee DC, et al. The effect of a sequential compression device on hemodynamics in arthroscopic shoulder surgery using beach-chair position. Arthroscopy 2010;26:729–33.
[65] Murphy GS, Szokol JW, Avram MJ, et al. Effect of ventilation on cerebral oxygenation in patients undergoing surgery in the beach chair position: a randomized controlled trial. Br J Anaesth 2014 May 23. pii: aeu109. [Epub ahead of print].
[66] Gillespie R, Shishani Y, Streit J, et al. The safety of controlled hypotension for shoulder arthroscopy in the beach-chair position. J Bone Joint Surg Am 2012;94:1284–90.

Advances in Anesthesia 32 (2014) 59–70

ADVANCES IN ANESTHESIA

Anesthesia for Endoscopic Procedures: The New Frontier

John E. Tetzlaff, MD[a,*], John Vargo, MD, MPH[b], Walter Maurer, MD[c]

[a]Department of General Anesthesia, Cleveland Clinic Lerner College of Medicine of Case Western Reserve University, Cleveland Clinic, 9500 Euclid Avenue, Cleveland, OH 44195, USA; [b]Department of Gastroenterology and Hepatology, Cleveland Clinic Lerner College of Medicine of Case Western Reserve University, Cleveland Clinic, 9500 Euclid Avenue, Cleveland, OH 44195, USA; [c]Ambulatory Anesthesia, Department of General Anesthesia, Cleveland Clinic, 9500 Euclid Avenue, Cleveland, OH 44195, USA

Keywords

• Anesthesia • Sedation • Endoscopy • Gastrointestinal diseases • Pulmonary diseases • Ultrasound

Key points

- The number and complexity of gastrointestinal procedures performed with the participation of an anesthesia team is rapidly increasing.
- Routine endoscopy is being performed on an increasingly complex patient population.
- The techniques and technology for endoscopy is dramatically expanding the scope of the practice, with many endoscopic techniques replacing the previous need for surgical intervention.
- The role of the anesthesia team is determined by the procedure, the technology, and the comorbidity of the patients.
- The anesthetic options include moderate sedation, deep sedation, and general anesthesia.
- Future expansion of the techniques performed in the endoscopy suite may result from natural orifice transluminal endoscopic surgery, which may allow cavity procedures to be performed endoscopically using natural orifice access (mouth, anus, vagina) and even potentially allowing thoracic, abdominal, and pelvic procedures to be performed without the traditional surgical approach.

The authors have nothing to disclose.

*Corresponding author. *E-mail address*: tetzlaj@ccf.org

0737-6146/14/$ – see front matter
http://dx.doi.org/10.1016/j.aan.2014.08.006

INTRODUCTION

The role of the anesthesia team in the gastrointestinal (GI) endoscopy suite is rapidly expanding with an increase in the number of patients and the number and types of endoscopic procedures being performed. Many of these procedures are partially or completely replacing the need for surgery or accomplishing tasks that were only possible with a surgical procedure. The level of participation by the anesthesia team is determined by the procedure, the urgency, and by the comorbidity of the patients. Both the technique and the technology of endoscopy are expanding the number of procedures being performed with the participation of the anesthesia service. Future developments including natural orifice transluminal endoscopic surgery (NOTES) will continue this trend for expansion of the scope of practice in the GI endoscopy suite. In this article, the authors outline many of these procedures with details about the endoscopic technique and the options for anesthetic management.

GASTROINTESTINAL ENDOSCOPIC PROCEDURES

Esophagogastroduodenoscopy

Routine esophagogastroduodenoscopy (EGD) is used for the diagnosis and treatment of pathologic findings in the esophagus, stomach, or proximal duodenum. Because GI bleeding can occur further into the GI tract, modifications of this technique have been developed to investigate the jejunum and further. Push enteroscopy involves the insertion of a longer endoscope 90 to 150 cm from the teeth, typically reaching the variable lengths of the jejunum but not the ileum. The diagnostic yield of diagnostic or therapeutic specimen retrieval of this technique is 25% to 40% [1]. Treatment of upper GI bleeding via EGD is facilitated by technical modifications that allow injection of vasoconstrictive or sclerosing agents (eg, epinephrine), thermal energy (eg, heater probe) electrocoagulation, heated probe insertion, application of mechanical devices (eg, metallic clips), and combinations of treatments [2]. Mucosal and submucosal lesions and gastric and duodenal lipomas can be completely resected with additional technical modifications of the EGD technique [3]. Additionally, radiation treatments for esophageal cancer are facilitated with insertion of plastic conduits for radiation pellets (brachytherapy).

To reach further into the small bowel, modifications of EGD have been introduced, including double-balloon endoscopy (DBE), single-balloon endoscopy (SBE), and spiral endoscopy, which are described in a subsequent section of this article.

Most patients for EGD receive conscious sedation, directed by the endoscopist and using midazolam and fentanyl. Anesthesia services are requested based on comorbidity, prior difficulty with sedation, or risk of aspiration. When anesthesia services are requested, propofol is the most commonly selected agent. When endotracheal intubation is chosen, the anesthetic technique focuses on rapid emergence because most of these patients are outpatients. When brachytherapy is the goal of EGD, it is particularly important to achieve excellent topical anesthesia, both for the procedure and for the hour after while patients go through the radiation treatment.

Colonoscopy

Colonoscopy is most often performed for colon cancer screening or repeated excision of polyps. With endoscopic mucosal resection techniques, extensive or sessile right-sided colon polyps can be removed without surgery [4]. Technical modifications allow for the treatment of lesions that are actively bleeding or are at risk to bleed, such as arteriovenous malformations. Strictures from inflammatory bowel disease, surgery, or radiation can be dilated via colonoscopy if they can be reached with conventional equipment or a deep endoscopy technique (described later).

Like EGD, most colonoscopy procedures are performed with conscious sedation directed by the endoscopist. When deep endoscopy techniques are used, deep sedation or general anesthesia by an anesthesia team may be necessary because of the length of the procedure. Any signs of bowel obstruction, subtotal colectomy, or surgical removal of the ileocecal valve should be considered an indication for endotracheal intubation via rapid sequence technique.

Endoscopic retrograde cholangiopancreatography

Endoscopic retrograde cholangiopancreatography (ERCP) is designed for the visualization of the patency of the biliary and pancreatic ducts (Fig. 1), identification of stones or masses obstructing either ductal system, as well as the identification and treatment of purulent cholangitis with irrigation and stenting. When combined with balloon techniques, strictures of these ductal systems can be dilated and stented. When combined with endoscopic ultrasonography (EUS) technology, it is possible to drain giant pancreatic pseudocysts. ERCP is also applied to the confirmatory tissue diagnosis of lesions of the ampulla, combined with EUS [5].

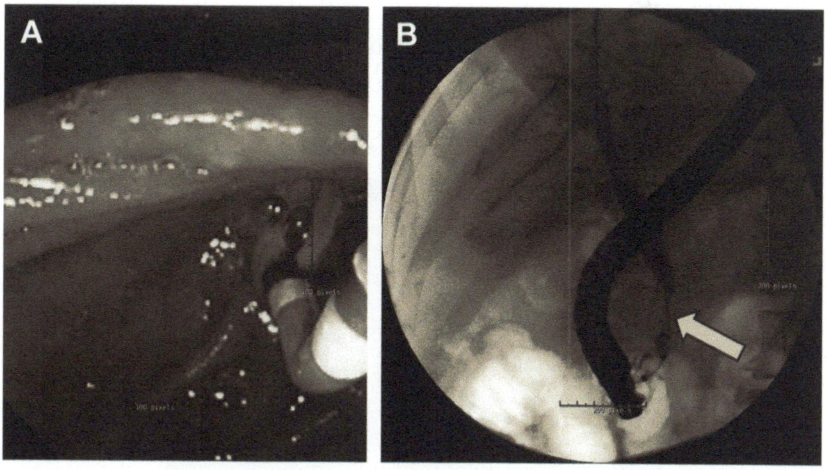

Fig. 1. ERCP. A 78-year-old woman with jaundice following an attack of acute pancreatitis. (*A*) Endoscopic photograph showing positioning of the catheter through the major papilla. (*B*) Injection of contrast (cholangiogram) reveals a stricture of the distal common bile duct (*arrow*). A stent was subsequently placed.

Because these patients are prone and often very sick, they receive either deep sedation or general anesthesia. Many anesthesia providers will choose to intubate all of these patients; others reserve intubation for indications, such as obstruction, bleeding, or obesity. Drainage of large pancreatic pseudocysts may require endotracheal intubation to prevent pulmonary soilage with potentially infectious material. When numerous or large stones are encountered in the biliary or pancreatic ducts, the volume of irrigation may also be an indication for endotracheal intubation, also to avoid pulmonary soilage. With repeat ERCP, the conditions of the prior procedure can influence the decision because difficulty in the previous procedure is likely to recur. Simple ERCP for stent removal can often be performed with deep sedation with propofol. Ketorolac has a role for ERCP because of the inflammatory nature of the pain.

Endoscopic ultrasonography

EUS is a modification of endoscopy that involves insertion of a modified endoscope into the esophagus, stomach, or intestine with an ultrasound probe at the tip [6]. There are 2 options, depending on the diagnostic target, either linear or radial. The linear scope provides a parallel view, which allows fine-needle aspiration (FNA) or other therapeutic modalities, such as the drainage of pseudocysts and abscesses. The radial view provides a 360° view, perpendicular to the long axis of the scope, favored for the diagnosis of unknowns. This platform does not have any additional diagnostic or therapeutic capabilities. EUS can aid in the identification of possible causes of acute pancreatitis (Fig. 2), with less risk of acute exacerbation compared with ERCP. It will often identify the cause of pancreatitis. Chronic pancreatitis can be confirmed with pancreatic histology, possible with EUS-FNA. Tissue diagnosis of lesions around the pancreas, liver, biliary tree, and other structures in the retroperitoneum and pelvis can be achieved with FNA, where previously surgical tissue harvest or percutaneous sampling was necessary [7].

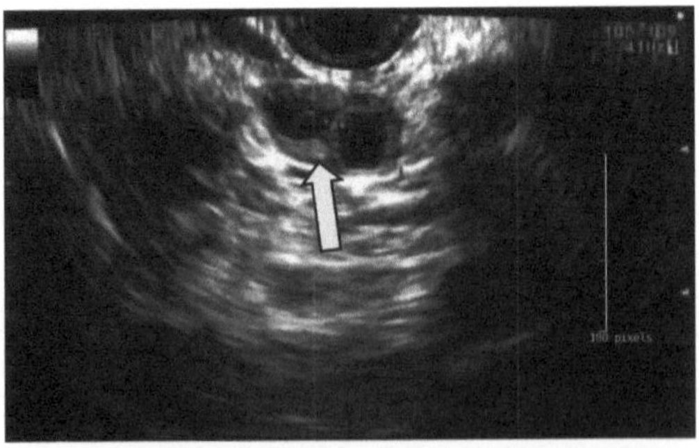

Fig. 2. EUS. A 64-year-old man with abnormal imaging of the pancreas on computed axial tomography. EUS of the pancreas revealed a focal process in the genu of the gland with both solid and cystic components. *Arrow* demonstrates a pancreatic mass identified by EUS.

Because of the complexity of these cases, deep sedation or general anesthesia is most often selected, with delivery by an anesthesia team. With EUS/FNA, there is some evidence that deep sedation improves the quality of the tissue diagnosis compared with conscious sedation [8]. In cases involving pancreatitis, ketorolac has a role because of the inflammatory quality of the pain. Many patients with chronic pancreatitis also have chronic pain, and there is an increasing role for ketamine in their care for deep sedation. Very small doses can be effective as a part of multimodal pain control.

Deep endoscopy

Deep enteroscopy is performed to reach lesions beyond the reach of the push technique and includes DBE, SBE, and spiral endoscopy. The oldest and most evaluated technique is DBE (Fig. 3), which uses an overtube with a balloon and an endoscope with a balloon (hence, the term *double balloon*), which allows a push-pull technique to telescope the gut and advance the enteroscopy beyond the jejunum, often completely viewing the entire ileum [1]. It can also be used both from above and below, viewing the entire GI tract. The reported ranges for the rate of the detection of lesions are from 38% to 68%. The complication rate (bleeding, perforation, acute pancreatitis) is low but higher compared with EGD with 1% for diagnostic procedures and about 5% for therapeutic procedures [9]. The most significant complication is acute pancreatitis [10] with a rate estimated at 0.2% to 0.3% [11,12].

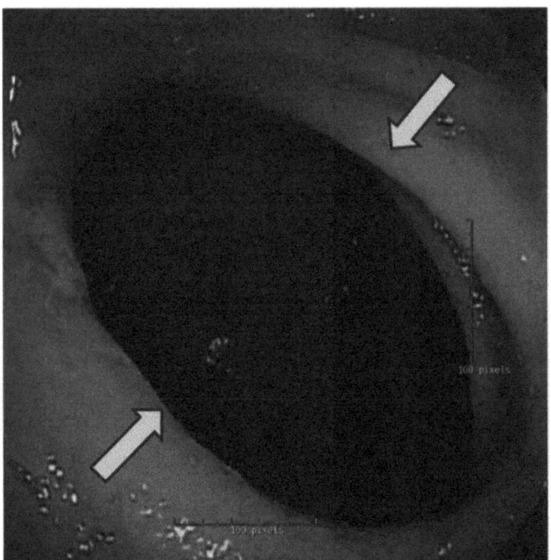

Fig. 3. Balloon enteroscopy. A 46-year-old woman with known Crohn disease, s/p ileocecectomy, who developed postprandial cramping abdominal pain. The neo-terminal ileum reveals a stricture with mild ulceration, consistent with Crohn disease. The stricture was serially dilated with a through-the-scope balloon device. *Arrows* demonstrate a stricture, prior to dilation with balloon enteroscopy. s/p, status post.

Because of issues with overtube use, SBE has been developed. This technique uses an angulated tip of the endoscope to fix the gut, in addition to a balloon tipped overtube and is comparable to the second balloon of DBE. As opposed to the DBE platform, the SBE system is latex free. The enteroscopy times are reported as faster [13] with a slightly lower complication rate, but a great decrease in the reaching the predetermined target of the procedure (total endoscopy rate) [14].

A newer modification of deep enteroscopy is the spiral enteroscopy technique. The overtube has a coupling device that fixes it to the endoscope while allowing rotation of the corkscrew or spiraled overtube. This technique is also known as *rotational enteroscopy*. With clockwise rotation, the intestine is pleated onto the overtube, allowing advancement of the endoscope [15]. Enteroscopy times are faster compared with DBE [16] although the technique may have increased risk of perforation in the presence of strictures [1].

With deep enteroscopy, a variety of procedures within the small bowel are possible, including coagulation, injections, contact cautery, gluing, clipping, endolooping, polypectomy, dilation, stenting, and ERCP for patients with altered small bowel anatomy after Roux-en-Y procedures [17].

For deep enteroscopy, most centers use an anesthesia team and either deep sedation or general anesthesia. With upper DBE, there is as strong preference for endotracheal anesthesia, which is a result of the mechanical reality of DBE. If there is an issue with the airway or obstruction, it takes some time to deflate both balloons and extract the endoscope. Combined with the often-long duration of the procedure, the anesthesia will very frequently elect to perform general endotracheal anesthesia before insertion of the scope.

Endoscopic mucosal resection

Endoscopic mucosal resection is a procedure used for the removal of gastric mucosal (endoscopic mucosal dissection [EMD])/submucosal (endoscopic submucosal dissection [ESD]) tissue for the diagnosis of lesions or curative resection of known gastric carcinoma [18]. The procedural steps include marking of the lesion, elevation of the lesion with injected fluid, and removal of the lesion using a specially adapted cap on the end of the endoscope that draws the lesion into the lumen and resected [19]. In the case of ESD, a host of specially designed devices are used to dissect the lesion.

The anesthesia considerations for EMD/ESD are similar to the approach (ie, EGD or colonoscopy), although the potential for complications is slightly higher. The main complications are bleeding (6%) and perforation, with many of the perforations being treated with endoscopic clipping versus surgery [20].

Esophageal ablation therapy

Many patients with Barrett esophagus have extensive surface lesions of the esophagus. These pathologic changes can undergo radiofrequency ablation with the Halo system (BARRX Medical, Inc, Sunnyvale, CA) without damage to underlying tissue layers. After identification by routine esophagoscopy, a sizing balloon is introduced to determine the correct sizing for the ablation catheter, with a total procedure time of 30 minutes or less [21].

The anesthesia considerations are similar to those for EGD, although the option to immediately remove the endoscope is not as available, with implications for airway management.

Chromoendoscopy

The use of dye and the alteration of light bands create chromoendoscopy, which allows the identification of abnormal surface lesions that otherwise would not be detected [22]. This use of dye has particular relevance combined with high resolution and magnifying endoscopy for routine screening for malignancy in the setting of inflammatory bowel disease and Barrett esophagus [23].

Endoscopic dilation and stenting

Esophageal strictures can be related to chronic reflux, malignancy, or radiation treatment of the esophagus for malignancy. Dilation with stenting can be therapeutic or palliative. Stenting alone can be used for the treatment of acute tracheoesophageal fistula (TEF) related to tracheal cancer or radiation treatment of this disease.

Small bowel strictures are typically seen after surgery with Crohn disease or with chronic use of nonsteroidal antiinflammatory drugs. The strictures can be modified or eliminated with balloon dilation [24]. The endoscope is used to identify the stricture, and a balloon dilator is introduced under direct vision and inflated. The result is confirmed with the endoscope before completion of the procedure.

Gastroduodenal stenting is performed for palliation of gastric or intestinal obstruction from advanced esophageal, gastric, biliary, small bowel, or colonic malignancy [25]. When the biliary or pancreatic ductal systems are also obstructed, they are first stented; then the gastroduodenal passage is stented with self-expanding metal stents [18]. The procedure involves passing a small endoscope through the narrowed lumen, marking the lesions, advancing a wire past the lesion, and deploying the stent through the scope and over the wire, with deployment controlled under fluoroscopic control [26]. Although more technically difficult, there have been reports of stents deployed via the DBE technique for stricture in the jejunum and ileum [27].

The anesthesia issues with dilation and stenting are related to the site. With dilation and stenting of strictures within the colon, the implications are no different from routine colonoscopy except that the procedure can be much longer. With upper endoscopy for dilation and stenting, the issues with rapid removal of the endoscope must be considered for airway management. With proximal esophageal stenting, particularly for TEF, there is very likely the need to secure the airway with endotracheal intubation because of proximal esophageal instrumentation.

Enteric feeding tubes

Enteric feeding tubes are placed for patients with a functional GI tract who are unable to consume enough calories to meet their metabolic needs because of difficulty with swallowing, malignancies of the upper GI tract, neurologic events, advanced dementia, and other indications [18]. The options include nasoenteric tubes, percutaneous endoscopic gastrostomy tubes (PEG), PEG tubes with jejunal extension, and percutaneous jejunostomy tubes. Jejunal placement is particularly indicated in patients at risk for aspiration.

Although placement of nasogastric tubes is routine, endoscopic assistance ensures their placement past the stomach and can identify lesions that would interfere with use or create complications with less procedure time and sedation compared with direct insertion [28]. PEG tube placement is facilitated endoscopically with transillumination to identify the best abdominal wall site, placement of a trocar, and then a guidewire, which is snared endoscopically and pulled through the mouth, followed by insertion of the tube with bumper and endoscopic confirmation [28]. J-PEG insertion involves the placement of the endoscope into the jejunum under direct vision and using the light to transilluminate to the abdominal wall where a trocar is inserted and a technique similar to PEG placement completes the procedure [29,30].

The anesthetic implication for endoscopic feeding tube placement is very similar to EGD. Many of these patients have functional or anatomic obstruction of either the stomach or proximal small bowel and are at risk for aspiration. Any history of bloating, fullness, nausea, or vomiting is a relative indication to secure the airway with endotracheal intubation before endoscopic intubation.

SEDATION FOR ADVANCED ENDOSCOPIC PROCEDURES

An important adjunct to sedation for EGD and other upper endoscopic procedures is topical anesthesia of the oropharynx [31]. There is evidence that the technical ease of endoscopic intubation and comfort are improved with properly applied topical local anesthetics, such as benzocaine or lidocaine [32]. In addition to the advantage of decreased secretions during the endoscopy, the antisialagogue properties of glycopyrrolate may improve the quality of topical anesthesia of the oropharynx if given a sufficient interval before application of the local anesthetic.

Propofol is clearly the gold standard as the principal or sole agent for moderate or deep sedation [21]. In addition to improved patient satisfaction, this technique provides sedation with the best control on depth of sedation and depression of respiration [33]. When moderate sedation is the goal, the combination of fentanyl and midazolam may be superior from the standpoint of the quality of the endoscopy achieved compared with either alone [34].

The starting point for decisions about sedation versus general anesthesia is whether to intubate the trachea or not. Simple endoscopy requires very little analgesia, and moderate sedation is adequate. Other endoscopies, such as EUS or ERCP, can be more complex and are associated with higher levels of stimulus. For these cases, the choice is between deep sedation and general anesthesia [31]. Deep sedation directed by an anesthesia team may actually improve the quality of the procedural outcome for EUS/FNA compared with conscious sedation directed by the gastroenterologist [8]. The decision to secure the airway involves several issues. For patients with chronic gastroparesis, symptomatic reflux, or esophageal food impaction, the risk of aspiration is high and intubation is relatively indicated. The prone position, which is frequently chosen by the endoscopist for ERCP, is an indication for endotracheal intubation for some anesthesia teams. A strong indication to intubate comes with the plan to drain giant pancreatic pseudocyst, purulent cholangitis, or high-volume irrigation to remove multiple small common duct stones. Obesity is an area where some anesthesia teams will choose endotracheal intubation, although, again, other providers will defer intubation until clinically indicated. In many cases, insertion of the endoscope is like an oral airway, pulling the tongue forward and improving the airway. If there is a concern about stomach contents, it is possible to create excellent topical anesthesia and anxiolysis and enter the stomach with a small endoscope with presumably intact airway reflexes. If empty, the planned endoscopy can proceed. If not, the stomach can be emptied before proceeding. If solids are encountered, the procedure can be aborted and rescheduled; if emergent, the endoscope is withdrawn and patients endotracheally intubated with a rapid sequence technique. When proper screening is deployed, propofol-based deep sedation with anesthesia coverage without intubation for a variety of complex endoscopic procedures was performed without airway compromise [35].

THE FUTURE

Natural orifice transluminal endoscopic surgery

NOTES procedures are a combination of general surgery and GI endoscopy. In the preliminary stages of being introduced, these procedures are performed with flexible video endoscopes, which are advanced through a natural orifice and allowed to create a visceral incision, creating access to the peritoneal cavity. Specially constructed devices are introduced via the channels of the endoscope, allowing surgical manipulation of abdominal or pelvic tissue [21]. Procedures that have been accomplished include gastrostomy, appendectomy, cholecystectomy, and liver biopsy via either transvaginal or transgastric approaches. A modification of the NOTES technique allows endoscopic full-thickness resection of early gastric carcinoma [36]. Future developments will allow application of robotic technology currently in use for laparoscopic surgery to create intraluminal robotic devices [37]. A modification of NOTES has evolved as an alternative to laparoscopic Heller myotomy-peroral endoscopic myotomy with excellent results in early reports [38]. A per-oral approach to gastric fundoplication is also under investigation [39].

Transgastric necrosectomy of the pancreas

One of the most serious complications of acute pancreatitis is infected necrotizing involvement of the body of the pancreas. Interventions are required, but there is hesitation to operate because of complications. Surgical necrosectomy has been modified by a laparoscopic technique but still has a high complication rate. A NOTES approach has been applied and involves an endoscopic approach via the stomach, using endoscopic ultrasound guidance [40]. The advantage is an endoscopic approach under sedation in this very sick patient population, with preliminary results superior to a surgical technique in a small number of patients.

Cholangioscopy

Traditional ERCP is performed with fluoroscopy, which delivers a 2-dimensional, black-and-white image. Cholangioscopy offers the potential advantage of direct visualization of the biliary and pancreatic ductal systems with improved diagnostic and therapeutic options [21].

Endoscopic bariatric procedures

Endoscopic alternatives to surgical bariatric procedures are being developed, including intragastric balloons, intragastric suturing, transoral stapling, transoral gastric restriction, intragastric sleeves, and a robotic operating platform to achieve gastric volume reduction [41]. There is also rapidly increasing interest in long-term management of bariatric procedures with endoscopic modifications [42].

Endoscopic treatment of postoperative leaks and fistula

Surgical management of leaks and fistula after surgery on the GI tract are associated with morbidity and mortality. Endoscopic interventions are being developed as an alternative, including stent placement, endoscopic suturing, and vacuum-assisted sponge closure of leaks/fistula, with rapidly expanding safety and efficacy data to support their use [43]. Endoscopic clips are also being studies for the closure of postoperative endoscopic defects [44] and for gastrostomy closure [45].

References

[1] Singh A, Baptista V, Stoicov C, et al. Evaluation of small bowel bleeding. Curr Opin Gastroenterol 2013;29:119–24.

[2] Kovacs TO, Jensen DM. Endoscopic therapy for severe ulcer bleeding. Gastrointest Endosc Clin N Am 2011;21:681–96.

[3] Aydin HN, Bertin P, Singh K, et al. Safe techniques for endoscopic resection of gastrointestinal lipomas. Surg Laparosc Endosc Percutan Tech 2011;21:218–22.

[4] Chandrasekhara V, Ginsberg GG. Endoscopic mucosal resection: not your father's polypectomy anymore. Gastroenterology 2011;141:42–9.

[5] El Hajj II, Cote G. Endoscopic diagnosis and management of ampullary lesions. Gastrointest Endosc Clin N Am 2013;23:95–109.

[6] Albashir S, Stevens T. Endoscopic ultrasonography to evaluate pancreatitis. Cleve Clin J Med 2012;79:202–6.

[7] Samarasena JB, Nakai Y, Chang KJ. Endoscopic ultrasonography-guided fine-needle aspiration of pancreatic cyst lesions: a practice approach to diagnosis and management. Gastrointest Endosc Clin N Am 2012;22:169–85.

[8] Ootaki C, Stevens T, Vargo J, et al. Does general anesthesia increase the diagnostic yield of endoscopic ultrasound-guided fine needle aspiration of pancreatic masses? Anesthesiology 2012;117:1044–50.

[9] Rondonotti E, Sunada K, Yano T, et al. Double-balloon endoscopy in clinical practice: where are we now? Dig Endosc 2012;24:209–19.

[10] Aktas H, Mensink PB. Small bowel diagnostics: current place of small bowel endoscopy. Best Pract Res Clin Gastroenterol 2012;26:209–20.
[11] Mensink PB, Haringsma J, Kucharzik T, et al. Complications of double balloon enteroscopy: a multicenter survey. Endoscopy 2007;39:613–5.
[12] Kopacova M, Tacheci I, Rejchrt S, et al. Double balloon enteroscopy and acute pancreatitis. World J Gastroenterol 2010;21:2331–40.
[13] Teshima CW. Small bowel endoscopy for obscure GI bleeding. Best Pract Res Clin Gastroenterol 2012;26:247–61.
[14] Takano N, Yamada A, Watabe H, et al. Single-balloon versus double-balloon endoscopy for achieving total enteroscopy: a randomized, controlled trial. Gastrointest Endosc 2011;73:734–9.
[15] Williamson JB, Judah JR, Gaidos JK, et al. Prospective evaluation of long term outcomes for spiral enteroscopy in patients with obscure GI bleeding. Gastrointest Endosc 2012;76:771–8.
[16] Akerman PA, Haniff M. Spiral enteroscopy: prime time or for the happy few? Best Pract Res Clin Gastroenterol 2012;26:293–301.
[17] Kaffes AJ. Advances in modern enteroscopy therapeutics. Best Pract Res Clin Gastroenterol 2012;26:235–46.
[18] Wassef W, Rullan R. Interventional endoscopy. Curr Opin Gastroenterol 2005;21:644–52.
[19] Soetikno RM, Gotoda T, Nakanishi Y, et al. Endoscopic mucosal resection. Gastrointest Endosc 2003;57:567–9.
[20] Ciocirlan M, Gincul R, Lepillicz V, et al. Non-Barrett's esophageal and gastric tumors: diagnosis and treatment. Gastrointest Endosc 2012;76:501–5.
[21] De Villiers WJ. Anesthesiology and gastroenterology. Anesthesiol Clin 2009;27:57–70.
[22] de Melo SW, Wallace MB. Endoscopic colorectal imaging and therapy. Curr Opin Gastroenterol 2010;27:54–60.
[23] Kiesslich R. Chromoendoscopy: what is its true value for ulcerative colitis surveillance? Dig Dis 2010;28:445–51.
[24] Pannala R, Ross A. Small bowel polyps, arteriovenous malformations, and miscellaneous lesions. Gastrointest Endosc Clin N Am 2013;23:111–21.
[25] Yates MR, Morgan DE, Baron TH. Palliation of malignant and intestinal strictures with self-expanding metal stents. Endoscopy 1998;30:266–72.
[26] Mergener K, Kozarek RA. Stenting of the gastrointestinal tract. Dig Dis 2002;20:173–81.
[27] Zhang F, Amateau SK, Khashab MA. Mid-gut stents. Curr Opin Gastroenterol 2012;28:451–60.
[28] DiSario JA, Baskin WN, Brown RD, et al. Endoscopic approaches to enteral nutrition support. Gastrointest Endosc 2002;55:901–8.
[29] Varadarajulu S, Delegge MH. Use of a 19-gauge injection needle as a guide for direct percutaneous endoscopic jejunostomy tube placement. Gastrointest Endosc 2003;57:942–5.
[30] Zhu Y, Shi L, Tang H, et al. Current considerations in direct percutaneous endoscopic jejunostomy. Can J Gastroenterol 2012;26:92–6.
[31] Goulson DT, Fragneto RY. Anesthesia for gastrointestinal endoscopic procedures. Anesthesiol Clin 2009;27:71–85.
[32] Evans LT, Saberi S, Kim HM, et al. Pharyngeal anesthesia during sedated EGDs: is "the spray" beneficial? A meta-analysis and systematic review. Gastrointest Endosc 2006;63:761–6.
[33] Aisenberg J, Cohen LB. Sedation in endoscopic practice. Gastrointest Endosc Clin N Am 2006;16:695–708.
[34] Barriga J, Sachdev MS, Royall L, et al. Sedation for upper endoscopy: comparison of midazolam versus fentanyl plus midazolam. South Med J 2008;101:362–6.

[35] Cote GA, Hovis RM, Ansstas MA, et al. The incidence of sedation-related complications with propofol use during advanced endoscopic procedures. Clin Gastroenterol Hepatol 2010;8:137–42.
[36] Garud SS, Willingham FF. Natural orifice transluminal endoscopic surgery. Gastrointest Endosc 2012;76:491–5.
[37] Kibansky D, Rothstein RI. Robotics in endoscopy. Curr Opin Gastroenterol 2012;28: 477–82.
[38] Rosch T. Progress in endoscopy: areas of current interest and topics to watch out for. Endoscopy 2012;44:1148–57.
[39] Testoni PA, Vailati C. Transoral incisionless fundoplication with EsophyX for treatment of gastro-oesophageal reflux disease. Dig Liver Dis 2012;44:631–5.
[40] Bakker OJ, van Santvoort HC, Brunschot S, et al. Endoscopic transgastric vs surgical necrosectomy for infected necrotizing pancreatitis. A randomized trial. JAMA 2012;307: 1053–61.
[41] Ryou M, Ryan MB, Thompson CC. Current status of endoluminal bariatric procedures for primary and revision indications. Gastrointest Endosc Clin N Am 2011;21:315–33.
[42] Levitzsky BE, Wassef WY. Endoscopic management in the bariatric surgical patient. Curr Opin Gastroenterol 2010;26:632–9.
[43] Kumar N, Thompson C. Endoscopic therapy for postoperative leaks and fistulae. Gastrointest Endosc Clin N Am 2013;23:123–36.
[44] Disibeyaz S, Koksal AS, Parlak E, et al. Endoscopic closure of gastrointestinal defects with an over-the-scope clip device. A case series and review of the literature. Clin Res Hepatol Gastroenterol 2012;36:614–21.
[45] Raju GS. Gastrointestinal perforations: role of endoscopic closure. Curr Opin Gastroenterol 2011;27:418–22.

Advances in Anesthesia 32 (2014) 71–87

ADVANCES IN ANESTHESIA

ELSEVIER
MOSBY

Anesthesia and Upper and Lower Airway Management for Advanced Diagnostic and Therapeutic Bronchoscopy

Basem Abdelmalak, MD[a,b,c,*], Sonali Sethi, MD[d], Thomas R. Gildea, MD, MS[e]

[a]Department of General Anesthesiology, Cleveland Clinic Lerner College of Medicine of Case Western Reserve University, Cleveland Clinic, 9500 Euclid Avenue, Cleveland, OH 44195, USA; [b]Anesthesia for Bronchoscopic Surgery, Department of General Anesthesiology, Anesthesiology Institute, Cleveland Clinic, 9500 Euclid Avenue, Cleveland, OH 44195, USA; [c]Department of Outcomes Research, Anesthesiology Institute, Cleveland Clinic, 9500 Euclid Avenue, Cleveland, OH 44195, USA; [d]Department of Pulmonary, Allergy and Critical Care Medicine, Respiratory Institute, Cleveland Clinic, Cleveland, OH, USA; [e]Section of Bronchoscopy, Department of Pulmonary, Allergy and Critical Care Medicine, Transplant Center, Respiratory Institute, Cleveland Clinic, 9500 Euclid Avenue, Cleveland, OH 44195, USA

Keywords

• Bronchoscopy • Lower airway management • Silicon stents • Metallic stents • EBUS • ENB • Anesthesia

Key points

- Advanced diagnostic and therapeutic bronchoscopy is evolving.
- Pulmonologists and anesthesiologists should stay abreast of these advances.
- Most patients having bronchoscopic surgery are high risk.
- Flexibility is needed to tailor and modify the anesthetic techniques to match patient and procedure needs.
- Bronchoscopic procedures take the concept of sharing the airway to a new level.
- The key to favorable outcomes lies in deep understanding of the underlying lung disorder, open 2-way communication between anesthesiologists and pulmonologists, understanding the nature of the procedure, and above all, vigilance and preparedness.

Financial Support: Support was provided solely from institutional and/or departmental sources.
Disclosure: The authors have no conflicts of interest to declare.

*Corresponding author. Department of General Anesthesiology, Cleveland Clinic, 9500 Euclid Avenue/E31, Cleveland, OH 44195. *E-mail address*: abdelmb@ccf.org

0737-6146/14/$ – see front matter
http://dx.doi.org/10.1016/j.aan.2014.08.011

INTRODUCTION

Advanced Diagnostic Bronchoscopy is a relatively new term that describes several new bronchoscopic techniques. Over the last decade advancements in the optical capabilities of the flexible bronchoscope and adjunctive catheter-based imaging tools have created new windows into the lung. Autofluorescence, Narrow-Band imaging (NBI), probe-based confocal light endomicroscopy (pCLE) are in various levels of clinical utility and investigation. Endobronchial Ultrasound (EBUS) is now replacing mediastinoscopy and combined with conventional or navigational bronchoscopy is now the preferred route for diagnosis and staging lung cancer [1–3]. Navigational Bronchoscopy is a group of similar technologies that incorporate additional image guidance. These can be in the form of virtual bronchoscopy, real-time CT guidance, and adjunctive peripheral endobronchial ultrasound. Electromagnetic guidance is combined with specific catheters and probes to reach peripheral lung lesions. While many studies regarding these technologies have used what is described as "moderate sedation", the evolving practice of multimodality bronchoscopy favors the use of general anesthesia [4,5]. This is because these techniques often require a longer duration than simple diagnostic bronchoscopy, precise positioning, and often a large diameter bronchoscope with complex instrumentation. We describe some of these advanced diagnostic procedures in more detail along with their anesthetic considerations and management.

Therapeutic bronchoscopic procedures aim at either relieving central airway obstruction, management of tracheobronchial defects such as fistulas and/or dehiscence of anastomosis (e.g post lung transplant), or endobronchial treatment of severe asthma. Central airway obstruction can result from relatively benign conditions like Wegner's granulomatosis (now known as granulomatosis with polyangiitis), a complication of tracheostomy or tracheal intubation related trauma, or as a result of a malignant process. However, the principles of management are somewhat similar; thus for the sake of simplicity we will focus on discussing malignant central airway obstruction to demonstrate principles of therapeutic interventional bronchoscopy and the anesthetic management.

ADVANCED DIAGNOSTIC BRONCHOSCOPY

Endobronchial optical advanced diagnostic techniques

Autofluorescence (AF) bronchoscopy is a technique that is based on the observation that dysplasia and carcinoma in situ show less fluorescence than normal tissue when stimulated with wavelengths of light between 380 and 460 nm. This so-called blue light bronchoscopy has been shown to be more sensitive than standard white light bronchoscopy for detecting malignant and premalignant endobronchial lesions [6]. However, this is a nonspecific test in that it can be abnormal with any inflammation or prior injury [7]. At present there are no available AF systems in the United States.

Narrow band imaging is another use of different wavelengths of light in the blue and green spectrum (415 nm and 540 nm) to enhance abnormal airway findings.

There are described patterns of abnormalities that indicate dysplasia and carcinoma to guide endobronchial biopsies [8–11]. Probe-based confocal light endomicroscopy is currently an experimental procedure. This procedure involves a catheter-based endoscopic microscope that uses the properties of autofluorescence to visualize living tissue. Based on the physician's understanding of the abnormalities investigated, it has been used to guide biopsies. It has not yet been declared as standard biopsy practice and a full understanding of pulmonary disease is still being investigated with this optical technology [12].

All of these optical techniques are typically performed under moderate sedation and without the use of an endotracheal tube to allow complete visualization of all airway structures. When these techniques are used for peripheral lung applications, general anesthesia with intubation may be necessary.

Endobronchial ultrasonography

Endobronchial ultrasonography (EBUS) describes several different techniques associated with bronchoscopy. The original description of EBUS involved catheter-based ultrasonography with a balloon used for assessing anatomic structures surrounding central airways. This device was also adopted for assessing airway wall structures for mucosal invasion of malignancy. Since then, a linear convex probe ultrasonography bronchoscope was developed specifically for transbronchial needle aspiration of mediastinal adenopathy. At present, the most common use of EBUS is sampling mediastinal masses, specifically in staging non–small cell lung cancer [2]. There is also now peripheral lung sampling using catheter-based ultrasonography for localizing peripheral lung lesions. Each of these techniques has been performed using either moderate sedation or general anesthesia and each requires a specific set of equipment and expertise, and has related risks to the patients.

Utility of radial probe EBUS has been noted in endobronchial disease even for radiographically invisible tumors [13]. This technique involves placing a balloon catheter with an embedded ultrasonography probe over suspicious areas and images are recorded. In general, this technique requires that clinicians only have to achieve tissue contact as shown in Fig. 1 but care must be maintained to avoid airway occlusion. Peripheral radial EBUS has been used to help localize, and in some cases detect, malignancy. There are several different probes made for this purpose and most of them are directed via guide sheath or some other catheter-based system. For radial EBUS, risks are associated with the biopsy and are not specifically associated with the imaging technique. The most common risk is pneumothorax, which theoretically may be accentuated with use of positive pressure ventilation; however, this has not definitely been proven [14]. Linear convex probe EBUS is a very specific procedure requiring a dedicated bronchoscope. The EBUS bronchoscope is slightly larger than the standard therapeutic bronchoscope. The distal tip has a 6.9-mm outer diameter, a 30° angle of vision, and slightly limited range of motion. Significant skills are required to perform this procedure beyond those required for standard conventional bronchoscopy [15]. There are 2 separate techniques: (1) mediastinal sampling and (2) systematic mediastinal staging. Depending on the indication, the procedure may be significantly longer in the case of systematic mediastinal staging (distinct nodal stations are identified and targeted for lymph nodes >5 mm). In known or suspected non–small cell lung cancer each of these nodal stations are sampled with multiple needle passes [1,2]. Procedure duration can be 120 minutes or longer depending on the complexity and number of nodal stations that require biopsy. This procedure is traditionally performed either via a large endotracheal tube (ideally 8.5 mm ID or larger) or via a supraglottic airway (SGA) under general anesthesia. It has also been described as being performed transorally with moderate sedation. This procedure is rapidly replacing mediastinoscopy as the primary modality of diagnosing and staging advanced-stage lung cancer. Overall this is a safe procedure in which the risks are mainly the same as those associated with other biopsy techniques or damage to the instruments [14,16].

Electromagnetic navigation bronchoscopy

Electromagnetic navigation bronchoscopy describes a platform for several different therapeutic and diagnostic techniques. A computed tomography scan of the patient is used as a virtual roadmap on which a target map is developed. The patient is placed inside an electromagnetic field with special care taken to minimize ferromagnetic interference. The flexible bronchoscope is used as a conduit to direct the catheter-based probe, which interacts with the electromagnetic field and generates real-time, directional information to the operator to direct the catheter toward a target [17,18]. This information allows additional confirmation with techniques like fluoroscopy or radial probe EBUS to facilitate transbronchial lung tissue acquisition. There are also established techniques for placing fiducial implants, directing high-dose radiation brachytherapy catheters, and placing dye marking on the pleural surface for assisting in video-assisted thoracoscopic surgery (VATS).

Considerable research is now being directed toward bronchoscopic ablative techniques [19–21]. This procedure has been described using both moderate sedation and general anesthesia [5,18]. In cases in which advanced-stage lung cancer may be suspected, mediastinal staging may also occur during this procedure using convex probe linear EBUS. In these cases general anesthesia is preferred because of the duration and complexity of the procedures.

ADVANCED THERAPEUTIC BRONCHOSCOPY

Central airway obstruction

Definition/pathogenesis

Malignant central airway obstruction is broadly defined as obstruction of the trachea, either mainstem bronchus, and/or the bronchus intermedius by tumor. In general, the airway must be obstructed at least 50% before the development of symptoms. However, any other airway compromise, such as secretions, edema, or hemoptysis, may result in the patient becoming symptomatic earlier. In some cases, a ball-valve phenomenon can exist whereby gas trapping distal to the lesion results in a mechanical disadvantage, thus increasing the work of breathing. In some patients, symptoms are acute in onset with severe respiratory distress and imminent failure. In other instances, the symptoms develop slowly. More than half of patients presenting acutely with malignant airway obstructions present in respiratory failure requiring an emergent airway intervention.

Patients often present with cough, stridor, wheezing, and recurrent or persistent postobstructive pneumonia. Stridor is usually attributable to impingement at the level of the trachea or larynx, whereas wheezing may be focal and as a result of obstruction distal to the main carina. Dyspnea in these patients is caused by airflow limitation and increased work of breathing.

Many patients are too ill to perform pulmonary function tests in the acute setting. However, in more stable patients, spirometry may provide information regarding the severity of disease and whether it is an intrathoracic or extrathoracic obstruction. The spirometric abnormalities are in 3 categories: (1) fixed airway obstruction with reduction of both inspiratory and expiratory flow rates, (2) variable intrathoracic obstruction with flow limitation of expiration, and (3) variable extrathoracic obstruction that shows inspiratory flow limitations [22].

The gold standard for diagnostic testing for malignant airway obstruction is bronchoscopy. The safety and efficacy of rigid versus flexible bronchoscopy as the initial tool remains controversial.

Classification of central airway obstruction

Central airway obstruction is generally classified into 3 types depending on whether the tumor is purely endoluminal, extraluminal, or mixed. If the tumor is confined to the airway lumen (endoluminal), it is considered intrinsic compression. In contrast, if the tumor is obstructing the airway because of mass effect and there is no endoluminal component, it is called extrinsic compression (extraluminal). Most central airway obstructions are in the final mixed category, in which there are elements of both intrinsic and extrinsic involvement. The tumor often originates adjacent to the airway and erodes through the airway wall, invading the lumen. This classification system provides the best therapeutic approach that can be used [23].

Bronchoscopic management of central airway obstruction

The management of central airway obstruction poses a unique challenge and requires a multidisciplinary approach. Bronchoscopy gives the most essential information in the preinterventional assessment of patients. Direct visualization identifies the location of the lesion, the extent of airway involvement, and the vascularity and fragility of the lesion. However, bronchoscopy in these patients has risks. There is potential for patients to develop complete airway obstruction caused by the presence of the bronchoscope in a critically narrowed central airway. In addition, local bleeding and mucosal trauma during bronchoscopy may further compromise the airway lumen. Therefore, it is essential that the procedure is performed with the utmost care. Rigid bronchoscopy has several advantages compared with flexible bronchoscopy when dealing with central airway obstruction. The major advantage is the ability to ventilate the patient while reestablishing airway patency. It has a wider working channel, which permits efficient suctioning and instrumentation. In addition, the rigid bronchoscope may also be used to tamponade any bleeding, selectively intubate one of the main stem bronchi, and/or mechanically debride the airway. The flexible bronchoscope may be used through the rigid barrel, allowing the evaluation of airways distal to the obstruction.

Relief of the obstruction should be expeditious and should initially focus on securing the airway. Once the airway is secured, a variety of airway interventions can be used to restore the patency of central airways. The most appropriate endobronchial management of a malignant airway stenosis is based on whether there is an intrinsic, extrinsic, or mixed stenosis. Purely intrinsic tumor involving the airway may simply be debrided and definitive treatment planned. Mechanical debulking using a rigid bronchoscope is an effective method to achieve rapid recanalization of central airways combined with ablative techniques. If there is concern about rapid regrowth or tumor pending response to treatment, an endobronchial stent may be considered.

Extrinsic airway compression nearly always results in recurrence within days to weeks if the airway is not stented following dilatation. As such, most of these cases require airway stents to prevent airway obstruction recurrence pending initiation of definitive treatment.

In a mixed stenosis, there is often a significant component of extrinsic compression and simply removing the endoluminal component is insufficient to maintain airway patency. A stent may be necessary both to prevent regrowth and to counteract the mass effect of the extrinsic component [24].

In the case of highly chemosensitive or radiosensitive tumors, such as small cell lung cancer or lymphoma, endobronchial management may be deferred until the patient shows clinical relapse of the malignant airway obstruction.

Tumor ablative techniques

Endobronchial tumors are often well vascularized and easily bleed; therefore, before considering tumor debridement, it is often necessary to devitalize the tumor. A host of techniques exist with some having immediate effects and other techniques being performed as staged procedures with ablative properties. Immediate ablative techniques include laser, argon plasma coagulation, and electrocautery, whereas the most common delayed techniques are cryotherapy, brachytherapy, and photodynamic therapy [25]. In most instances, a combination of several interventional procedures is needed for best results.

Airway stents

Once the airway has been debrided, the clinician must estimate the risk of airway recollapse. Airway stents (Fig. 1) have a critical role in maintaining airway patency. If there is a concern regarding postprocedure patency, clinicians must consider placement of an airway stent. However, complications related to stents may themselves result in airway obstruction; these include formation of granulation tissue, obstruction secondary to secretions, bacterial

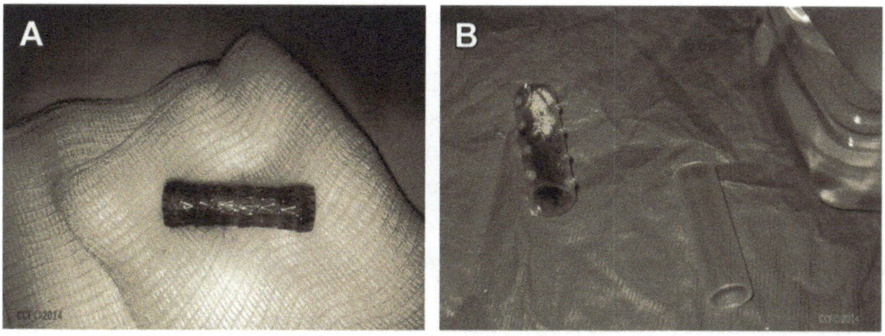

Fig. 1. (*A*) A self-expanding metallic stent used to relieve central airway obstruction; these are available in 2 forms: covered and uncovered. (*B*) A silicon stent used to relieve central airway obstruction: these are available in 2 forms: tubular (for trachea and/or main stem bronchi) or Y shaped (for carinal support). (*Courtesy of* Cleveland Clinic Center for Medical Art and Photography. © 2014. All rights reserved; with permission.)

overgrowth, and migration. Such complications may necessitate additional interventions later that require a specially trained pulmonologist and carry several risks; they may result in severe consequences like total airway obstruction or loss of airway integrity [26].

Other examples of therapeutic bronchoscopic procedures

A variety of procedures are currently being performed endobronchially, including placing fiducial implants, directing high-dose brachytherapy catheters, and placing dye marking on the pleural surface for assisting in VATS using the endoscopic navigational bronchoscopy capabilities as discussed earlier. Additional procedures include foreign body removal; inserting valves for treating persistent bronchopleural fistulas; post–lung transplant airway dehiscence restoration, as well as the procedure newly approved by the US Food and Drug Administration; and thermoplasty for asthma, which is discussed in more detail later because of its novelty.

ENDOBRONCHIAL TREATMENT OF SEVERE ASTHMA

Bronchial thermoplasty is a procedure in which controlled heat is applied endobronchially to reduce the mass of the airway smooth muscle as a treatment of severe asthma despite maximal medical therapy [27]. This procedure is performed over 3 sessions, targeting the right lower lobe, the left lower lobe, and bilateral upper lobes respectively in each session. This treatment modality has been shown to reduce asthma symptoms and emergency room visits as well as lost days of work [28,29]. These procedures are done with conscious sedation after premedication with bronchodilators and systemic steroids. However, in select cases when patients experience severe intraprocedural bronchospasm, general anesthesia is indicated to complete the 3 sessions. We have noticed that the benefits of the bronchodilatory effect of sevoflurane assists in these cases but data are needed to validate this observation. Although severe asthma is considered a relative contraindication to both bronchoscopy and elective surgery, it is reasonably well tolerated. The main complications associated with this procedure are in the immediate postoperative period with exacerbation of airflow obstruction. The patient is not discharged from observation until postprocedure forced expiratory volume in 1 second is within 20% of baseline.

ANESTHETIC CONSIDERATIONS AND MANAGEMENT

Preoperative assessment

Preoperative assessment is conducted in the customary fashion, the same as for any other surgical procedure. However, because of the urgency and the airway compromise already being experienced by many of these patients, clinicians may end up proceeding with care for patients with less than ideal optimization of some coexisting conditions. Special attention is needed during airway evaluation, symptoms of compromise, and review of the pulmonologist's evaluation regarding the size of the lesion or tumor and its location within the bronchial tree and the degree of impact on ventilation, as discussed earlier for central airway obstruction. The incidence of the so-called difficult airway, which is a term used to identify difficulty to mask ventilate, intubate the trachea, difficulty with ventilation using a supraglottic airway, and/or difficulty with surgical airway [30], may not be any higher than the general surgical population. However, lower airway–related difficulties can be encountered, such as airway bleeding, obstruction, and loss of airway integrity from lesions such as fistulas. However, because of an aging population and advances in treatment, the authors have encountered many patients who survived their head and neck cancers after undergoing a resection, a flap reconstruction, and/or neck radiation. These patients lived long enough to develop lung cancer and related lower airway stenosis/obstruction, and thus had upper and lower airway challenges and required some modifications and custom management that are beyond the scope of this article. Note that judicious use of premedication sedatives and anxiolytics is advised in this patient population because many of them have limited respiratory reserve [31].

Type of anesthetic

For most of the advanced diagnostic and therapeutic bronchoscopy procedures, a general anesthetic is preferred rather than moderate sedation. General anesthesia not only provides a comfortable and amnestic experience for the patient, it allows better control of ventilation through an airway and use of muscle relaxants, which has many advantages as detailed later. General anesthesia also arguably reduces procedure time, and allows faster recovery because of the use of the faster onset and shorter acting anesthetics compared with sedation medications used for moderate sedation; such procedures would require sedation medication doses that are higher than those used for moderate sedation for conventional simple airway examination bronchoscopy. Moreover, the involvement of the anesthesia team focusing on monitoring and managing patients' ventilation and homeostasis allows pulmonology teams to focus on the procedure at hand. When general anesthesia is used, a total intravenous anesthetic technique (TIVA), usually an infusion of propofol, is preferred rather than an inhalational anesthetic technique. Compared with an inhalational anesthetic technique, TIVA ensures continuous delivery of the anesthetic and prevents the pollution of the operating room by inhalational anesthetic that can be caused by circuit leaks because of the nature of the procedure [26]. Sarkiss and colleagues [32], also reported observing more bleeding at the needle biopsy site when inhalation anesthetics were used compared with the TIVA technique, presumably because of the vascular dilatory effects of inhalational anesthetics. Inhalational anesthetics may have some advantages in certain situations. We previously described our anesthetic technique [33] for the management of mediastinal mass, when inhalational anesthetics were used to augment the amnestic properties of dexmedetomidine while still maintaining spontaneous ventilation. The potent bronchodilating effect of inhalational anesthetics can be helpful in overcoming the severe bronchospasm often encountered in the third session of thermoplasty for endobronchial treatment of severe asthma, as discussed earlier [5].

When TIVA is used, the continuous flow of the anesthetic through the intravenous line should be monitored throughout the procedure. In addition, a hypnosis/anesthesia monitor (eg, the Bispectral index monitor [BIS Monitor] Covidien, Dublin, Ireland) should be used to help monitor the depth of anesthesia and possibly avoid intraoperative recall [34].

Anesthetic adjuvants

Muscle relaxants are commonly used in these procedures (regardless of the airway used: endotracheal tube [ETT] or SGA). They facilitate ETT insertion and/or SGA placement and improve overall lung compliance by eliminating the chest wall component and thus making positive pressure ventilation easier and more effective. Moreover, when an SGA is used (vs ETT) paralyzed vocal cords in an abducted position are potentially exposed to less trauma caused by the large-diameter operating bronchoscope. In addition, they provide a motionless patient, which is advantageous because unexpected patient movement can have serious consequences [35]. An example of such a situation is when trying to sample a node that is very close to the great vessels adjacent to hilar area. Irritation of the tracheobronchial tree during needle insertion for biopsy in a nonparalyzed patient may result in patient movement, which may lead to missing the target, especially if it is a small node, requiring the process to be repeated, multiplied by the number of attempts at each location, which can considerably prolong the procedure time. However, avoiding muscle relaxation and maintaining spontaneous ventilation may have some advantages in managing patients with very large mediastinal masses [33], as well as in avoiding positive pressure ventilation in cases associated with loss of airway integrity; for example, tracheoesophageal fistula, and post–lung transplant main stem dehiscence.

It is wise to restrict all administered fluids to the minimum needed for these patients, because many of them present with very limited lung reserve. Any pulmonary congestion may aggravate their condition.

Many anesthesiologists and pulmonologists use corticosteroids, in particular dexamethasone, as a prophylactic measure to decrease airway edema after airway surgery so that residual postoperative swelling can be minimized. Steroids are also used in cases of extensive surgical tracheobronchial tissue trauma. However, this practice is defended only because of its perceived clinical advantage, but evidence of its real advantage is controversial at best [36–39]. Furthermore, steroids are a known effective antiemetic for prophylaxis against postoperative nausea and vomiting [40]. In addition, corticosteroids can shorten recovery time [41].

Airway control and fresh gas flow

Intubation with a large-diameter ETT (eg, size 8.5 or 9.0 mm ID) facilitates ventilation around the large-diameter flexible bronchoscope (Fig. 2A) and the ETT is generally cut short to facilitate the maneuverability of the fiberoptic bronchoscope and decrease the resistance to its insertion and removal through the ETT (see Fig. 2B). We cautiously maintain the original length of the ETT in procedures involving management of tumors that are highly vascular and for which the chances of bleeding are high, to be able to advance the ETT to one

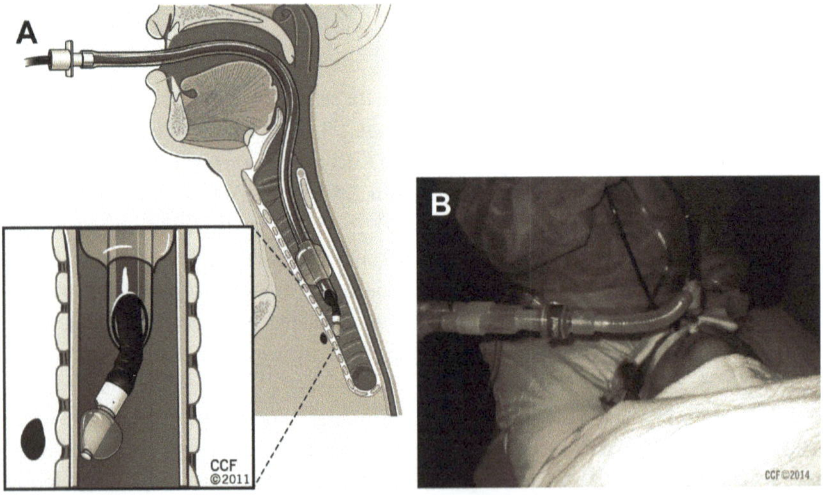

Fig. 2. (*A*) The operating EBUS bronchoscope inserted through a large 8.5-mm internal diameter (ID) ETT to biopsy a paratracheal lymph node [35]. (*B*) A large 8.5-mm ID ETT cut short with the operating bronchoscope inserted through it. Simultaneous ventilation is made possible by attaching the circuit to the blue swivel adapter. The flexible corrugated connector allows tube stability as the bronchoscope is inserted and removed from the airway. (*Courtesy of* Cleveland Clinic Center for Medical Art and Photography. © 2014. All rights reserved; with permission.)

main stem for the purpose of lung isolation should bleeding ensue from either of the lungs. Use of a fiberoptic swivel connector/adaptor allows continuous ventilation, thereby avoiding circuit disconnection during flexible bronchoscopy (see Fig. 2B) [5]. The ETT provides a secure airway to facilitate adequate ventilation, especially in such patients as those who are obese or have severe lung compromise, and it protects the airway in those with very high risk for aspiration. The ETT also protects the vocal cords (VCs) from rubbing against the large-diameter operating bronchoscope as it goes in and out of the airway, which could result in VC edema.

In cases in which the site of the lesion to be treated is subglottic (Fig. 3A), an SGA for example, a laryngeal mask airway or an i-gel can be effective [42,43]. They also allow better apposition of the scope in the mid and upper trachea (see Fig. 3B) and offer a means of ventilation as well. Another situation in which an SGA might be helpful is when caring for small patients (eg, a patient weighing 40 kg). The use of a large-diameter ETT might be a challenge, whereas the use of small SGA, like a size 3 i-gel, is feasible, but still provides a large-diameter airway that allows the easy passage of the large-diameter operating bronchoscope and ventilation around it. However, SGAs do not guarantee reliable protection against aspiration.

Administering a fraction of inspired oxygen (FiO_2) of 1.0 (100%) in such procedures is common. Also, maintaining a high fresh gas flow rate (12–15 L/min

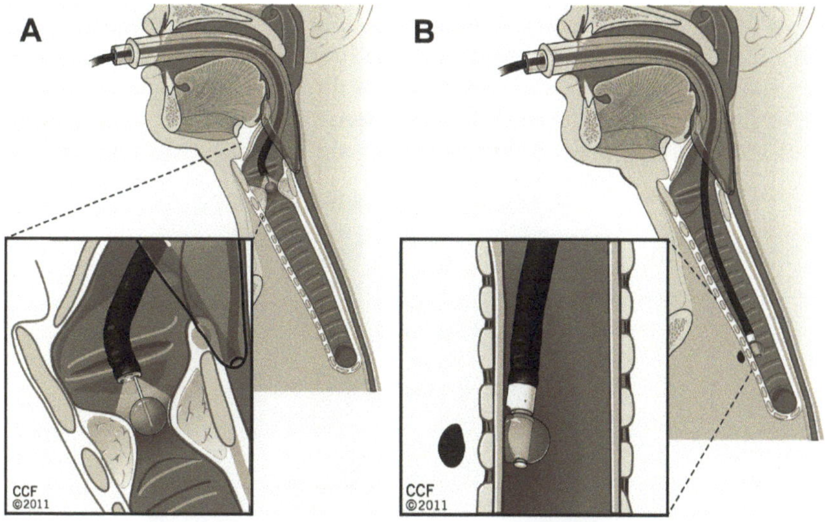

Fig. 3. The operating EBUS bronchoscope inserted through a supraglottic airway (i-gel shown here) to treat a subglottic stenosis (*A*) or to biopsy a paratracheal lymph node (*B*). (*Courtesy of* Cleveland Clinic Center for Medical Art and Photography. © 2014. All rights reserved; with permission; *Data from* Abdelmalak B, Sarkiss M. Anesthesia for diagnostic bronchoscopic procedures, anesthesia for otolaryngologic surgery. Abdelmalak B, DD, editors. London: Cambridge University Press; 2013. p. 297–308.)

of oxygen) is essential to compensate for the circuit leaks caused by the nature of the procedure. This high FiO_2 needs to be titrated down to less than 40%, preferably around 30% if tolerated, when using laser energy in the airway, and/or electrocautery. Reducing FiO_2 should also be achieved while maintaining a high fresh gas flow rate. An example of flow rate used at the authors' institution is 12 L/min of air mixed with 1.5 L/min of oxygen, resulting in an FiO_2 around 32%. In patients who do not tolerate such a low FiO_2, an alternative treatment strategy should be considered, like the use of cryoablation when FiO_2 of 1.0 can be maintained.

The techniques described earlier require clear communication between the anesthesiologist and the pulmonologist. Such advanced diagnostic pulmonary procedures are currently being performed in bronchoscopy laboratories attached to a main hospital (Fig. 4). However, with increased training and experience in providing this service on the part of the pulmonologists and anesthesiologists, it is expected to become a common procedure at ambulatory surgery centers [44].

Rigid bronchoscopy and anesthesia

A rigid bronchoscope is preferred for major airway interventions (ie, insertion and removal of silicon stents) because of its size and its noncompressible material; for removal of large broncholiths and granulation tissue; as part of treating a central airway obstruction as detailed earlier; and, in some instances, to support airway patency when a large mediastinal mass is compressing the airway. When the rigid bronchoscope is used, ventilation can be accomplished through either attaching the anesthetic circuit to the bronchoscope ventilating port for conventional positive pressure ventilation or through jet ventilation for which the jetting device is attached through a special adaptor to the bronchoscope ventilating port. When positive pressure conventional ventilation is used

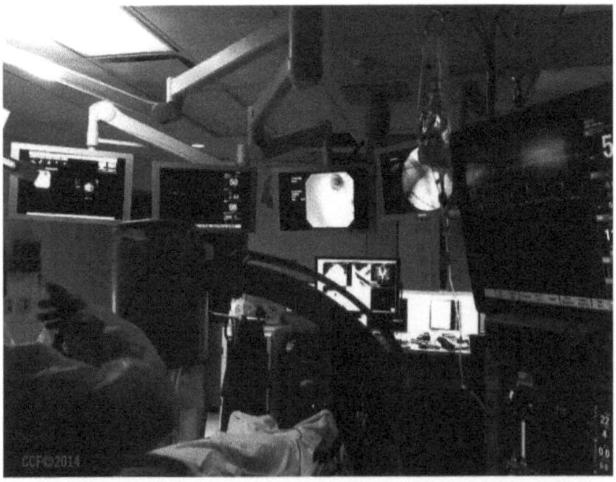

Fig. 4. Electromagnetic navigation bronchoscopy in a modern bronchoscopy suite. (*Courtesy of* Cleveland Clinic Center for Medical Art and Photography. © 2014. All rights reserved; with permission.)

(Fig. 5), it is important to minimize leaks around the rigid bronchoscope, which can easily be accomplished through maximizing the fresh gas flow, using rubber plugs to cover all unused rigid bronchoscopy ports, using fenestrated caps to introduce various rigid bronchoscopy tools and suction, and packing the mouth with saline-soaked gauze. At the authors' institution this is the preferred modality for ventilation with rigid bronchoscopy because of its simplicity, ease, safety, and low cost. Whenever a rigid bronchoscope is used, special attention should be given to protecting the lips and teeth and assessing them at the end of the procedure, as well as removing all the gauze to avoid subsequent airway obstruction from retained gauze pieces when the bronchoscope is removed.

When rigid bronchoscopy is used in the context of a very difficult airway, especially in patients with minimal reserve who cannot tolerate even a brief apnea, we often start the anesthetic with ETT awake intubation. Following the induction of general anesthesia and complete muscle relaxation, the rigid bronchoscope intubation is then inserted next to the ETT; when the VCs come into view, the ETT is withdrawn and the rigid bronchoscope is advanced into the trachea. At the end of the procedure, a tube exchange catheter is used to change the rigid bronchoscope to a single-lumen ETT (see Fig. 5).

Complex bronchoscopic procedures

The more advanced the referral center, and the more experienced the providers, the greater the complexity of the case mix for which they are caring. Thus, it is common for specialized centers to care for certain high-risk subpopulations, such as those having tracheomalacia, having tracheal reconstruction after airway fires (usually present with recurrent airway stenosis caused by buildup of fibrous tissue and scars), and patients with complications related

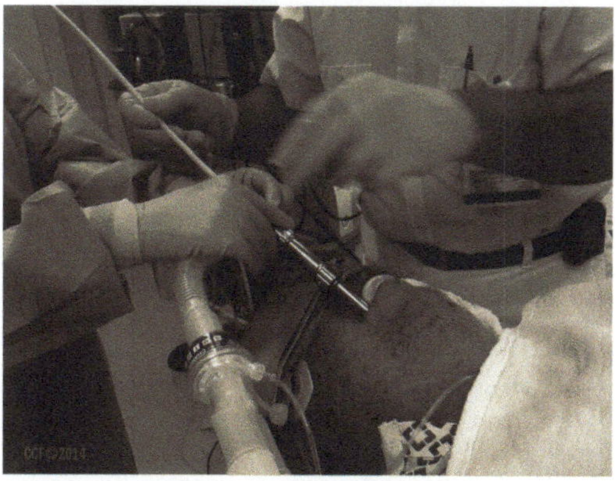

Fig. 5. Conventional positive pressure ventilation using a breathing circuit. Note the gauze coming out of the mouth to pack around the scope in the hypopharyngeal area. An airway exchange catheter is introduced through the rigid bronchoscope as a first step in an exchange process to a single-lumen tube in case of airways that are extremely difficult to intubate. (*Courtesy of* Cleveland Clinic Center for Medical Art and Photography. © 2014. All rights reserved; with permission.)

to T tubes. Such complex airway procedures may require alternative techniques of management, and they may require the anesthesiologist to improvise, which often means the continued change of airway devices and ventilation modes from SGA, endotracheal tubes, rigid bronchoscopy, to no airway, and

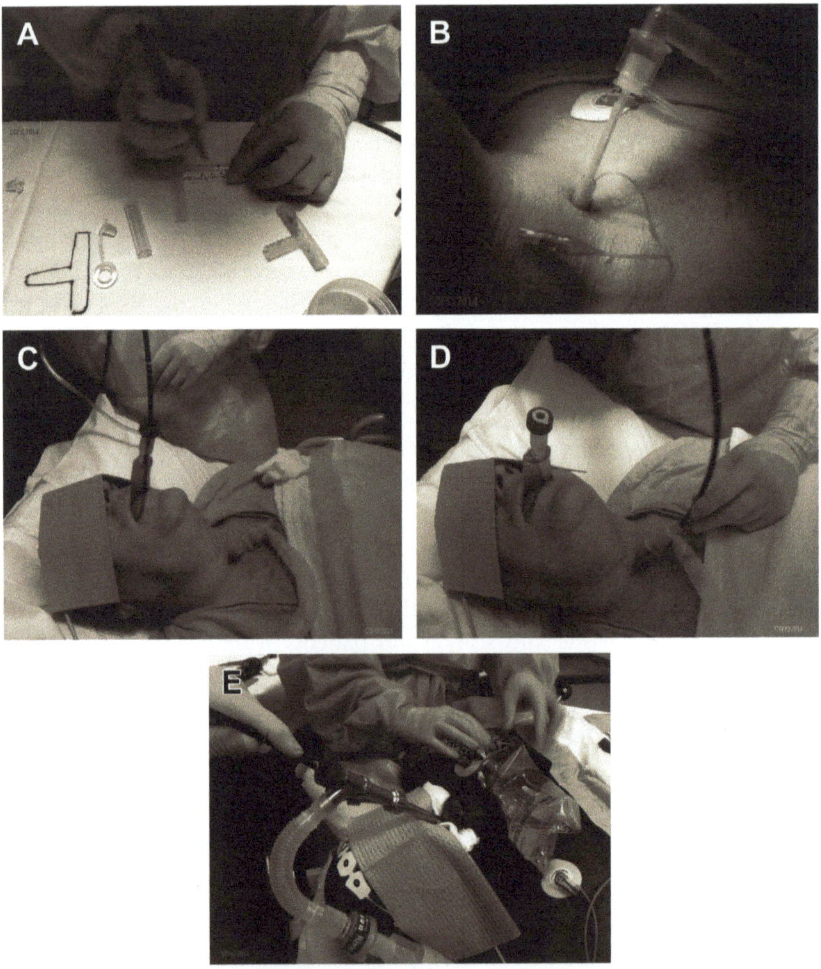

Fig. 6. (*A*) T tube being measured and cut to fit the patient's measurements. (*B*) Ventilation through a T tube using a size #4 pediatric ETT. (*C*) Ventilation and bronchoscopic examination through an ETT connector, attached to the T tube while the upper end of the T tube is sealed by the presence of the SGA with its connector opening capped. (*D*) Ventilation through an ETT connector, attached to the T tube while the upper end of the T tube is sealed by the presence of the SGA with its connector opening capped while a bronchoscope is passed through it for upper airway examination. (*E*) Ventilation through a circuit attached to the rigid scope side port while the T tube is removed and the site is sealed with Vaseline gauze, and a 500-mL fluid bag. (*Courtesy of* Cleveland Clinic Center for Medical Art and Photography. © 2014. All rights reserved; with permission.)

intermittent apnea technique. Detailed discussion of such scenarios is beyond the scope of this article. However, as an example of a complex scenario, the management of patients with a T tube, may require the use of different airways and ventilation techniques depending on the stage of the procedure and whether it is a replacement, or dilatation of the stoma and/or the trachea below and/or above the stoma, as shown in Fig. 6.

Postanesthesia care

Patients typically go home immediately following a short recovery time of 45 minutes to 1 hour [35]. This recovery period compares favorably with that of invasive thoracic surgery such as mediastinoscopy or open or minimally invasive lung biopsy, which may require postoperative hospital admission, and potentially intensive care unit admission in cases of lung biopsy or mediastinal staging.

COMPLICATIONS

As discussed earlier, potential complications of bronchoscopic procedures range from hypercapnia and minor levels of hypoxemia and/or cough to pneumothorax [14], major bleeding, and even loss of the airway. These complications should always be considered when patients rapidly deteriorate during and/or after the procedure.

The most commonly seen complications include varying degrees of sore throat that may last up to a day or so and severe cough that usually improves and returns to baseline levels in about 20 to 30 minutes after conclusion of the procedure.

SUMMARY

Advanced diagnostic and therapeutic bronchoscopy is evolving. Pulmonologists and anesthesiologists should stay abreast of these advances. Flexibility is needed to tailor and modify the anesthetic techniques to match patient and procedure needs. The key to favorable outcomes lies in deep understanding of the underlying lung disorder; open 2-way communication between the anesthesiologist and pulmonologist; understanding the nature of the procedure; and, above all, vigilance and preparedness.

References

[1] Almeida FA. Bronchoscopy and endobronchial ultrasound for diagnosis and staging of lung cancer. Cleve Clin J Med 2012;79(Electronic Suppl 1):eS11–6.

[2] Kinsey CM, Arenberg DA. Endobronchial ultrasound-guided transbronchial needle aspiration for non-small cell lung cancer staging. Am J Respir Crit Care Med 2014;189:640–9.

[3] Rivera MP, Mehta AC, Wahidi MM. Establishing the diagnosis of lung cancer: diagnosis and management of lung cancer, 3rd ed: American College of Chest Physicians evidence-based clinical practice guidelines. Chest 2013;143:e142S–65S.

[4] Yarmus LB, Akulian JA, Gilbert C, et al. Comparison of moderate versus deep sedation for endobronchial ultrasound transbronchial needle aspiration. Ann Am Thorac Soc 2013;10: 121–6.

[5] Abdelmalak BB, Gildea TR, Doyle DJ. Anesthesia for bronchoscopy. Curr Pharm Des 2012;18:6314–24.
[6] Sun J, Garfield DH, Lam B, et al. The value of autofluorescence bronchoscopy combined with white light bronchoscopy compared with white light alone in the diagnosis of intraepithelial neoplasia and invasive lung cancer: a meta-analysis. J Thorac Oncol 2011;6:1336–44.
[7] Gildea TR. Autofluorescence bronchoscopy: a far rising. J Bronchol Intervent Pulmonol 2006;13:52–3.
[8] Zaric B, Stojsic V, Sarcev T, et al. Advanced bronchoscopic techniques in diagnosis and staging of lung cancer. J Thorac Dis 2013;5:S359–70.
[9] Zaric B, Perin B, Stojsic V, et al. Relation between vascular patterns visualized by Narrow Band Imaging (NBI) videobronchoscopy and histological type of lung cancer. Med Oncol 2013;30:374.
[10] Shibuya K, Nakajima T, Fujiwara T, et al. Narrow band imaging with high-resolution bronchovideoscopy: a new approach for visualizing angiogenesis in squamous cell carcinoma of the lung. Lung Cancer 2010;69:194–202.
[11] Herth FJ, Eberhardt R, Anantham D, et al. Narrow-band imaging bronchoscopy increases the specificity of bronchoscopic early lung cancer detection. J Thorac Oncol 2009;4:1060–5.
[12] Yserbyt J, Dooms C, Ninane V, et al. Perspectives using probe-based confocal laser endomicroscopy of the respiratory tract. Swiss Med Wkly 2013;143:w13764.
[13] Herth F, Becker H, LoCicero J, et al. Endobronchial ultrasound improves classification of suspicious lesions detected by autofluorescence bronchoscopy. J Bronchology Interv Pulmonol 2003;10:249–52.
[14] Eapen GA, Shah AM, Lei X, et al. Complications, consequences, and practice patterns of endobronchial ultrasound-guided transbronchial needle aspiration: results of the AQuIRE registry. Chest 2013;143:1044–53.
[15] Jantz MA, McGaghie WC. It's time for a STAT assessment of bronchoscopy skills: the endobronchial ultrasound bronchoscopy (EBUS)-STAT and EBUS-transbronchial needle aspiration skill evaluation. Am J Respir Crit Care Med 2012;186:703–5.
[16] Asano F, Aoe M, Ohsaki Y, et al. Complications associated with endobronchial ultrasound-guided transbronchial needle aspiration: a nationwide survey by the Japan Society for Respiratory Endoscopy. Respir Res 2013;14:50.
[17] Schwarz Y, Greif J, Becker HD, et al. Real-time electromagnetic navigation bronchoscopy to peripheral lung lesions using overlaid CT images: the first human study. Chest 2006;129:988–94.
[18] Gildea TR, Mazzone P, Karnak D, et al. Electromagnetic navigation diagnostic bronchoscopy: a prospective study. Am J Respir Crit Care Med 2006;174:982–9.
[19] Eberhardt R, Kahn N, Herth FJ. 'Heat and destroy': bronchoscopic-guided therapy of peripheral lung lesions. Respiration 2010;79:265–73.
[20] Anantham D, Feller-Kopman D, Shanmugham LN, et al. Electromagnetic navigation bronchoscopy guided fiducial placement for robotic stereotactic radiosurgery of lung tumors: a feasibility study. Chest 2007;132:930–5.
[21] Harley DP, Krimsky WS, Sarkar S, et al. Fiducial marker placement using endobronchial ultrasound and navigational bronchoscopy for stereotactic radiosurgery: an alternative strategy. Ann Thorac Surg 2010;89:368–73 [discussion: 373–4].
[22] Miller RD, Hyatt RE. Evaluation of obstructing lesions of the trachea and larynx by flow-volume loops. Am Rev Respir Dis 1973;108:475–81.
[23] Ernst A, Feller-Kopman D, Becker HD, et al. Central airway obstruction. Am J Respir Crit Care Med 2004;169:1278–97.
[24] Chen K, Varon J, Wenker OC. Malignant airway obstruction: recognition and management. J Emerg Med 1998;16:83–92.
[25] Lee P, Kupeli E, Mehta AC. Therapeutic bronchoscopy in lung cancer. Laser therapy, electrocautery, brachytherapy, stents, and photodynamic therapy. Clin Chest Med 2002;23:241–56.

[26] Doyle DJ, Abdelmalak B, Machuzak M, et al. Anesthesia and airway management for removing pulmonary self-expanding metallic stents. J Clin Anesth 2009;21:529–32.
[27] Cox G, Miller JD, McWilliams A, et al. Bronchial thermoplasty for asthma. Am J Respir Crit Care Med 2006;173:965–9.
[28] Gildea TR, Khatri SB, Castro M. Bronchial thermoplasty: a new treatment for severe refractory asthma. Cleve Clin J Med 2011;78:477–85.
[29] Castro M, Rubin AS, Laviolette M, et al. Effectiveness and safety of bronchial thermoplasty in the treatment of severe asthma: a multicenter, randomized, double-blind, sham-controlled clinical trial. Am J Respir Crit Care Med 2010;181:116–24.
[30] Apfelbaum JL, Hagberg CA, Caplan RA, et al. Practice guidelines for management of the difficult airway: an updated report by the American Society of Anesthesiologists Task Force on Management of the Difficult Airway. Anesthesiology 2013;118:251–70.
[31] Abdelmalak B, Riad I. Monitored anesthesia care and anesthesia outside the operating room. In: Longnecker DE, Brown DL, Newman MD, Zapol WM, editors. Anesthesiology. New York: The McGraw-Hill Medical; 2013. p. 1260–74.
[32] Sarkiss M, Kennedy M, Riedel B, et al. Anesthesia technique for endobronchial ultrasound-guided fine needle aspiration of mediastinal lymph node. J Cardiothorac Vasc Anesth 2007;21:892–6.
[33] Abdelmalak B, Marcanthony N, Abdelmalak J, et al. Dexmedetomidine for anesthetic management of anterior mediastinal mass. J Anesth 2010;24:607–10.
[34] Avidan MS, Zhang L, Burnside BA, et al. Anesthesia awareness and the bispectral index. N Engl J Med 2008;358:1097–108.
[35] Abdelmalak B, Sarkiss M. Anesthesia for diagnostic bronchoscopic procedures. In: Abdelmalak B, Doyle DJ, editors. Anesthesia for otolaryngologic surgery. London: Cambridge University Press; 2013. p. 297–308.
[36] Weber CR, Griffin JM. Evaluation of dexamethasone for reducing postoperative edema and inflammatory response after orthognathic surgery. J Oral Maxillofac Surg 1994;52:35–9.
[37] Blair E, Montgomery AV, Swan H. Posthypothermic circulatory failure. I. Physiologic observations on the circulation. Circulation 1956;13:909–15.
[38] Gersema L, Baker K. Use of corticosteroids in oral surgery. J Oral Maxillofac Surg 1992;50:270–7.
[39] Hughes R, McGuire G, Montanera W, et al. Upper airway edema after carotid endarterectomy: the effect of steroid administration. Anesth Analg 1997;84:475–8.
[40] Gan TJ, Diemunsch P, Habib AS, et al. Consensus guidelines for the management of postoperative nausea and vomiting. Anesth Analg 2014;118:85–113.
[41] Coloma M, Duffy LL, White PF, et al. Dexamethasone facilitates discharge after outpatient anorectal surgery. Anesth Analg 2001;92:85–8.
[42] Abdelmalak B, Ryckman JV, AlHaddad S, et al. Respiratory arrest after successful neodymium:yttrium-aluminum-garnet laser treatment of subglottic tracheal stenosis. Anesth Analg 2002;95:485–6.
[43] Hung WT, Liao SM, Su JM. Laryngeal mask airway in patients with tracheal stents who are undergoing non-airway related interventions: report of three cases. J Clin Anesth 2004;16:214–6.
[44] Abdelmalak B. Anesthesia for interventional pulmonology. In: Urman R, Gross W, Philip B, editors. Anesthesia outside of the operating room. New York: Oxford University Press; 2011. p. 167–74.

Advances in Anesthesia 32 (2014) 89–117

ADVANCES IN ANESTHESIA

Advances in Perioperative Pulmonary Protection Strategies

J. Kyle Bohman, MD*, Daryl J. Kor, MD

Division of Critical Care Medicine, Department of Anesthesiology, Mayo Clinic, 200 First Street Southwest, Rochester, MN 55905, USA

Keywords

• Perioperative • Pulmonary protection • Postoperative pulmonary complications
• Acute respiratory distress syndrome

Key points

- Postoperative pulmonary complications (PPCs) significantly affect patient-important outcomes and utilization of health care resources.
- Identification of risk factors that portend risk for PPCs is an essential first step in mitigating these adverse events.
- Prevention strategies specifically targeting those with modifiable risk factors for PPCs are likely to have the largest impact on patients' outcomes.
- Prevention of PPCs requires an awareness of risk factors and implementation of prevention strategies during all phases of the perioperative experience.
- Unless specifically contraindicated, lung-protective ventilation should be used for all mechanically ventilated patients.
- Although early smoking cessation is preferred, it is recommended for all patients who are to receive general anesthesia regardless of the duration of cessation.

INTRODUCTION

Postoperative pulmonary complications (PPCs) are a significant cause of morbidity and mortality in modern surgical practice. Although published definitions frequently vary, PPCs generally include respiratory infections, respiratory failure, pleural effusions, atelectasis, pneumothorax, bronchospasm, and aspiration pneumonitis [1,2]. A recent review of PPCs reported a composite frequency of 5.0%, with more specific risk rates for respiratory failure (2.6%),

Disclosures: The authors have nothing to disclose.

*Corresponding author. *E-mail address*: bohman.john@mayo.edu

0737-6146/14/$ – see front matter
http://dx.doi.org/10.1016/j.aan.2014.08.005 Published by Elsevier Inc.

bronchospasm (1.8%), pleural effusion (1.7%), respiratory infection (1.6%), atelectasis (1.4%), aspiration pneumonia (0.4%), and pneumothorax (0.3%) during the in-hospital postoperative period [1]. Specific complications, such as respiratory infection and respiratory failure, likely have a more significant impact on patient-oriented outcomes, including length of stay in hospital and mortality [3].

A large study using the National Surgical Quality Improvement Project (NSQIP) database found that independent of preoperative risk, PPCs were associated with a significant increase in mortality from 2% to 22% [4]. The impact of PPCs on mortality is similar in other studies; one of which showed an overall incidence of PPC of 5% and a 30-day mortality of 19.5% in patients with a PPC versus only 0.5% in patients without a PPC [1]. Furthermore, PPCs have a dramatic impact on health care costs, with NSQIP data suggesting that each PPC may have an attributable cost of US$50,000 and may extend the length of stay in hospital by as much as 20 days [5].

In an early review of PPCs in 1920, the term "ether pneumonia" was used demonstrating the long-standing association between anesthesia, surgical procedures, and pulmonary complications [6]. Anesthesiologists and other perioperative care providers have the potential to affect many of the modifiable risk factors for PPCs and, therefore, enhance the safety of surgical patients.

In this review a broad range of general PPC prevention measures are discussed. Specific topics include smoking cessation, mechanical ventilation, anesthetic and analgesic techniques, pulmonary hygiene, aspiration, fluid and blood products, and some monitoring techniques. Additional discussion centers on specific high-risk patients including those with obstructive lung disease, obesity, obstructive sleep apnea, and patients undergoing high-risk surgical procedures such as intrathoracic operations. In an effort to keep this review concise, the impact of baseline neuromuscular weakness is not discussed, nor are thoracic anatomic abnormalities (such as scoliosis) that may portend risk for PPCs. Likewise, prevention strategies for venous thromboembolism are not addressed, nor is the management of perioperative pleural effusions and pneumothoraces.

RISK FACTORS AND CAUSES OF POSTOPERATIVE PULMONARY COMPLICATIONS

Risk factors for postoperative pulmonary complications

Whether reflecting true causation or simply association, the identification of potential risk factors for PPCs is an essential first step as we work toward mitigating these undesirable postoperative outcomes. Indeed, strategies aiming to prevent PPCs are presumed to be most effective when directed toward the population at highest risk. To this end, a large systematic review by Smetana and colleagues [7] previously outlined patient-related and procedure-related risk factors associated with PPCs (Table 1). Specifically, patient-related factors associated with the highest risk of PPCs included advanced age, American Society of Anesthesiologists (ASA) class II or greater, congestive heart failure (CHF), functional dependence (not able to perform activities of daily living without

Table 1
Risk factors for perioperative pulmonary complications

Patient-related risk factors	Procedural risk factors
Advanced age (>80 y)	Open aortic aneurysm repair
ASA class II or greater	Thoracic surgery
Congestive heart failure	Abdominal surgery
Chronic obstructive pulmonary disease	Neurosurgery
Functional dependence	Head and neck surgery
Hypoalbuminemia (<3.5 mg/dL)	Prolonged anesthesia
Frailty	Emergency surgery
	General anesthesia

Data from Refs. [1,7,8]

assistance or medical equipment), chronic obstructive pulmonary disease (COPD), and hypoalbuminemia (<3.5 g/dL, likely a marker of general health status). Procedural factors associated with the highest risk of PPCs included open aortic aneurysm repair, thoracic surgery, abdominal surgery, neurosurgery, prolonged surgery, head and neck surgery, emergency surgery, vascular surgery, and general anesthesia. In a related study, there appeared to be a significant increase in PPCs for patients older than 80 years [1]. Similar risk factors were identified in a study of more than 180,000 Veterans Affairs Medical Center patients, including surgical type (abdominal aortic aneurysm, intrathoracic, neurosurgical, upper abdominal, and neck), emergency surgery, albumin less than 3.0 g/dL, COPD, and advanced age (see Table 1) [8]. More recently, preoperative functional status, often quantified by a frailty index (such as the Canadian Study of Health and Aging Clinical Frailty Scale), has also been associated with PPCs and mortality [9,10].

Causes of perioperative respiratory impairment

There are numerous specific pulmonary insults and mechanisms of pulmonary impairment that may occur during the perioperative period which are commonly associated with the development of PPCs. Common perioperative sources of pulmonary impairment associated with PPCs are listed in Box 1 and described in detail here.

A common insult that may portend risk for PPCs is mechanical ventilation. Associated complications may include ventilator-induced lung injury (VILI) and resultant acute respiratory distress syndrome (ARDS). Our current understanding of VILI is based on the concepts of excessive tidal volume (volutrauma), elevated airway pressures (barotrauma), and injury related to repeated collapse and opening of alveoli (atelectrauma) [11].

Barotrauma is an infrequent complication of mechanical ventilation, typically manifesting with pneumothoraces or pneumomediastinum. Volutrauma is believed to be the primary cause of VILI. Such injury results from the application of large tidal volumes causing alveolar overdistension, epithelial injury, and resultant local and systemic inflammation. The importance of limiting tidal

Box 1: Causes of perioperative respiratory injury or impairment

Mechanical ventilation
Gastric-to-pulmonary aspiration
Allogeneic blood product transfusion
Direct surgical injury
Smoking
General anesthesia
Neuromuscular blockade and inadequate reversal
Atelectasis
Excessive oxygen
Sedation and opioids
Excessive intravenous fluids

volumes and plateau airway pressures with the goal of mitigating the presence or severity of VILI is supported by a large body of both basic science and clinical data.

The application of positive end-expiratory pressure (PEEP) to prevent alveolar collapse and resultant atelectrauma is generally endorsed as well. However, optimal PEEP strategies are somewhat more controversial, with recent reviews suggesting the potential for benefit with higher PEEP levels in those with severe ARDS, but harm with the application of such strategies in patients with milder forms of ARDS [12]. Of note, volutrauma can also be a self-perpetuating phenomenon when lung injury leads to the loss of functional lung units. The remaining functional alveoli then face a relative increase in local tidal volume resulting from the reduced overall lung volume. Ventilator strategies intended to reduce PPCs are discussed in more detail later.

Although believed to be uncommon, gastric-to-pulmonary aspiration is associated with significant morbidity and mortality. Patients at high risk for aspiration and its associated lung injury include: those presenting for emergency surgery; the presence of nonfasting status at the time of endotracheal intubation; or esophageal abnormality, gravid status, bowel obstruction, chronic alcohol consumption, or malnutrition. Key factors of an aspiration event that have been associated with injury to the lung parenchyma include a larger volume of aspirate, lower pH, and the presence of particulate matter [13]. Methods of reducing the risk of aspiration and its associated PPCs are discussed later.

General anesthesia and neuromuscular blockade leads to changes in diaphragmatic function and chest wall shape and motion. This alteration of pulmonary mechanics may contribute to the development of some PPCs [14]. In theory, minimizing these changes (and the extent of sedation or anesthesia provided) by using regional anesthetic techniques may reduce the risk of PPCs (see later discussion).

Residual neuromuscular blockade is a likely contributor to PPCs. A large case-control study demonstrated that residual neuromuscular blockade is clinically significant and is associated with acute respiratory failure postoperatively [15]. A prospective study demonstrated a reduced forced vital capacity (FVC) in patients despite adequate (train-of-four [TOF] ≥0.9) reversal (FVC = 62% baseline) and a significantly greater reduction in FVC in patients with residual (TOF <0.9) neuromuscular blockade (FVC = 49% baseline) [16]. It has been shown that even after adequate neuromuscular blockade reversal (TOF ≥0.9), patients remain at risk of upper airway obstruction [17]. Of note, these findings may be confounded by residual sedation and anesthetic.

Transfusion-related acute lung injury (TRALI) and transfusion-associated circulatory overload (TACO) are 2 PPCs caused by administration of blood products. Pathophysiologic mechanisms underlying TACO are believed to include volume overload and elevated left atrial filling pressures, resulting in hydrostatic pulmonary edema and associated hypoxemia. Risk factors for developing TACO include advanced age, ventricular dysfunction, and total volume of blood product transfused [18]. The pathophysiology of TRALI is believed to be more complex and is thought to be primarily related to donor antibodies interacting with cognate antigens on recipient leukocytes, resulting in neutrophil activation and subsequent injury to pulmonary endothelium [19]. The end result of this process is the development of nonhydrostatic pulmonary edema and hypoxemia. The primary risk factor for the development of TRALI appears to be the receipt of plasma-rich blood products (such as fresh frozen plasma or apheresis platelets), particularly when donated by multiparous women [20,21]. Additional risk factors have also been identified and include liver transplantation surgery, chronic alcohol abuse, shock, higher peak airway pressures while being mechanically ventilated, active smoking, and positive fluid balance [22]. Methods to reduce the risk of TRALI are discussed later.

Paralleling an increase in the prevalence of obesity in the American population is an increase in patients with obstructive sleep apnea (OSA). OSA is an independent risk factor for PPCs including aspiration, pulmonary embolism, and requirement for mechanical ventilation [23]. The likely mechanisms for PPCs in the OSA population include an increased risk of hypoxic and hypercapneic responses to anesthetics, sedatives and analgesics, and microaspiration.

GENERAL PREVENTION STRATEGIES

- Smoking cessation
- Mechanical ventilation strategies
- Pulmonary hygiene and early ambulation
- Anesthetic and analgesic technique
- Prevention of gastric-to-pulmonary aspiration
- Management of intravenous fluids
- Prevention of TRALI
- Avoiding hyperoxia

- Management of neuromuscular blockade
- Use of postoperative pulse oximetry
- Minimizing perioperative sedation
- Prevention of ventilator-associated pneumonia (VAP)

Smoking cessation

Smoking is a major modifiable risk factor not only for PPCs but also for many other surgical complications [24]. The perioperative period is an invaluable opportunity to help patients start the smoking cessation process. Although previous reports had suggested no benefit or even potential harm from smoking cessation within 2 months preoperatively [25], new evidence shows an overall benefit of smoking cessation at any point preoperatively [26,27].

A large retrospective database analysis illustrated a marked association between preoperative smoking and PPCs, with a relative risk of PPCs of 1.8 in all smokers and 6.3 in young, obese smokers [28]. For patients undergoing noncardiac surgery, smoking increases 30-day mortality by as much as 40% [29]. The primary mechanisms of harm include reduced oxygen delivery caused by the impact of carbon monoxide on oxygen uptake and release, endothelial dysfunction, atherosclerosis, and increased sympathetic tone [24].

Smoking cessation has a clear benefit for a reduction in both surgical complications and PPCs. A multicenter, randomized controlled trial of a smoking intervention (either cessation or at least 50% reduction) 6 to 8 weeks preoperatively compared with no intervention demonstrated a significant reduction in overall postoperative complications, including wound-related complications (5% vs 31%) and cardiovascular complications (0% vs 10%) [30]. A systematic review and meta-analysis of studies on preoperative smoking cessation showed a significant difference in PPCs when comparing previous with current smokers (15% vs 20%), with a larger effect seen with a longer duration of abstinence [26].

Previously there was a persistent concern that smoking cessation within 2 months of the surgical procedure might actually lead to pulmonary complications because of impaired mucociliary clearance of secretions [25]. However, more recent evidence has shifted recommendations to encourage preoperative smoking cessation regardless of the proximity to the surgical procedure. Although there appears to be greater benefit from a prolonged course of smoking abstinence, there is no evidence of harm from cessation immediately preoperatively. To help address the important issues of perioperative tobacco abuse, associated PPCs, and the potential for improved outcomes with smoking cessation, the ASA has launched a "Stop Smoking Initiative" to provide anesthesia providers with the necessary resources to help patients quit smoking [31].

Mechanical ventilation strategies

Lung-protective ventilation

With more than a decade of accumulating evidence supporting the use of lung-protective ventilation (LPV) strategies for the treatment of ARDS, more recent evidence has also begun to support its use in patients without ARDS.

The primary objectives with LPV are to avoid injury resulting from lung overdistension (volutrauma) in addition to the repeated opening and closing of lung segments at low lung volumes (atelectrauma) during mechanical ventilation. Key interventions include limiting tidal volume (and consequently also plateau pressures) and applying PEEP to prevent atelectasis. A landmark ARDS-net trial randomized ARDS patients to low tidal volume ventilation (6 mL/kg ideal body weight [IBW]) versus "traditional" tidal volumes (12 mL/kg IBW), and demonstrated a significant morality benefit (31% vs 39.8%) and more ventilator-free days with the low tidal volume strategy [32]. Using IBW to calculate recommended tidal volumes (in place of actual body weight) is essential for ensuring LPV. It must be emphasized that lung size is best estimated with consideration of sex and height (IBW) rather than actual body weight.

Since this study, there has been growing interest in the potential benefit of LPV in patients without ARDS. By the time of a large meta-analysis in 2012, there had already been at least 40 studies on LPV in patients without ARDS [33]. Studies conducted in the operating room and in the intensive care unit (ICU) were included in this meta-analysis, which showed a statistically and clinically significant reduction in the development of ARDS with LPV strategies (relative risk = 0.33, number needed to treat = 11). This study also demonstrated an association between LPV and both decreased pulmonary infections and length of stay in hospital.

Initially there was concern that given the short duration of mechanical ventilation in the operating theater, LPV may not be associated with the benefits seen in the ICU populations with longer exposures to mechanical ventilation. However, a recent meta-analysis demonstrated the benefit (lower risk of developing ARDS or pulmonary infection) of LPV for patients receiving mechanical ventilation only for the duration of their operation [34]. This study also showed an association between higher levels of PEEP and lower rates of ARDS and pulmonary infections. In a prospective, randomized trial of patients undergoing open abdominal procedures, a LPV strategy (tidal volumes of 7 mL/kg with 10 cm H_2O PEEP) was compared with traditional ventilation (9 mL/kg tidal volume without PEEP). This configuration of LPV led to decreased pulmonary infections, improved postoperative oxygenation, and a decrease in postoperative atelectasis [35].

Positive end-expiratory pressure

A small randomized trial evaluating an "open-lung" ventilator strategy during general anesthesia in elderly patients demonstrated significantly improved respiratory mechanics and oxygenation intraoperatively but not postoperatively [36]. This study compared intraoperative mechanical ventilation with 6 mL/kg tidal volumes and 12 cm H_2O of PEEP with 6 mL/kg tidal volumes and no PEEP. However, the study was not powered to detect differences in more meaningful outcomes such as mortality and PPCs.

A Cochrane review was conducted to evaluate the impact of PEEP during general anesthesia. This study showed an association between intraoperative

PEEP and oxygenation (increased partial pressure of arterial oxygen/fraction of inspired oxygen [FiO_2] on postoperative day 1) and decreased postoperative atelectasis [37]. The investigators concluded that there was not enough statistical power to demonstrate a mortality benefit of PEEP, because there were only 172 patients with mortality data in the final analysis.

Recruitment maneuvers

Recruitment maneuvers are intended to recruit collapsed alveoli to improve oxygenation and prevent low-volume lung injury. Various methods have been described regarding how to perform a recruitment maneuver [38]. There is a positive effect of recruitment maneuvers on oxygenation and compliance during abdominal laparoscopic procedures. A randomized trial comparing PEEP with PEEP plus recruitment maneuvers in the setting of pneumoperitoneum demonstrated improved intraoperative oxygenation and compliance with PEEP plus recruitment maneuvers [39]. Unfortunately, postoperative pulmonary outcomes were not recorded in this study, and the aggregate of data have not consistently shown improvements in patient-important outcomes, thus precluding the endorsement of such strategies more broadly (Table 2).

Pulmonary hygiene

Respiratory physiotherapy

Perioperative chest physiotherapy has been shown to improve pulmonary outcomes following procedures with a high risk for PPCs. Chest physiotherapy is generally considered the use of incentive spirometry or deep breathing exercises with a respiratory therapist. A systematic review concluded that preoperative chest physiotherapy is effective at reducing PPCs following major abdominal surgery [40]. A large study examining PPCs before and after implementation of a perioperative chest physiotherapy program demonstrated a reduction of PPCs with physiotherapy from 15.5% to 4.7% [41]. Physiotherapy for the postoperative care of lung-resection patients has been widely accepted and implemented, and is included in the British Thoracic Society guidelines for pulmonary resection [42].

Preoperative exercise capacity is the most reliable predictor of pulmonary complications following lung resection [43]. It is not clear whether initiating

Table 2
Mechanical ventilation strategies to prevent PPCs

Strategy	Rationale and evidence
Lung-protective ventilation[a]	For ARDS, significant mortality benefit [32] If no ARDS, prevents ARDS and pneumonia [33]
Positive end-expiratory pressure	Improves oxygenation [37] Inadequate data on PPCs
Recruitment maneuvers	Improves oxygenation [39] Inadequate data on PPCs

[a]Lung-protective ventilation is generally defined as tidal volumes 6 to 8 mL/kg IBW and maintaining plateau pressures less than 30 cm H_2O.

physiotherapy to increase preoperative exercise capacity leads to a decrease in PPCs. A small but well-designed randomized trial suggests that preoperative physiotherapy for patients with moderate or severe COPD undergoing lung cancer resection leads to shorter postoperative hospital stays and fewer PPCs following lung resection surgery [44]. This finding is consistent with those of other randomized trials of intensive preoperative pulmonary physiotherapy for high-risk patients undergoing intrathoracic procedures [45,46].

A protocolized, or bundled, multispecialty approach to PPC prevention also showed favorable results. Specifically, institution of a postoperative protocol including incentive spirometry, coughing, deep breathing, ambulation, and head-of-bed elevation reduced the incidence of postoperative pneumonia and reintubation following general and vascular surgical procedures. The rate of pneumonia fell from 2.6% to 1.6% and the rate of reintubation decreased from 2.0% to 1.2% [47]. This result is consistent with findings following implementation of similar pulmonary physiotherapy protocols in patients undergoing lung resection [41]. It is not possible to ascertain from this study which element of the protocol or bundle contributed the most benefit.

Incentive spirometry

The bulk of available data regarding the effectiveness of incentive spirometry and deep breathing exercises suggest that they each significantly reduce the risk of PPCs [48]. However, despite its widespread use, there is a paucity of data to support the use of incentive spirometry over alternative pulmonary physiotherapy modalities. A randomized trial comparing incentive spirometry with deep breathing exercises did not show any difference in PPCs [49]. A systematic review and meta-analysis of studies comparing the effectiveness of incentive spirometry, intermittent positive pressure breathing, and deep breathing exercises found no significant difference among the modalities [48]. Two Cochrane reviews have suggested a lack of benefit in terms of a reduction of PPCs following abdominal surgery [50] and coronary artery bypass grafting (CABG) [51] when comparing postoperative incentive spirometry with deep breathing exercises. A systematic review of randomized controlled trials comparing incentive spirometry with physiotherapy or noninvasive positive pressure ventilation failed to show any reduction in PPCs [52]. Incentive spirometry seems to be effective, but only if there is adequate patient education regarding its use and if there is a lack of pulmonary physiotherapy (deep breathing exercises and ambulation).

Early ambulation

There are a limited number of investigations evaluating the impact of early postoperative ambulation on PPCs other than pulmonary embolism [53,54]. Observational data suggest that early postoperative ambulation may prevent PPCs [55–57]. Postoperatively, early ambulation, as part of a fast-track protocol, has been shown to reduce PPCs [47,58]. However, there are no large clinical trials directly and specifically investigating the impact of early ambulation on PPCs.

Anesthetic and analgesic techniques

Neuraxial and regional anesthesia

Several large, multicenter studies have demonstrated an association between neuraxial and regional anesthetic techniques and decreased pulmonary complications in comparison with general anesthesia. A recent observational study of patients undergoing primary joint arthroplasty demonstrated a significant association between neuraxial anesthesia and reduced pulmonary complications (including pneumonia, pulmonary embolism, and "pulmonary compromise") when compared with general anesthesia [59]. In a large multicenter, prospective observational comparison, neuraxial anesthesia was strongly associated with a reduction in PPCs compared with general anesthesia [1]. A large, multicenter retrospective study showed a reduction in pulmonary complications with neuraxial anesthesia in comparison with general anesthesia for hip fractures, despite having a higher baseline prevalence of COPD in the neuraxial group [60]. Studies specifically evaluating epidural anesthesia and analgesia have also reported a reduction in postoperative pneumonia [61]. In addition, a large meta-analysis demonstrated a reduction in postoperative respiratory depression with neuraxial anesthesia when compared with general anesthesia (odds ratio [OR] = 0.66) [62]. Randomized controlled trials of epidural anesthesia for intra-abdominal procedures demonstrate similar, beneficial effects on PPCs, perhaps secondary to improved postoperative analgesia [63,64]. A multicenter, retrospective cohort study comparing spinal anesthesia with general anesthesia for hip fracture repairs failed to show a difference in postoperative incidence of pneumonia, but this study was likely confounded by significant baseline differences in comorbidities [65].

The benefits of neuraxial anesthesia may be at least partially explained by their mitigated effect on respiratory mechanics and respiratory drive in comparison with general anesthesia. The respiratory effects of lumbar and low-thoracic neuraxial anesthesia are negligible, and only a 20% to 30% decrease in FVC and forced expiratory volume in 1 second (FEV_1) are observed with higher thoracic blockade [66]. With these relatively minor impairments in respiratory parameters, it is perhaps not surprising that spinal anesthesia may improve immediate postoperative oxygenation compared with general anesthesia [67], and that epidural anesthesia and analgesia improve postoperative lung function parameters [68].

Caution should be taken when considering neuraxial anesthesia and certain regional anesthetic techniques in patients with severe preoperative pulmonary dysfunction. Patients with limited respiratory reserve may decompensate if their baseline compensatory mechanisms are inhibited. For example, respiratory failure has been reported in patients with severe COPD or contralateral phrenic nerve dysfunction following interscalene nerve block or cervical plexus block caused by phrenic nerve blockade [69]. Neuraxial anesthetic techniques are generally acceptable and are often preferred for patients with severe pulmonary disease, unless the neuraxial anesthetic level rises high enough to inhibit accessory respiratory muscle function.

Postoperative analgesia

Several postoperative analgesic approaches have been used with varying effects on PPCs. Broadly speaking, analgesic regimens that are able to reduce sedation and facilitate a more physiologic respiratory state (persistence of deep breathing and coughing) appear to have a favorable effect on the incidence of PPCs. Epidural analgesia has been shown to improve vital capacity (18% increase) and functional residual capacity (5.8% increase) following major abdominal surgery [70]. It seems that limiting both general anesthesia and opioids (while adequately controlling pain) may be the common element in analgesic regimens associated with a reduction in PPCs.

Neuraxial and regional analgesia generally reduce systemic opioid consumption, and may therefore reduce the risk of PPCs [71]. Following CABG, epidural analgesia (with a wide variety of epidural local anesthetic and opioid mixtures) has been shown to decrease the incidence of PPCs [72,73]. Similar results were seen with morphine-based epidural analgesia and local anesthetic–based epidural analgesia for major abdominal procedures [63,74]. A randomized clinical trial comparing a fast-track protocol (using epidural ropivacaine/sufentanil analgesia, nonsteroidal anti-inflammatory drugs [NSAIDs], early ambulation, and no opioids) with conservative treatment (intercostal nerve blocks, intravenous opioids, NSAIDs, and ambulation on postoperative day 1) following thoracotomy showed a reduction of pulmonary complications in the fast-track group [75]. A meta-analysis of randomized controlled trials demonstrated a reduction in PPCs with epidural opioid analgesia when compared with systemic opioids for mainly thoracotomy and upper abdominal procedures [76].

The addition of regional analgesia to general anesthesia has not consistently been shown to decrease the risk of PPCs [77]. One large observational study of lower extremity joint replacements showed a significant difference in PPCs for patients receiving general anesthesia with neuraxial analgesia in comparison with general anesthesia alone [59]. The addition of a single-shot femoral nerve block to general anesthesia for total knee arthroplasty has been shown to increase oxygen saturation in the immediate postoperative period, although a full analysis of PPCs was not completed in this study [78].

Inhalational versus intravenous anesthesia

There does not appear to be sufficient evidence to support either inhalational or total intravenous anesthesia (TIVA) for preventing PPCs. In a recent study, comparison of a sevoflurane inhalational anesthetic versus a TIVA (with propofol and remifentanil) during esophagectomy did not demonstrate a significant difference in PPCs [79].

Prevention of gastric-to-pulmonary aspiration

Gastric-to-pulmonary aspiration carries a significant risk of morbidity and mortality [80,81]. Patients receiving any degree of sedation are at risk for aspiration because of reduced airway-protective reflexes and alterations in esophageal tone. Several standard interventions are used to reduce the risk of aspiration during anesthesia, including preoperative fasting, nonparticulate antacid consumption, cricoid pressure, head-of-bed elevation, gastric decompression, and rapid (or modified rapid) sequence induction and intubation.

The risk of aspiration persists throughout the anesthetic period, so it is important that continuous efforts are made to avoid aspiration at the end of an anesthetic as well as at induction. The 2011 ASA practice guidelines outline several recommendations regarding aspiration prevention. Patients with nonfasting status, bowel obstruction, esophageal or gastric disorders including achalasia, hiatal hernia, strictures, diverticulum, preoperative altered level of consciousness, and gravid status are designated as at high risk for aspiration. For those not at high risk for aspiration, the use of antacids, promotility agents, and antiemetic medications are not recommended for routine use [82]. Preoperative gastric decompression is controversial and is not consistently effective [83]. Based on ICU ventilator studies, head-of-bed elevation appears to reduce the risk of aspiration [84]. There is great debate over the necessity and effectiveness of cricoid pressure, yet it remains common practice in many institutions [85]. Rapid sequence induction and intubation is a widely accepted method of reducing the risk of aspiration, because it minimizes the time between loss of protective airway reflexes and endotracheal intubation, and limits the amount of gastric insufflation from mask ventilation. However, a recent review found a lack of evidence to support current rapid sequence induction and intubation practices [86].

In addition to macroaspiration (gross evidence on visual inspection of the airway), data are accumulating to suggest significant morbidity associated with microaspiration. Microaspiration has been strongly associated with ARDS and is a presumptive mechanism of VAP [87,88]. Methods to prevent microaspiration are presumed to be the same as those used to prevent macroaspiration. However, such interventions for microaspiration prevention are used with wide variability among practicing anesthesiologists [89].

Management of intravenous fluids

Based on the rationale that excessive intravenous fluids rapidly extravasate into the interstitium (including the lungs), the hypothesis that a conservative intraoperative fluid-management strategy results in fewer PPCs has been tested. Several studies have shown that limiting intraoperative crystalloid infusion may decrease PPCs. A randomized clinical trial of patients undergoing intra-abdominal procedures demonstrated a reduction of PPCs with a conservative intravenous fluid regimen (4 mL/kg/h) compared with a liberal intravenous fluid infusion (10 mL/kg crystalloid bolus followed by 12 mL/kg/h) strategy [90]. During esophageal resection, a conservative intravenous fluid strategy, compared with a historical cohort, was associated with shorter times to extubation and hospital length of stay [91]. In a randomized clinical trial in the setting of laparoscopic cholecystectomy, liberal intravenous fluids (40 mL/kg lactated Ringer solution) led to a reduction in pulmonary function parameters (FVC and FEV_1) when compared with a conservative intravenous fluid strategy

(15 mL/kg lactated Ringer). However, this study did not specifically report the incidence of PPCs or many potential confounders (specifically blood product transfusion) [92]. In addition, it is important to recognize that the ideal fluid strategy may change over a patient's course of care. For example, early septic shock typically mandates aggressive fluid resuscitation, whereas more conservative fluid strategies have been associated with improved outcomes in the later stages of sepsis management, particularly when complicated by ARDS [93].

Preventing transfusion-related acute lung injury

As discussed earlier, TRALI is believed to be largely the result of interactions between donor antibodies found in plasma-rich blood products (particularly plasma and pooled platelets) and cognate antigens located on recipient leukocytes. The most effective method of preventing TRALI is to simply avoid (or at least limit) unnecessary administration of blood products. However, as this is not always possible, alternative strategies for TRALI prevention have also been investigated. The most effective TRALI mitigation strategy is believed to have been the transition to male-only plasma donation. This intervention was recently associated with a significant reduction in TRALI incidence when compared with a historical cohort (OR = 0.21) [94]. Observational data have also suggested prolonged duration of red blood cell (RBC) storage may portend a risk of adverse respiratory outcomes [95]. However, in a randomized clinical trial evaluating single-unit RBC transfusion in stable but critically ill patients, fresh RBC transfusion was not shown to improve respiratory outcomes when compared with standard-issue RBCs (median storage of 4 vs 26.5 days) [96]. The impact of fresh versus standard-issue RBC transfusion in those who receive a greater volume of RBCs will be borne out in ongoing large clinical trials.

Avoiding hyperoxia

Anesthesiologists routinely use hyperoxia to delay the onset of hypoxia following apnea during the induction of anesthesia [97]. Hyperoxia is defined as providing more oxygen than is required to maintain adequate arterial saturations and end-organ oxygen delivery. Numerous studies suggest the potential for pulmonary toxicity with sustained hyperoxia [98,99]. Although the threshold of oxygen toxicity in terms of the administered Fio_2 and duration of administration are not known, some suggest an Fio_2 greater than 0.6 can result in pulmonary toxicity [100]. Prolonged exposure to high oxygen concentrations has also been shown to lead to absorption atelectasis, decreased mucociliary clearance, decreased surfactant production, and free radical formation [101]. It is unclear how, or if, these observations translate into clinically relevant acute PPCs.

Clinical data regarding the effects of hyperoxia are mixed. In a randomized trial of obese surgical patients, high Fio_2 led to worsened postoperative lung function and arterial oxygenation [102]. In a large randomized trial of high Fio_2, in which pulmonary outcomes were a secondary aim, there was no statistically significant difference detected in PPCs including atelectasis, pneumonia, and respiratory failure [103].

Bleomycin exposure presents a unique scenario that has historically been considered a contraindication for hyperoxia. A case series of patients with a history of bleomycin exposure received an Fio_2 greater than 0.3 and later developed ARDS. However, further studies failed to confirm these findings [104,105]. A short interval between the last bleomycin dose and exposure to hyperoxia likely increases the risk of pulmonary injury [106]. However, in the largest study of patients with a history of bleomycin exposure, no association between median Fio_2 and postoperative ARDS was found [107]. In fact, in a series of patients with a history of bleomycin exposure who subsequently required hyperbaric oxygen therapy, there were no reported cases of ARDS [108].

Management of neuromuscular blockade reversal

As described earlier, neuromuscular blockade is associated with a reduction in postoperative FVC, which is suggested to increase the risk for PPCs [109]. In addition to changes in respiratory mechanics, residual neuromuscular blockade has a significant impact on oropharyngeal muscle tone, and increases the risk of upper airway obstruction or aspiration postoperatively. Long-acting neuromuscular blocking agents have consistently been linked with PPCs, presumably because of residual neuromuscular blockade, and should generally be avoided [110,111].

There has been a gradual evolution of the criteria that define adequate neuromuscular blockade reversal. Train-of-four ratio measured subjectively at the adductor pollicis with mechanomyography has traditionally been used to assess the adequacy of neuromuscular blockade reversal. The goal TOF ratio has gradually increased over time from at least 0.7 to at least 0.9, in light of recognition that even mild and difficult-to-detect residual neuromuscular blockade increases the risk of PPCs [15]. A TOF ratio of 0.7 correlates with normal tidal volumes, sustained eye opening, tongue protrusion, and handgrip. A TOF ratio of 0.7 to 0.9 correlates with sustained head lift and sustained leg lift, but still does not guarantee an adequate degree of neuromuscular recovery to prevent PPCs [112]. More recently, acceleromyography has been introduced as a more quantitative method of ensuring adequate neuromuscular blockade [113]. However, further studies will be needed to better understand the impact of this monitoring technique on prevention of PPCs.

Postoperative pulse oximetry

Despite clear rationale to support the use of postoperative pulse oximetry for preventing PPCs, there are very limited data to demonstrate its effectiveness. In theory, early detection and prompt treatment of hypoxia should decrease the incidence and severity of associated PPCs. Studies have shown that perioperative pulse oximetry reduces the incidence and severity of hypoxemia [114]. In a randomized trial of more than 20,000 patients, perioperative pulse oximetry was shown to change clinical management (including more oxygen and more naloxone), but was not shown to reduce the incidence of PPCs [115]. In a randomized trial, the use of continuous pulse oximetry in a general care postsurgical ward did not significantly affect the rate of transfer to the ICU, mortality, or total hospitalization cost in comparison with general postoperative monitoring without continuous pulse oximetry [116]. The surprising lack of evidence to show an improvement in PPCs with perioperative pulse oximetry is summarized in a recent Cochrane review [117].

Minimizing perioperative sedation

Opioid analgesics and many sedating medications cause a dose-dependent inhibition of protective airway reflexes, and both hypercarbic and hypoxic respiratory drive [118,119]. By inhibiting these reflexes, perioperative sedation may increase the risk for PPCs. Prolonged sedation is also associated with delirium, which may further complicate extubation efforts. Evidence from studies on ICU patients has shown that deeper sedation is associated with delayed extubation and increased mortality [120]. The avoidance of benzodiazepines in the ICU is associated with shorter duration of intubation, which may translate into less pulmonary complications, but this remains unproven [121]. Dexmedetomidine has opioid-sparing characteristics, and therefore may have the potential to reduce the risk of some PPCs [122].

Prevention of ventilator-associated pneumonia

The Institution for Healthcare Improvement has endorsed the implementation of a "ventilator bundle" for ICU patients with the goal of preventing VAP [123]. The bundle includes 5 components: elevation of the head of bed, daily sedation disruption with evaluation for extubation potential, peptic ulcer prophylaxis, thromboembolism prophylaxis, and daily oral hygiene with chlorhexidine [124–126]. Drainage of subglottic secretion and use of closed-circuit suctioning systems should be considered for the prevention of VAP [127]. However, studies of VAP prevention must be interpreted with caution, as many of the proposed interventions seem to reduce the rate of VAP without any impact on clinical outcomes, such as length of stay in hospital and mortality [128].

POPULATION-SPECIFIC PREVENTION STRATEGIES

- Obstructive lung disease
- OSA and obesity
- Intrathoracic surgical procedures
- Specialized care of ARDS and refractory hypoxia

Certain patient populations are at particular risk for PPCs. The following are specific preventive measures designed to reduce the risk of PPCs for selected high-risk populations.

Obstructive lung disease

The risk for PPCs in patients with COPD has been associated with baseline hypercapnia, preoperative wheezing, and objective evidence of reactive airway disease [129,130]. Prevention of PPCs in patients with obstructive lung disease is primarily focused on preoperative optimization. Care providers must recognize that those with obstructive lung disease (COPD or asthma) may quickly develop clinically significant respiratory decompensation caused by bronchoconstriction and dynamic hyperinflation (or auto-PEEP) during the perioperative period.

It is generally thought that preoperative optimization of any reversible aspects of obstructive lung disease may prevent PPCs. To this end, preoperative respiratory infections should be fully treated, smoking cessation should be accomplished whenever possible, and medication regimens for obstructive lung disease should be optimized before the onset of the surgical procedure.

Prevention of perioperative bronchospasm and secondary dynamic hyperinflation may be accomplished through several methods. Bronchospasm may be prevented by avoiding airway instrumentation and using regional or neuraxial anesthesia [131,132]. In patients with COPD, neuraxial anesthesia has been associated with decreased mortality in comparison with general anesthesia [133]. If general anesthesia is used, one should avoid medications that can exacerbate bronchial reactivity, including some volatile anesthetics (eg, desflurane), histamine-releasing opioids, certain neuromuscular blocking agents, and thiopental (Table 3). Treatment with β2-agonists and anticholinergics before airway instrumentation and before extubation is recommended. Utilization of neuraxial analgesia in addition to general anesthesia for major abdominal procedures in patients with COPD has been shown to decrease the incidence of PPCs and mortality [134].

Dynamic hyperinflation is primarily caused by inadequate expiratory time to allow lung emptying to reach a normal functional residual capacity. Dynamic hyperinflation can be prevented by decreasing the ratio of inspiratory to expiratory time (I:E ratio) i.e. increasing the expiratory time and avoiding tachypnea. In cases of severe limitation of expiratory flow, one may be forced to tolerate a degree of permissive hypercapnia. In the perioperative period, dynamic hyperinflation may cause PPCs by increasing work-of-breathing. Application of PEEP during spontaneous breathing can decrease work-of-breathing and, in theory, may prevent PPCs. In addition, in the setting of severe airflow obstruction, inhalation of helium-oxygen (heliox) improves airflow because of decreased density and, therefore, less turbulent flow.

Noninvasive positive pressure ventilation can facilitate extubation and prevent reintubation of patients with severe COPD. Because of underlying severe

Table 3
Anesthetic medications associated with bronchospasm

Intravenous anesthetics	Thiopental
Neuromuscular blockers, via histamine release	Mivacurium
	Atracurium
Opioids, via histamine release	Morphine
	Meperidine
Irritating volatile anesthetics	Isoflurane (during inhalational induction)
	Desflurane
Antiarrhythmics	Adenosine
Cholinesterase inhibition	Neostigmine

airway obstruction compounded by the added airflow obstruction from an endotracheal tube, many patients may not appear appropriate for extubation even if they are neurologically appropriate. There is evidence to support the use of extubation and continuous positive airway pressure (CPAP) for patients with severe COPD reducing the rate of reintubation, pneumonia, and 60-day mortality in ICU patients [135].

Obstructive sleep apnea and obesity

OSA is a significant risk factor for PPCs, particularly aspiration and pulmonary embolism [23]. In 2013, it was estimated that approximately 1 in 4 men and 1 in 10 women had OSA [136]. Equally concerning is the suggestion that up to 90% of cases are believed to be undiagnosed [137].

Several clinical scoring tools (including STOP-BANG and SACS) can be used to identify patients who are at high risk for OSA [138–140]. Use of a focused patient history and physical examination to identify those with OSA or at high risk of OSA is supported by the 2006 ASA guidelines for the perioperative management of OSA [141]. With adequate preoperative diagnosis of OSA, its contribution as a risk factor for PPCs can be greatly mitigated. Preoperative evaluation with polysomnography before bariatric surgical procedures and noninvasive positive pressure ventilation (such as CPAP) as indicated seem to have the potential to decrease the risk of OSA-related PPCs [142,143].

The preoperative and intraoperative recommendations for preventing PPCs in patients with known or suspected OSA include preoperative screening for OSA, avoidance of sedative premedication, using regional anesthesia and analgesia if possible, and vigilance and preparation for difficult airway situations [144]. Postoperatively, the primary intervention used to prevent PPCs in the setting of OSA is CPAP. For outpatient or ambulatory surgery, it is recommended that patients with or at high risk for OSA should be observed with continuous pulse oximetry for at least 6 hours to demonstrate the absence of significant respiratory events before discharge [145].

Data also suggest that avoiding supranormal intraoperative hyperoxia may improve postoperative pulmonary function in the obese population. Specifically, obese patients who were randomized to 40% oxygen while in the operating room environment had significantly greater arterial oxygenation levels and forced expiratory flows in the postoperative period when compared with those randomized to 80% oxygen [102].

Intrathoracic procedures

Intrathoracic procedures have been consistently associated with PPCs [1,7,8]. In this population, frailty appears to be a particularly important risk factor, as it has been specifically associated with PPCs and mortality following lobectomy [146]. Owing to their increased risk of developing PPCs, this patient population is often targeted for PPC-prevention interventions.

Procedures requiring thoracotomy are also frequently associated with significant postoperative pain, which alters normal respiratory mechanics [147]. Limiting the size of thoracotomy through the use of video-assisted thoracoscopy and other minimally invasive surgical approaches is associated with a reduction in PPCs [148,149].

For patients undergoing thoracotomy, perioperative analgesia strategies can have a marked impact on the risk for PPCs. As previously discussed, neuraxial and regional analgesia can prevent PPCs in various surgical populations, especially those undergoing thoracic procedures. Thoracic epidural analgesia leads to a lower rate of PPCs following thoracotomy in comparison with intravenous opioids [66]. There is also evidence to suggest that paravertebral blocks are as effective as thoracic epidurals for preventing PPCs and analgesia [150]. In general, thoracic epidural (with local anesthetic and opioid) or paravertebral block (with long-acting liposomal bupivacaine or continuous-infusion local anesthetic) is preferred for thoracic procedures. When these approaches are contraindicated, intercostal blocks should be considered [151].

Patients undergoing procedures requiring cardiopulmonary bypass (CPB) are at high risk of PPCs because of their exposure to several risk factors for lung injury. Specific examples include administration of blood products, reperfusion injury of the lungs, systemic inflammation following exposure to the nonbiological surfaces of the CPB circuit, chest wall defects, prolonged sedation, and postoperative mechanical ventilation [152].

Epidural analgesia has been shown to improve pulmonary function following CABG with CPB [72]. In a randomized trial, epidural analgesia (local anesthetic–based) led to a reduction in pain scores, a 16% increase in FEV_1, and a reduction in atelectasis on postoperative day 1 when compared with intravenous morphine [73]. However, considering the incidence of significant coagulopathy following major cardiac procedures, neuraxial analgesia may not always be feasible.

In addition to specific analgesic techniques, several other methods have been proposed to reduce PPCs following cardiac surgery. Heparin-coated CPB circuits are less proinflammatory and may reduce the risk of lung injury [153]. Intraoperative hemofiltration to attenuate hypervolemia may reduce the risk of PPCs [154]. Limiting pulmonary ischemic time during CPB or eliminating ischemia altogether with bilateral extracorporeal circulation can attenuate ischemia-reperfusion lung injury. In a randomized trial, bilateral extracorporeal circulation (maintaining pulmonary circulation) during CABG showed decreased systemic inflammatory markers and increased systemic oxygen saturations [155]. Prophylactic CPAP has also been studied in a randomized trial following cardiac surgery, and appeared to decrease the incidence of PPCs, including pneumonia and reintubation following cardiac surgery [156].

Data are scarce regarding the impact of postcardiac surgery fast-track protocols on PPCs. The only consistently reported PPC in studies of postcardiac surgery fast-track protocols appears to be the rate of reintubation. Several studies reported earlier extubation and no significant change in the rate of reintubation following fast-track management [157,158]. The decrease in time to extubation resulting from fast-track management may in theory reduce the risk of developing PPCs. Overall, fast-track protocols aimed at limiting the duration of sedation and mechanical ventilation appear to be safe following low-risk and moderate-risk cardiac surgery [159].

Specialized care of acute respiratory distress syndrome and refractory hypoxemia

Treatment of patients with severe ARDS and refractory hypoxemia often requires extensive resources and an intimate knowledge of rescue therapies. The breadth of this topic is too extensive for this review, but a brief introduction is included. In some cases, it becomes difficult or impossible to maintain normal arterial oxygen saturations, normocapnia, and normal hemodynamics without exceeding the limits of LPV. In such cases, advanced techniques are often required to support the patient and prevent further lung injury.

An emerging theme in the management of severe ARDS is the necessity of maximizing lung-protective therapies early. Examples of this include early neuromuscular blockade, early initiation of prone positioning, and early consideration of extracorporeal membrane oxygenation (ECMO) [160]. In general, these modalities are believed to attenuate the risk of VILI [161]. There are accumulating data to support the early use of both prone positioning and ECMO in the setting of severe ARDS [162,163]. On the other hand, recent studies have failed to support the use of high-frequency oscillatory ventilation in the setting of ARDS [164]. Inhaled pulmonary vasodilators, including alprostadil and nitric oxide, improve ventilation-perfusion matching and can improve arterial oxygen saturations. However, the impact of inhaled pulmonary vasodilators on clinical outcomes has not been encouraging [165].

PREOPERATIVE EVALUATION

- Evaluation of obstructive lung disease
- Evaluation of OSA
- Preoperative pulmonary function testing
- Preoperative evaluation before lung resection

Obstructive lung disease

Preoperative evaluation and management of patients with obstructive lung disease is a key step in preventing PPCs. In the setting of severe COPD, one must remain vigilant for pulmonary hypertension and right ventricular dysfunction, because its presence increases perioperative risk [166]. In the case of elective procedures, patients with obstructive lung disease should be on an adequate medical regimen as directed by their primary care physician or pulmonary specialist, with adequately controlled symptoms preoperatively. Without evidence of an acute COPD exacerbation, prophylactic antibiotics are not recommended. Chest radiographs should only be obtained if there is specific acute concern [167,168].

Obstructive sleep apnea

Identification of patients with OSA may facilitate prevention of PPCs. Evaluation for OSA should include review of the medical record, focused history and physical examination, collateral history from family or roommates, and sleep studies. Several clinical scoring tools (including STOP-BANG and SACS) can be used to identify patients who are at high risk for OSA [138–140]. These screening tools include measurements of neck circumference, history of hypertension, and history of snoring or gasping while sleeping. It is preferable for OSA evaluation (and initiation of treatment) to begin before the day of surgery [141]. Specifically for the bariatric surgery population, there is evidence to support routine polysomnography preoperatively [169]. Preoperative evaluation and, if indicated, prescription of a CPAP regimen appears to greatly reduce the risk of PPCs in those with OSA [142].

Preoperative pulmonary function testing

The role of preoperative pulmonary functions tests (PFTs), in general, is limited. A systematic review of preoperative PFTs failed to demonstrate any clinically significant benefit [170]. With the exception of preoperative evaluation of lung resection candidates, clinical guidelines recommend against the routine use of preoperative PFTs [168].

Preoperative evaluation before lung resection

Thorough preoperative evaluation before lung-resection surgery is necessary to prevent mortality and severe postoperative respiratory morbidity. Evaluating patients before lung resection should begin with lung spirometry including diffusing capacity. Using the results from spirometry, predicted postoperative (ppo) lung function can and should be calculated, as it is strongly associated with morbidity and mortality following lung resection [171]. Determining eligibility for lung resection is commonly assessed by a "3-legged stool" approach, which quantifies pulmonary mechanics, parenchymal function, and cardiopulmonary capacity: $ppoFEV_1$, ppo diffusion capacity of carbon monoxide (DLCO), and preoperative maximum oxygen consumption (Vo_{2max}) [172]. $ppoFEV_1$ less than 30%, ppoDLCO less than 30%, and Vo_{2max} less than 10 mL/kg/min are predictive of mortality and PPCs following lung resection [173]. It is worth noting that preoperative predictions of postoperative lung function may overestimate the effect of lung resection [174]. It has been suggested that with modern anesthetic techniques and postoperative care, outcomes for those deemed to be very high risk for lung resection may be improving [175].

SUMMARY

- PPCs significantly affect patient-important outcomes and utilization of health care resources.
- Identification of risk factors that portend risk for PPCs is an essential first step in mitigating these adverse events.
- Prevention strategies specifically targeting those with modifiable risk factors for PPCs are likely to have the largest impact on patients' outcomes.
- Prevention of PPCs requires an awareness of risk factors and implementation of prevention strategies during all phases of the perioperative experience.

- Unless specifically contraindicated, LPV should be used for all mechanically ventilated patients.
- Although early smoking cessation is preferred, it is recommended for all patients who are to receive general anesthesia, regardless of the interval preceding surgery.

References

[1] Canet J, Gallart L, Gomar C, et al. Prediction of postoperative pulmonary complications in a population-based surgical cohort. Anesthesiology 2010;113(6):1338–50.

[2] Smetana GW. Postoperative pulmonary complications: an update on risk assessment and reduction. Cleve Clin J Med 2009;76(Suppl 4):S60–5.

[3] Melsen WG, Rovers MM, Groenwold RH, et al. Attributable mortality of ventilator-associated pneumonia: a meta-analysis of individual patient data from randomised prevention studies. Lancet Infect Dis 2013;13(8):665–71.

[4] Khuri SF, Henderson WG, DePalma RG, et al. Determinants of long-term survival after major surgery and the adverse effect of postoperative complications. Ann Surg 2005;242(3): 326–41 [discussion: 341–3].

[5] Dimick JB, Chen SL, Taheri PA, et al. Hospital costs associated with surgical complications: a report from the private-sector National Surgical Quality Improvement Program. J Am Coll Surg 2004;199(4):531–7.

[6] Cutler EC, Hunt A. Postoperative pulmonary complications. Arch Surg 1920;1(1): 114–57.

[7] Smetana GW, Lawrence VA, Cornell JE. Preoperative pulmonary risk stratification for noncardiothoracic surgery: systematic review for the American College of Physicians. Ann Intern Med 2006;144(8):581–95.

[8] Arozullah AM, Daley J, Henderson WG, et al. Multifactorial risk index for predicting postoperative respiratory failure in men after major noncardiac surgery. The National Veterans Administration Surgical Quality Improvement Program. Ann Surg 2000;232(2): 242–53.

[9] Tsiouris A, Horst HM, Paone G, et al. Preoperative risk stratification for thoracic surgery using the American College of Surgeons National Surgical Quality Improvement Program data set: functional status predicts morbidity and mortality. J Surg Res 2012;177(1):1–6.

[10] Rockwood K, Song X, MacKnight C, et al. A global clinical measure of fitness and frailty in elderly people. CMAJ 2005;173(5):489–95.

[11] Carney D, DiRocco J, Nieman G. Dynamic alveolar mechanics and ventilator-induced lung injury. Crit Care Med 2005;33(Suppl 3):S122–8.

[12] Briel M, Meade M, Mercat A, et al. Higher vs lower positive end-expiratory pressure in patients with acute lung injury and acute respiratory distress syndrome: systematic review and meta-analysis. JAMA 2010;303(9):865–73.

[13] Roberts RB, Shirley MA. Reducing the risk of acid aspiration during cesarean section. Anesth Analg 1974;53(6):859–68.

[14] Warner DO. Anaesthesia and chest wall function. Ann Acad Med Singapore 1994;23(4): 566–71.

[15] Murphy GS, Szokol JW, Marymont JH, et al. Residual neuromuscular blockade and critical respiratory events in the postanesthesia care unit. Anesth Analg 2008;107(1):130–7.

[16] Kumar GV, Nair AP, Murthy HS, et al. Residual neuromuscular blockade affects postoperative pulmonary function. Anesthesiology 2012;117(6):1234–44.

[17] Eikermann M, Blobner M, Groeben H, et al. Postoperative upper airway obstruction after recovery of the train of four ratio of the adductor pollicis muscle from neuromuscular blockade. Anesth Analg 2006;102(3):937–42.

[18] Li G, Rachmale S, Kojicic M, et al. Incidence and transfusion risk factors for transfusion-associated circulatory overload among medical intensive care unit patients. Transfusion 2011;51(2):338–43.

[19] Triulzi DJ. Transfusion-related acute lung injury: current concepts for the clinician. Anesth Analg 2009;108(3):770–6.
[20] Gajic O, Yilmaz M, Iscimen R, et al. Transfusion from male-only versus female donors in critically ill recipients of high plasma volume components. Crit Care Med 2007;35(7): 1645–8.
[21] Gajic O, Rana R, Winters JL, et al. Transfusion-related acute lung injury in the critically ill: prospective nested case-control study. Am J Respir Crit Care Med 2007;176(9):886–91.
[22] Toy P, Gajic O, Bacchetti P, et al. Transfusion-related acute lung injury: incidence and risk factors. Blood 2012;119(7):1757–67.
[23] Memtsoudis S, Liu SS, Ma Y, et al. Perioperative pulmonary outcomes in patients with sleep apnea after noncardiac surgery. Anesth Analg 2011;112(1):113–21.
[24] Warner DO. Perioperative abstinence from cigarettes: physiologic and clinical consequences. Anesthesiology 2006;104(2):356–67.
[25] Warner MA, Offord KP, Warner ME, et al. Role of preoperative cessation of smoking and other factors in postoperative pulmonary complications: a blinded prospective study of coronary artery bypass patients. Mayo Clin Proc 1989;64(6):609–16.
[26] Mills E, Eyawo O, Lockhart I, et al. Smoking cessation reduces postoperative complications: a systematic review and meta-analysis. Am J Med 2011;124(2):144–54.e8.
[27] Myers K, Hajek P, Hinds C, et al. Stopping smoking shortly before surgery and postoperative complications: a systematic review and meta-analysis. Arch Intern Med 2011;171(11):983–9.
[28] Schwilk B, Bothner U, Schraag S, et al. Perioperative respiratory events in smokers and nonsmokers undergoing general anaesthesia. Acta Anaesthesiol Scand 1997;41(3): 348–55.
[29] Turan A, Mascha EJ, Roberman D, et al. Smoking and perioperative outcomes. Anesthesiology 2011;114(4):837–46.
[30] Moller AM, Villebro N, Pedersen T, et al. Effect of preoperative smoking intervention on postoperative complications: a randomised clinical trial. Lancet 2002;359(9301):114–7.
[31] America Society of Anesthesiologists. ASA stop smoking initiative for providers. 2014. Available at: http://www.asahq.org/for-members/clinical-information/asa-stop-smoking-initiative.aspx. Accessed April 4, 2014.
[32] Ventilation with lower tidal volumes as compared with traditional tidal volumes for acute lung injury and the acute respiratory distress syndrome. The Acute Respiratory Distress Syndrome Network. N Engl J Med 2000;342(18):1301–8.
[33] Serpa Neto A, Cardoso SO, Manetta JA, et al. Association between use of lung-protective ventilation with lower tidal volumes and clinical outcomes among patients without acute respiratory distress syndrome: a meta-analysis. JAMA 2012;308(16):1651–9.
[34] Hemmes SN, Serpa Neto A, Schultz MJ. Intraoperative ventilatory strategies to prevent postoperative pulmonary complications: a meta-analysis. Curr Opin Anaesthesiol 2013;26(2):126–33.
[35] Severgnini P, Selmo G, Lanza C, et al. Protective mechanical ventilation during general anesthesia for open abdominal surgery improves postoperative pulmonary function. Anesthesiology 2013;118(6):1307–21.
[36] Weingarten TN, Whalen FX, Warner DO, et al. Comparison of two ventilatory strategies in elderly patients undergoing major abdominal surgery. Br J Anaesth 2010;104(1):16–22.
[37] Imberger G, McIlroy D, Pace NL, et al. Positive end-expiratory pressure (PEEP) during anaesthesia for the prevention of mortality and postoperative pulmonary complications. Cochrane Database Syst Rev 2010;(9):CD007922.
[38] Pelosi P, Gama de Abreu M, Rocco PR. New and conventional strategies for lung recruitment in acute respiratory distress syndrome. Crit Care 2010;14(2):210.
[39] Futier E, Constantin JM, Pelosi P, et al. Intraoperative recruitment maneuver reverses detrimental pneumoperitoneum-induced respiratory effects in healthy weight and obese patients undergoing laparoscopy. Anesthesiology 2010;113(6):1310–9.

[40] Pouwels S, Stokmans RA, Willigendael EM, et al. Preoperative exercise therapy for elective major abdominal surgery: a systematic review. Int J Surg 2014;12(2):134–40.
[41] Novoa N, Ballesteros E, Jimenez MF, et al. Chest physiotherapy revisited: evaluation of its influence on the pulmonary morbidity after pulmonary resection. Eur J Cardiothorac Surg 2011;40(1):130–4.
[42] Lim E, Baldwin D, Beckles M, et al. Guidelines on the radical management of patients with lung cancer. Thorax 2010;65(Suppl 3):iii1–27.
[43] Benzo R, Kelley GA, Recchi L, et al. Complications of lung resection and exercise capacity: a meta-analysis. Respir Med 2007;101(8):1790–7.
[44] Benzo R, Wigle D, Novotny P, et al. Preoperative pulmonary rehabilitation before lung cancer resection: results from two randomized studies. Lung Cancer 2011;74(3):441–5.
[45] Hulzebos EH, Helders PJ, Favie NJ, et al. Preoperative intensive inspiratory muscle training to prevent postoperative pulmonary complications in high-risk patients undergoing CABG surgery: a randomized clinical trial. JAMA 2006;296(15):1851–7.
[46] Nomori H, Kobayashi R, Fuyuno G, et al. Preoperative respiratory muscle training. Assessment in thoracic surgery patients with special reference to postoperative pulmonary complications. Chest 1994;105(6):1782–8.
[47] Cassidy MR, Rosenkranz P, McCabe K, et al. I COUGH: reducing postoperative pulmonary complications with a multidisciplinary patient care program. JAMA Surg 2013;148(8):740–5.
[48] Thomas JA, McIntosh JM. Are incentive spirometry, intermittent positive pressure breathing, and deep breathing exercises effective in the prevention of postoperative pulmonary complications after upper abdominal surgery? A systematic overview and meta-analysis. Phys Ther 1994;74(1):3–10 [discussion: 10–6].
[49] Agostini P, Naidu B, Cieslik H, et al. Effectiveness of incentive spirometry in patients following thoracotomy and lung resection including those at high risk for developing pulmonary complications. Thorax 2013;68(6):580–5.
[50] do Nascimento P Jr, Modolo NS, Andrade S, et al. Incentive spirometry for prevention of postoperative pulmonary complications in upper abdominal surgery. Cochrane Database Syst Rev 2014;(2):CD006058.
[51] Freitas ER, Soares BG, Cardoso JR, et al. Incentive spirometry for preventing pulmonary complications after coronary artery bypass graft. Cochrane Database Syst Rev 2012;(9):CD004466.
[52] Overend TJ, Anderson CM, Lucy SD, et al. The effect of incentive spirometry on postoperative pulmonary complications: a systematic review. Chest 2001;120(3):971–8.
[53] White RH, Gettner S, Newman JM, et al. Predictors of rehospitalization for symptomatic venous thromboembolism after total hip arthroplasty. N Engl J Med 2000;343(24): 1758–64.
[54] Geerts WH, Heit JA, Clagett GP, et al. Prevention of venous thromboembolism. Chest 2001;119(Suppl 1):132S–75S.
[55] Haines KJ, Skinner EH, Berney S. Association of postoperative pulmonary complications with delayed mobilisation following major abdominal surgery: an observational cohort study. Physiotherapy 2013;99(2):119–25.
[56] Rawal N, Sjostrand U, Christoffersson E, et al. Comparison of intramuscular and epidural morphine for postoperative analgesia in the grossly obese: influence on postoperative ambulation and pulmonary function. Anesth Analg 1984;63(6):583–92.
[57] Kamel HK, Iqbal MA, Mogallapu R, et al. Time to ambulation after hip fracture surgery: relation to hospitalization outcomes. J Gerontol A Biol Sci Med Sci 2003;58(11): 1042–5.
[58] Olsen MF, Wennberg E. Fast-track concepts in major open upper abdominal and thoracoabdominal surgery: a review. World J Surg 2011;35(12):2586–93.
[59] Memtsoudis SG, Sun X, Chiu YL, et al. Perioperative comparative effectiveness of anesthetic technique in orthopedic patients. Anesthesiology 2013;118(5):1046–58.

[60] Neuman MD, Silber JH, Elkassabany NM, et al. Comparative effectiveness of regional versus general anesthesia for hip fracture surgery in adults. Anesthesiology 2012;117(1):72–92.
[61] Yeager MP, Glass DD, Neff RK, et al. Epidural anesthesia and analgesia in high-risk surgical patients. Anesthesiology 1987;66(6):729–36.
[62] Rodgers A, Walker N, Schug S, et al. Reduction of postoperative mortality and morbidity with epidural or spinal anaesthesia: results from overview of randomised trials. BMJ 2000;321(7275):1493.
[63] Park WY, Thompson JS, Lee KK. Effect of epidural anesthesia and analgesia on perioperative outcome: a randomized, controlled Veterans Affairs cooperative study. Ann Surg 2001;234(4):560–9 [discussion: 569–71].
[64] Rigg JR, Jamrozik K, Myles PS, et al. Epidural anaesthesia and analgesia and outcome of major surgery: a randomised trial. Lancet 2002;359(9314):1276–82.
[65] O'Hara DA, Duff A, Berlin JA, et al. The effect of anesthetic technique on postoperative outcomes in hip fracture repair. Anesthesiology 2000;92(4):947–57.
[66] Groeben H. Epidural anesthesia and pulmonary function. J Anesth 2006;20(4):290–9.
[67] McKenzie PJ, Wishart HY, Dewar KM, et al. Comparison of the effects of spinal anaesthesia and general anaesthesia on postoperative oxygenation and perioperative mortality. Br J Anaesth 1980;52(1):49–54.
[68] Panaretou V, Toufektzian L, Siafaka I, et al. Postoperative pulmonary function after open abdominal aortic aneurysm repair in patients with chronic obstructive pulmonary disease: epidural versus intravenous analgesia. Ann Vasc Surg 2012;26(2):149–55.
[69] Urmey WF, McDonald M. Hemidiaphragmatic paresis during interscalene brachial plexus block: effects on pulmonary function and chest wall mechanics. Anesth Analg 1992;74(3):352–7.
[70] Wahba WM, Don HF, Craig DB. Post-operative epidural analgesia: effects on lung volumes. Can Anaesth Soc J 1975;22(4):519–27.
[71] Macfarlane AJ, Prasad GA, Chan VW, et al. Does regional anesthesia improve outcome after total knee arthroplasty? Clin Orthop Relat Res 2009;467(9):2379–402.
[72] Liu SS, Block BM, Wu CL. Effects of perioperative central neuraxial analgesia on outcome after coronary artery bypass surgery: a meta-analysis. Anesthesiology 2004;101(1):153–61.
[73] Tenenbein PK, Debrouwere R, Maguire D, et al. Thoracic epidural analgesia improves pulmonary function in patients undergoing cardiac surgery. Can J Anaesth 2008;55(6):344–50.
[74] Hasenbos M, van Egmond J, Gielen M, et al. Post-operative analgesia by high thoracic epidural versus intramuscular nicomorphine after thoracotomy. Part III. The effects of per- and post-operative analgesia on morbidity. Acta Anaesthesiol Scand 1987;31(7):608–15.
[75] Muehling BM, Halter GL, Schelzig H, et al. Reduction of postoperative pulmonary complications after lung surgery using a fast track clinical pathway. Eur J Cardiothorac Surg 2008;34(1):174–80.
[76] Ballantyne JC, Carr DB, deFerranti S, et al. The comparative effects of postoperative analgesic therapies on pulmonary outcome: cumulative meta-analyses of randomized, controlled trials. Anesth Analg 1998;86(3):598–612.
[77] Stundner O, Rasul R, Chiu YL, et al. Peripheral nerve blocks in shoulder arthroplasty: how do they influence complications and length of stay? Clin Orthop Relat Res 2014;472(5):1482–8.
[78] Wiesmann T, Steinfeldt T, Wagner G, et al. Supplemental single shot femoral nerve block for total hip arthroplasty: impact on early postoperative care, pain management and lung function. Minerva Anestesiol 2014;80(1):48–57.
[79] Lee JJ, Kim GH, Kim JA, et al. Comparison of pulmonary morbidity using sevoflurane or propofol-remifentanil anesthesia in an Ivor Lewis operation. J Cardiothorac Vasc Anesth 2012;26(5):857–62.

[80] Warner MA, Warner ME, Weber JG. Clinical significance of pulmonary aspiration during the perioperative period. Anesthesiology 1993;78(1):56–62.
[81] Pepe PE, Potkin RT, Reus DH, et al. Clinical predictors of the adult respiratory distress syndrome. Am J Surg 1982;144(1):124–30.
[82] American Society of Anesthesiologists Committee. Practice guidelines for preoperative fasting and the use of pharmacologic agents to reduce the risk of pulmonary aspiration: application to healthy patients undergoing elective procedures: an updated report by the American Society of Anesthesiologists Committee on Standards and Practice Parameters. Anesthesiology 2011;114(3):495–511.
[83] Jensen AG, Callesen T, Hagemo JS, et al. Scandinavian clinical practice guidelines on general anaesthesia for emergency situations. Acta Anaesthesiol Scand 2010;54(8): 922–50.
[84] Orozco-Levi M, Torres A, Ferrer M, et al. Semirecumbent position protects from pulmonary aspiration but not completely from gastroesophageal reflux in mechanically ventilated patients. Am J Respir Crit Care Med 1995;152(4 Pt 1):1387–90.
[85] Lerman J. On cricoid pressure: "may the force be with you". Anesth Analg 2009;109(5): 1363–6.
[86] Neilipovitz DT, Crosby ET. No evidence for decreased incidence of aspiration after rapid sequence induction. Can J Anaesth 2007;54(9):748–64.
[87] Bice T, Li G, Malinchoc M, et al. Incidence and risk factors of recurrent acute lung injury. Crit Care Med 2011;39(5):1069–73.
[88] Safdar N, Crnich CJ, Maki DG. The pathogenesis of ventilator-associated pneumonia: its relevance to developing effective strategies for prevention. Respir Care 2005;50(6): 725–39 [discussion: 739–41].
[89] Ehrenfeld JM, Cassedy EA, Forbes VE, et al. Modified rapid sequence induction and intubation: a survey of United States current practice. Anesth Analg 2012;115(1):95–101.
[90] Nisanevich V, Felsenstein I, Almogy G, et al. Effect of intraoperative fluid management on outcome after intraabdominal surgery. Anesthesiology 2005;103(1):25–32.
[91] Kita T, Mammoto T, Kishi Y. Fluid management and postoperative respiratory disturbances in patients with transthoracic esophagectomy for carcinoma. J Clin Anesth 2002;14(4): 252–6.
[92] Holte K, Hahn RG, Ravn L, et al. Influence of "liberal" versus "restrictive" intraoperative fluid administration on elimination of a postoperative fluid load. Anesthesiology 2007;106(1):75–9.
[93] Murphy CV, Schramm GE, Doherty JA, et al. The importance of fluid management in acute lung injury secondary to septic shock. Chest 2009;136(1):102–9.
[94] Eder AF, Herron RM Jr, Strupp A, et al. Effective reduction of transfusion-related acute lung injury risk with male-predominant plasma strategy in the American Red Cross (2006-2008). Transfusion 2010;50(8):1732–42.
[95] Koch CG, Li L, Sessler DI, et al. Duration of red-cell storage and complications after cardiac surgery. N Engl J Med 2008;358(12):1229–39.
[96] Kor DJ, Kashyap R, Weiskopf RB, et al. Fresh red blood cell transfusion and short-term pulmonary, immunologic, and coagulation status: a randomized clinical trial. Am J Respir Crit Care Med 2012;185(8):842–50.
[97] Edmark L, Kostova-Aherdan K, Enlund M, et al. Optimal oxygen concentration during induction of general anesthesia. Anesthesiology 2003;98(1):28–33.
[98] Kafer ER. Pulmonary oxygen toxicity. A review of the evidence for acute and chronic oxygen toxicity in man. Br J Anaesth 1971;43(7):687–95.
[99] Fisher AB, Forman HJ, Glass M. Mechanisms of pulmonary oxygen toxicity. Lung 1984;162(5):255–9.
[100] Dos Santos CC. Hyperoxic acute lung injury and ventilator-induced/associated lung injury: new insights into intracellular signaling pathways. Crit Care 2007;11(2):126.
[101] Bryan CL, Jenkinson SG. Oxygen toxicity. Clin Chest Med 1988;9(1):141–52.

[102] Zoremba M, Dette F, Hunecke T, et al. The influence of perioperative oxygen concentration on postoperative lung function in moderately obese adults. Eur J Anaesthesiol 2010;27(6): 501–7.
[103] Meyhoff CS, Wetterslev J, Jorgensen LN, et al. Effect of high perioperative oxygen fraction on surgical site infection and pulmonary complications after abdominal surgery: the PROXI randomized clinical trial. JAMA 2009;302(14):1543–50.
[104] Goldiner PL, Carlon GC, Cvitkovic E, et al. Factors influencing postoperative morbidity and mortality in patients treated with bleomycin. Br Med J 1978;1(6128):1664–7.
[105] Goldiner PL, Schweizer O. The hazards of anesthesia and surgery in bleomycin-treated patients. Semin Oncol 1979;6(1):121–4.
[106] Hulbert JC, Grossman JE, Cummings KB. Risk factors of anesthesia and surgery in bleomycin-treated patients. J Urol 1983;130(1):163–4.
[107] Aakre BM, Efem RI, Wilson GA, et al. Postoperative acute respiratory distress syndrome in patients with previous exposure to bleomycin. Mayo Clin Proc 2014;89(2):181–9.
[108] Torp KD, Carraway MS, Ott MC, et al. Safe administration of hyperbaric oxygen after bleomycin: a case series of 15 patients. Undersea Hyperb Med 2012;39(5):873–9.
[109] Murphy GS, Szokol JW, Avram MJ, et al. Postoperative residual neuromuscular blockade is associated with impaired clinical recovery. Anesth Analg 2013;117(1):133–41.
[110] Bissinger U, Schimek F, Lenz G. Postoperative residual paralysis and respiratory status: a comparative study of pancuronium and vecuronium. Physiol Res 2000;49(4): 455–62.
[111] Berg H, Roed J, Viby-Mogensen J, et al. Residual neuromuscular block is a risk factor for postoperative pulmonary complications. A prospective, randomised, and blinded study of postoperative pulmonary complications after atracurium, vecuronium and pancuronium. Acta Anaesthesiol Scand 1997;41(9):1095–103.
[112] Plaud B, Debaene B, Donati F, et al. Residual paralysis after emergence from anesthesia. Anesthesiology 2010;112(4):1013–22.
[113] Capron F, Fortier LP, Racine S, et al. Tactile fade detection with hand or wrist stimulation using train-of-four, double-burst stimulation, 50-hertz tetanus, 100-hertz tetanus, and acceleromyography. Anesth Analg 2006;102(5):1578–84.
[114] Moller JT, Jensen PF, Johannessen NW, et al. Hypoxaemia is reduced by pulse oximetry monitoring in the operating theatre and in the recovery room. Br J Anaesth 1992;68(2): 146–50.
[115] Moller JT, Johannessen NW, Espersen K, et al. Randomized evaluation of pulse oximetry in 20,802 patients: II. Perioperative events and postoperative complications. Anesthesiology 1993;78(3):445–53.
[116] Ochroch EA, Russell MW, Hanson WC 3rd, et al. The impact of continuous pulse oximetry monitoring on intensive care unit admissions from a postsurgical care floor. Anesth Analg 2006;102(3):868–75.
[117] Pedersen T, Nicholson A, Hovhannisyan K, et al. Pulse oximetry for perioperative monitoring. Cochrane Database Syst Rev 2014;(3):CD002013.
[118] Forster A, Gardaz JP, Suter PM, et al. I.V. midazolam as an induction agent for anaesthesia: a study in volunteers. Br J Anaesth 1980;52(9):907–11.
[119] Barash PG, editor. Clinical anesthesia. 7th edition. Philadelphia, PA: Lippincott Williams and Wilkins; 2013.
[120] Shehabi Y, Bellomo R, Reade MC, et al. Early intensive care sedation predicts long-term mortality in ventilated critically ill patients. Am J Respir Crit Care Med 2012;186(8): 724–31.
[121] Jakob SM, Ruokonen E, Grounds RM, et al. Dexmedetomidine vs midazolam or propofol for sedation during prolonged mechanical ventilation: two randomized controlled trials. JAMA 2012;307(11):1151–60.
[122] Hofer RE, Sprung J, Sarr MG, et al. Anesthesia for a patient with morbid obesity using dexmedetomidine without narcotics. Can J Anaesth 2005;52(2):176–80.

[123] Institute for Healthcare Improvement. Implement the IHI ventilator bundle. 2014. Available at: http://www.ihi.org/resources/Pages/Changes/ImplementtheVentilatorBundle.aspx. Accessed April 23, 2014.
[124] Drakulovic MB, Torres A, Bauer TT, et al. Supine body position as a risk factor for nosocomial pneumonia in mechanically ventilated patients: a randomised trial. Lancet 1999;354(9193):1851–8.
[125] Kress JP, Pohlman AS, O'Connor MF, et al. Daily interruption of sedative infusions in critically ill patients undergoing mechanical ventilation. N Engl J Med 2000;342(20):1471–7.
[126] Chan EY, Ruest A, Meade MO, et al. Oral decontamination for prevention of pneumonia in mechanically ventilated adults: systematic review and meta-analysis. BMJ 2007;334(7599):889.
[127] Muscedere J, Dodek P, Keenan S, et al. Comprehensive evidence-based clinical practice guidelines for ventilator-associated pneumonia: prevention. J Crit Care 2008;23(1):126–37.
[128] Klompas M. The paradox of ventilator-associated pneumonia prevention measures. Crit Care 2009;13(5):315.
[129] Milledge JS, Nunn JF. Criteria of fitness for anaesthesia in patients with chronic obstructive lung disease. Br Med J 1975;3(5985):670–3.
[130] Saad IA, De Capitani EM, Toro IF, et al. Clinical variables of preoperative risk in thoracic surgery. Sao Paulo Med J 2003;121(3):107–10.
[131] Licker M, Schweizer A, Ellenberger C, et al. Perioperative medical management of patients with COPD. Int J Chron Obstruct Pulmon Dis 2007;2(4):493–515.
[132] Groeben H. Strategies in the patient with compromised respiratory function. Best Pract Res Clin Anaesthesiol 2004;18(4):579–94.
[133] Regan EA, Radcliff TA, Henderson WG, et al. Improving hip fractures outcomes for COPD patients. COPD 2013;10(1):11–9.
[134] van Lier F, van der Geest PJ, Hoeks SE, et al. Epidural analgesia is associated with improved health outcomes of surgical patients with chronic obstructive pulmonary disease. Anesthesiology 2011;115(2):315–21.
[135] Ferrer M, Esquinas A, Arancibia F, et al. Noninvasive ventilation during persistent weaning failure: a randomized controlled trial. Am J Respir Crit Care Med 2003;168(1):70–6.
[136] Memtsoudis SG, Besculides MC, Mazumdar M. A rude awakening–the perioperative sleep apnea epidemic. N Engl J Med 2013;368(25):2352–3.
[137] Finkel KJ, Searleman AC, Tymkew H, et al. Prevalence of undiagnosed obstructive sleep apnea among adult surgical patients in an academic medical center. Sleep Med 2009;10(7):753–8.
[138] Chung F, Yegneswaran B, Liao P, et al. STOP questionnaire: a tool to screen patients for obstructive sleep apnea. Anesthesiology 2008;108(5):812–21.
[139] Flemons WW, Whitelaw WA, Brant R, et al. Likelihood ratios for a sleep apnea clinical prediction rule. Am J Respir Crit Care Med 1994;150(5 Pt 1):1279–85.
[140] Gali B, Whalen FX, Schroeder DR, et al. Identification of patients at risk for postoperative respiratory complications using a preoperative obstructive sleep apnea screening tool and postanesthesia care assessment. Anesthesiology 2009;110(4):869–77.
[141] Gross JB, Bachenberg KL, Benumof JL, et al. Practice guidelines for the perioperative management of patients with obstructive sleep apnea: a report by the American Society of Anesthesiologists Task Force on perioperative management of patients with obstructive sleep apnea. Anesthesiology 2006;104(5):1081–93 [quiz: 1117–8].
[142] Weingarten TN, Flores AS, McKenzie JA, et al. Obstructive sleep apnoea and perioperative complications in bariatric patients. Br J Anaesth 2011;106(1):131–9.
[143] McGlinch BP, Que FG, Nelson JL, et al. Perioperative care of patients undergoing bariatric surgery. Mayo Clin Proc 2006;81(Suppl 10):S25–33.
[144] Connolly LA. Anesthetic management of obstructive sleep apnea patients. J Clin Anesth 1991;3(6):461–9.

[145] Porhomayon J, Nader ND, Leissner KB, et al. Respiratory perioperative management of patients with obstructive sleep apnea. J Intensive Care Med 2014;29:145–53.
[146] Tsiouris A, Hammoud ZT, Velanovich V, et al. A modified frailty index to assess morbidity and mortality after lobectomy. J Surg Res 2013;183(1):40–6.
[147] Warner DO. Preventing postoperative pulmonary complications: the role of the anesthesiologist. Anesthesiology 2000;92(5):1467–72.
[148] Jeon JH, Kang CH, Kim HS, et al. Video-assisted thoracoscopic lobectomy in non-small-cell lung cancer patients with chronic obstructive pulmonary disease is associated with lower pulmonary complications than open lobectomy: a propensity score-matched analysis. Eur J Cardiothorac Surg 2014;45(4):640–5.
[149] Briez N, Piessen G, Torres F, et al. Effects of hybrid minimally invasive oesophagectomy on major postoperative pulmonary complications. Br J Surg 2012;99(11):1547–53.
[150] Scarci M, Joshi A, Attia R. In patients undergoing thoracic surgery is paravertebral block as effective as epidural analgesia for pain management? Interact Cardiovasc Thorac Surg 2010;10(1):92–6.
[151] Joshi GP, Bonnet F, Shah R, et al. A systematic review of randomized trials evaluating regional techniques for postthoracotomy analgesia. Anesth Analg 2008;107(3): 1026–40.
[152] Carvalho EM, Gabriel EA, Salerno TA. Pulmonary protection during cardiac surgery: systematic literature review. Asian Cardiovasc Thorac Ann 2008;16(6):503–7.
[153] Redmond JM, Gillinov AM, Stuart RS, et al. Heparin-coated bypass circuits reduce pulmonary injury. Ann Thorac Surg 1993;56(3):474–8 [discussion: 479].
[154] Nagashima M, Shin'oka T, Nollert G, et al. High-volume continuous hemofiltration during cardiopulmonary bypass attenuates pulmonary dysfunction in neonatal lambs after deep hypothermic circulatory arrest. Circulation 1998;98(Suppl 19):II378–84.
[155] Richter JA, Meisner H, Tassani P, et al. Drew-Anderson technique attenuates systemic inflammatory response syndrome and improves respiratory function after coronary artery bypass grafting. Ann Thorac Surg 2000;69(1):77–83.
[156] Zarbock A, Mueller E, Netzer S, et al. Prophylactic nasal continuous positive airway pressure following cardiac surgery protects from postoperative pulmonary complications: a prospective, randomized, controlled trial in 500 patients. Chest 2009;135(5): 1252–9.
[157] Engoren MC, Kraras C, Garzia F. Propofol-based versus fentanyl-isoflurane-based anesthesia for cardiac surgery. J Cardiothorac Vasc Anesth 1998;12(2):177–81.
[158] Silbert BS, Santamaria JD, O'Brien JL, et al. Early extubation following coronary artery bypass surgery: a prospective randomized controlled trial. The Fast Track Cardiac Care Team. Chest 1998;113(6):1481–8.
[159] Zhu F, Lee A, Chee YE. Fast-track cardiac care for adult cardiac surgical patients. Cochrane Database Syst Rev 2012;(10):CD003587.
[160] Papazian L, Forel JM, Gacouin A, et al. Neuromuscular blockers in early acute respiratory distress syndrome. N Engl J Med 2010;363(12):1107–16.
[161] Shekar K, Davies AR, Mullany DV, et al. To ventilate, oscillate, or cannulate? J Crit Care 2013;28(5):655–62.
[162] Guerin C, Reignier J, Richard JC, et al. Prone positioning in severe acute respiratory distress syndrome. N Engl J Med 2013;368(23):2159–68.
[163] Peek GJ, Mugford M, Tiruvoipati R, et al. Efficacy and economic assessment of conventional ventilatory support versus extracorporeal membrane oxygenation for severe adult respiratory failure (CESAR): a multicentre randomised controlled trial. Lancet 2009;374(9698):1351–63.
[164] Ferguson ND, Cook DJ, Guyatt GH, et al. High-frequency oscillation in early acute respiratory distress syndrome. N Engl J Med 2013;368(9):795–805.
[165] Taylor RW, Zimmerman JL, Dellinger RP, et al. Low-dose inhaled nitric oxide in patients with acute lung injury: a randomized controlled trial. JAMA 2004;291(13):1603–9.

[166] Ramakrishna G, Sprung J, Ravi BS, et al. Impact of pulmonary hypertension on the outcomes of noncardiac surgery: predictors of perioperative morbidity and mortality. J Am Coll Cardiol 2005;45(10):1691–9.
[167] Joo HS, Wong J, Naik VN, et al. The value of screening preoperative chest x-rays: a systematic review. Can J Anaesth 2005;52(6):568–74.
[168] Qaseem A, Snow V, Fitterman N, et al. Risk assessment for and strategies to reduce perioperative pulmonary complications for patients undergoing noncardiothoracic surgery: a guideline from the American College of Physicians. Ann Intern Med 2006;144(8):575–80.
[169] O'Keeffe T, Patterson EJ. Evidence supporting routine polysomnography before bariatric surgery. Obes Surg 2004;14(1):23–6.
[170] Lawrence VA, Page CP, Harris GD. Preoperative spirometry before abdominal operations. A critical appraisal of its predictive value. Arch Intern Med 1989;149(2):280–5.
[171] Ferguson MK, Watson S, Johnson E, et al. Predicted postoperative lung function is associated with all-cause long-term mortality after major lung resection for cancer. Eur J Cardiothorac Surg 2014;45(4):660–4.
[172] Slinger PD, Johnston MR. Preoperative assessment: an anesthesiologist's perspective. Thorac Surg Clin 2005;15(1):11–25.
[173] Brunelli A, Kim AW, Berger KI, et al. Physiologic evaluation of the patient with lung cancer being considered for resectional surgery: diagnosis and management of lung cancer, 3rd ed: American College of Chest Physicians evidence-based clinical practice guidelines. Chest 2013;143(Suppl 5):e166S–90S.
[174] Larsen KR, Svendsen UG, Milman N, et al. Cardiopulmonary function at rest and during exercise after resection for bronchial carcinoma. Ann Thorac Surg 1997;64(4):960–4.
[175] Cerfolio RJ, Allen MS, Trastek VF, et al. Lung resection in patients with compromised pulmonary function. Ann Thorac Surg 1996;62(2):348–51.

Advances in Anesthesia 32 (2014) 119–131

ELSEVIER MOSBY

ADVANCES IN ANESTHESIA

Perioperative Frailty

Definitions, Evaluation, Implications for Management, Impact on Outcomes After Anesthesia

Sheila Ryan Barnett, MD

Department of Anesthesiology, Beth Israel Deaconess of Medical Center, Harvard Medical School, 330 Brookline Avenue, Boston, MA 02215, USA

Keywords

• Frailty • Perioperative • Anesthesia • Outcomes

Key points

- Frailty is an important syndrome in the geriatric population.
- The occurrence of frailty has important prognostic implications, for patients in general and in particular at the time of surgery.
- Anesthesiologists should be able to recognize and diagnose frailty in older patients and understand the implications for outcomes.
- Measuring frailty may contribute to decision-making capability for patients and their families, as well as anesthesiologists and surgeons.
- Future research should be directed toward strategies to reverse frailty and reduce complications and readmissions in frail patients undergoing surgery.

INTRODUCTION

Advanced age is not considered a contraindication to surgery, and the elderly represent a significant proportion of the patients undergoing surgical and invasive procedures. In the United States more than 40% of surgery is performed in patients more than 65 years of age. As the volume of geriatric patients continues to grow, so does the understanding that older patients represent a special population for anesthesiologists, carrying inherently high risks from complications and even mortality. A major challenge encountered when caring for older patients is evaluating physiologic versus chronologic age, and estimating the consequences of aging and morbidity on a patient's functional reserve. It has recently been recognized that frailty is an important and increasingly common condition in the geriatric population that predisposes patients to adverse outcomes following anesthesia and surgery [1–6].

E-mail address: sbarnett@bidmc.harvard.edu

0737-6146/14/$ – see front matter
http://dx.doi.org/10.1016/j.aan.2014.08.012

WHY STUDY FRAILTY?

It is well known that, as people age, organ function declines and patients' reserve functions are diminished. In addition, common comorbidities such as hypertension, diabetes, coronary disease, and pulmonary disease are all more common in older patients and further reduce an elderly person's reserve function. However, the impact of aging or age-related diseases can vary considerably and the older population is by nature heterogeneous. Frailty is now a well-accepted concept that seems to provide a global assessment of the combined impact of aging and comorbidity on reserve function.

The preoperative identification of frailty ideally leads to strategies to reverse the frailty or improve baseline functional reserve [7–9]. Although the time available before surgery may often preclude the implementation of any preemptive measures, there may be circumstances in which early identification of frailty could affect decision making or lead to strategies to improve outcomes. It is known that exercise programs in very old patients may lead to improvements in several domains including strength, cognitive well-being, and balance. Physical activity programs may also lead to reduction in inflammatory activation, production of free radical scavengers, metabolic modulation, and improvement of insulin resistance [10]. Both muscle weakness and poor nutrition are hallmarks of frailty and low albumin has been associated with negative perioperative outcomes [11–14]. However, the data on preoperative nutrition in frail patients are still insufficient, likely in part because of the often limited period of time available before scheduled surgery in frail patients.

DEFINING FRAILTY

Frailty is a state of reduced physiologic reserve and consequent increased vulnerability from challenges that threaten homeostatic balance [11,12,15]. Frailty is not a disease state in and of itself, but instead represents a constellation of symptoms or conditions that lead to a recognizable decline in physical and cognitive function and general endurance [1,2,14,16]. Frailty is associated with an increased risk of adverse events such as falls, delirium and general morbidity. In the surgical domain, frailty has been increasingly recognized as an important geriatric syndrome that is associated with increased risk of complications, length of stay, discharge disposition and mortality [8,16–19].

The prevalence of frailty is not fully known, but for community-dwelling elders it is estimated at 3%–7% for 65–75 years, 20%–26% for 80–90 years and around 33% for people more than 90 years [20,21]. Frailty is especially prevalent in patients with cardiovascular disease, and the presence of frailty is becoming recognized as an important variable when considering appropriate treatment strategies for cardiovascular patients [22–25].

PATHOPHYSIOLOGY

The causes leading to the development of frailty are not fully understood. During 'normal' aging, gradual cell and molecular damage occur through multiple mechanisms. At some point the overall effect/affect of age-related damage is enough to negatively influence organ function, ultimately reducing reserve function in the older patient. In frail patients the rate and extent of decline is accelerated and the accumulation of deficits in multiple organs systems lead more rapidly to a global decline in function [11,15,26,27]. There is increasing evidence that the pathophysiology of frailty involves an interconnection between inflammatory changes and alterations in endocrine and immune modulation [28]. Inflammatory markers such as C-reactive protein and interleukin-6 (IL6), and immune alterations characterized by higher neutrophil and monocyte cell counts, have been found in frail elderly populations. Endocrine abnormalities, including insulin resistance, and declines in IGF-1 and testosterone have also been identified in frail populations [29]. The role of vitamin D deficiency is not clear, although increasing evidence supports an association with low vitamin D and decreased muscle mass and strength in elderly patients, both hallmarks of frailty. It is not known what the role of extrinsic factors such as smoking, and low physical activity play in the development of frailty [13,29].

Part of the difficulty in defining the pathophysiology of frailty is the lack of specific markers and symptoms associated with frailty. An increase in inflammatory markers and many of the mediators associated with frailty are also found in other conditions, including normal senescence, cancer, and Alzheimer's type dementia (Box 1) [11,12,22].

IDENTIFYING FRAILTY

There is no single test or tool that can be used to diagnose frailty, instead there are multiple scales and tools available [14,30,31]. Amongst accepted scales, the

Box 1: Nonspecific biomarkers associated with frailty

C-reactive protein
Interleukin-6
Tumor necrosis factor alpha
Neutrophil count
D-dimer
Plasminogen activator inhibitor-1
Testosterone
Insulinlike growth factor-1
Albumin
Vitamin D
Lymphocyte count
Memory/naive CD8 T-cell ratio

Data from Afilalo J, Alexander KP, Mack MJ, et al. Frailty assessment in the cardiovascular care of older adults. J Am Coll Cardiol 2014;63(8):747–62.

thresholds for identifying frailty may differ depending on the population [1,3]. Screening tools may be quite broad, as opposed to more specific scales used to measure a treatment effect following intervention. Despite the multitude of scales, there are 2 main approaches commonly used to define frailty. These are the clinical phenotype method and the accumulation deficit model; each approach has advantages and disadvantages [32,33].

Clinical phenotype

Fried and colleagues [32] first established the 'phenotype' of frailty, using data from more than 5000 patients in the Cardiovascular Health Study in 2001 (Box 2). The 5 variables associated with the frailty phenotype are:

1. Unintentional weight loss greater than 4.5 kg (10 lb) in prior year
2. Symptoms of exhaustion
3. Low physical activity
4. Poor handgrip strength
5. Slow walking speed

Patients are assigned a frailty score of 0–5 based on the presence or absence of symptoms of weight loss or exhaustion, a description of their activity, or a predetermined cut off for the hand grip or walking speed. These variables are weighted equally, and each 1 is equal to 1 point. Patients with a score of zero are considered robust or nonfrail, those with 1 or 2 points out of the possible 5 are considered 'prefrail'. Patients who have total score of 3, 4 or 5 of the factors are considered frail. Although easy to use, this model has been criticized as it relies heavily on the identification of a decline in muscle mass (sarcopenia) as the central feature of frailty, and excludes any inclusion of cognitive assessment or mood. Other tests that rely on a physical assessment include gait speed and handgrip measurements [31,34,35].

Deficit accumulation

The frailty index (FI) was initially created using data from the Canadian Study of Health and Aging (CSHA), a 5-year prospective cohort study including 10,263 patients (Box 3). Ninety 2 patient variables were identified that included a variety of symptoms, abnormal laboratory values, comorbidities, and a

Box 2: Fried frailty phenotype

1. Unintentional weight loss greater than 4.5 kg (10 lb) in prior year
2. Self-reported exhaustion or lack of energy
3. Diminished grip strength adjusted for sex and size
4. Low physical activity
5. Slow walking speed

From Fried LP, Tangen CM, Walston J, et al. Frailty in older adults: evidence for a phenotype. J Gerontol A Biol Sci Med Sci 2001;56:M146–56; with permission.

Box 3: Modified Canadian Frailty Index: accumulation deficit model

1. Diabetes mellitus
2. Chronic obstructive pulmonary disease
3. Congestive heart failure
4. Myocardial infarction
5. Hypertension treated with medication
6. Angina or prior coronary intervention including stent or coronary artery bypass grafting
7. Peripheral vascular disease
8. Impaired sensorium
9. Prior transient ischemic attack or stroke without residual deficit
10. Cerebrovascular accident with residual symptoms
11. Dependent function status

disability assessment. The FI is the number of variables identified, divided by the total possible (92 for the original test) [1,6,19,30,36]. The higher the score (reflecting more deficits) the more likely it is that a patient is frail. Because the development of the original model using 92 deficits, several modified FIs have been described, including only 70, 30, or even 11 variables. These modified frailty scales are much simpler to calculate and probably have greater utility in clinical practice. Because the accumulation deficit model (and variants) does not require a physical examination of the patient, this approach has also gained popularity for research, using data extraction from medical records. In the USA, the National Surgical Quality Improvement Program (NSQIP) collects data from surgical patients in more than 450 hospitals. NSQIP data were compared with the CSHA data and 11 preoperative variables were identified common to both programs. These 11 variables were incorporated into a modified FI (mFI) and, when applied to NSQIP data, a positive correlation between frailty and morbidity and mortality following surgery has been found [37–41].

There are other simple 'bedside' tests that can be used to assess the functional capacity of elderly patients before surgery, many of these are regularly used by geriatricians but rarely by anesthesiologists. Examples include the timed get up and go, grip strength and overall walking speed [31,42]. A simple history of falls is also an important marker of possible deterioration in independence that has been associated with increased complications following surgery. These tests may be important additions to the anesthesia preoperative evaluation especially when there are lingering questions regarding recovery options or choice of surgery [36].

THE ROLE OF THE COMPREHENSIVE GERIATRIC ASSESSMENT

As described earlier, there are multiple scales used to identify frailty, but these may only represent a limited evaluation of a patient's total functional capacity and health. The Comprehensive Geriatric Assessment (CGA) is a multidimensional evaluation process covering several distinct domains of an older person's health, and can provide a measure of frailty [23,24,40]. The CGA generally involves a team-based evaluation including an in-depth assessment of medical, cognitive, psychological, and functional status. A major goal of the CGA is to identify treatable aspects of health issues. The CGA seems to be particularly valuable for the assessment of life expectancy and survival. The CGA was not developed as a preoperative screening tool, although recently it has been used in the presurgical setting with mixed success.

The CGA provides an extensive evaluation of an older patient; the components may vary depending on the providers, institutions, and the situation. In one of its most complete forms, the CGA includes an evaluation in as many as 11 distinct domains, and involving several types of caregivers, including physicians, physical therapists, and social workers. The types of assessment areas range from screening for dementia and delirium to an assessment of sensory perception (hearing and vision). An essential part of all CGAs is an evaluation of mobility and independence. As stated earlier, the timed get-up-and-go test is a validated tool used to assess mobility and fall risk. The patient is asked to sit in a chair, walk a distance, make a full turn, and return to the chair. Although simple, this test requires strength and balance to execute without falling or requiring extra assistance. An assessment of the patient's independence includes an assessment of the activities of daily living (ADLs) using, for example, the Barthel index of ADLs, which includes questions about bladder and bowel continence, feeding, dressing, and the ability to go up and down stairs independently. In addition, the CGA may include an evaluation of the caregiver burden, detailing the support available and required by the patient on a regular basis.

In older patients who have cancer, studies have found that the CGA adds predictive power for morbidity and mortality associated with not only the cancer but also the treatment. These studies suggest that the CGA may have particular value for planning cancer treatments in patients who may be facing a complex course of treatments. However, when applied to the surgical setting, the value-added nature of the CGA has been variable. In one small study, Suh and colleagues [43] studied 60 patients undergoing elective surgery for gynecologic cancer who underwent extensive preoperative evaluations using the CGA. They then compared the utility of the complete CGA and all its components with a simple performance status assessment and instrumental ADLs. The complexity of the surgery predicted the occurrence of major and minor complications and the performance status assessment was useful at identifying patients at risk of any complication, in contrast with the CGA, which was not valuable in predicting complications. In contrast, Kim and colleagues [44] performed CGA in 140 patients undergoing surgery. The cumulative impairment identified within the CGA was independently associated with adverse surgical outcomes in elderly patients.

In a study of elderly patients presenting for laparoscopic cholecystectomy, Lasithiotakis and colleagues [37] divided patients into fit or frail groups using a CGA. The CGA comprised a comprehensive assessment including functional assessment tools of independence, an assessment of comorbidity using the Charlson comorbidity index, a nutritional appraisal and a cognitive screen using the mini–mental state examination. If patients had any criteria that were frail they were considered frail; to be considered fit they had to meet all the predefined criteria. The main outcome examined was the occurrence of postoperative complications within 30 days. Fifty-seven patients completed the preoperative CGA, and of these 56% were considered frail versus 44% who were fit. Postoperative complications, including length of stay, were significantly higher in frail patients than in fit patients: 85% versus 15%, respectively ($P < .022$). This study supports the theory that frail patients have more complications and potentially longer lengths of stay and therefore greater costs. Other studies have also shown that identifying frailty, using an individual test or the CGA approach, can provide an improved estimate of risk compared with a patient's age or the American Society of Anesthesiology (ASA) classification alone [16,19,38,45].

STRENGTH AND GAIT SPEED

The phenotype frailty evaluation and the CGA may both include a test of gait speed and mobility. For the Fried phenotype, a slow gait speed is the strongest predictor of chronic disability and institutionalization. In community-dwelling elders, slow gait speed is also associated with greater risk of cognitive impairment and disability. Although a valuable marker, gait speed is nonspecific and multiple disorders can contribute to a slow gait speed [31,34,42]. In most studies the time to walk 5 m on a flat surface is measured. Hand grip, another strength-related marker, also has good predictive value on outcomes [35].

SARCOPENIA

Normal aging is associated with a decrease in skeletal muscle quality and mass, and with associated strength and function. This condition is known as sarcopenia, which can be primary or secondary. Primary sarcopenia seems to be associated with age-related inactivity, and is associated with weakening and impaired function; secondary sarcopenia is more active and is associated with alterations in metabolism, referred to as cachexia. After the seventh decade of life, the rate of loss of function versus muscle mass is accelerated, which has important implications for mobility and functional independence [1,4,12]. In addition, the length of time to recovery of muscle function is impaired in older patients, and even a few days of bed rest or immobility can lead to a significant loss of muscle function [46,47]. Sarcopenia is an important feature of frailty and a predictor of mortality and complications after surgery. Although classic sarcopenia and frailty are characterized by weight loss and a low body mass index (BMI), sarcopenic obesity has also recently been recognized in older obese patients with high BMI but low muscle mass.

CARDIOVASCULAR DISEASE AND FRAILTY

General increases of inflammatory biomarkers such as interleukin-6, C-reactive protein, and various cytokines, and other alterations in immune modulation contribute to the development of atherosclerosis and damage to the cardiovascular system [22]. The frailty condition shares many of these markers, and subclinical cardiovascular disease (CVD) is commonly found in frail patients [48,49]. Frailty is becoming an increasingly important consideration in cardiovascular patients, affecting prognosis and treatment choices [27,40,45,48]. Estimates suggest that frailty occurs in 25% to 50% of patients with CVD. Khan and colleagues [21] found that in community-dwelling elders, moderate to severe frailty was associated with a greater than 30% risk of developing clinical heart failure. The underlying risk and association of CVD and frailty is important to the preoperative risk for patients undergoing anesthesia and surgery, especially in patients with congestive heart failure [12,22,45,49–51].

PREOPERATIVE IDENTIFICATION OF VULNERABLE PATIENTS

As described earlier, frailty is associated with increased complications following surgery, and preoperative identification of the frail patient ideally leads to effective preventative interventions. Using the mFI to assess the degree of frailty present in patients undergoing laparoscopic colorectal surgery, Keller and colleagues [39] found that higher frailty score was associated with longer length of stay, and that patients with a 0 score on the frailty assessment were discharged the earliest. The modified Hopkins Score criteria include a measure of shrinking or weight loss, decreased grip strength, exhaustion, low activity, and slow walking speed. The advantage of the modified frailty score described by Keller is the simplicity to perform, requiring little or no additional expense. The Hopkins Score alone is a robust predictor of postoperative complications. Adding other predictors of postoperative complications such as albumin, C-reactive protein, the glomerular filtration rate alone, and classic ADLs did not improve the predictive power of the mFI. At present there is little to do to reverse frailty before surgery, but this study and others like it suggest that a frailty assessment before surgery can predict who will need additional resources after surgery and which are the most vulnerable populations [19,38].

Robinson and colleagues [6] studied the incidence of postoperative complications in elderly patients after colorectal and cardiovascular surgery. They used an array of 7 different frailty tests and categorized patients as nonfrail, prefrail, and frail (Box 4). For colorectal patients, complications occurred in 21% of the nonfrail, 40% of the prefrail, and 58% of the frail groups ($P = .016$). The incidence of complications in patients having cardiac surgery was 17% for nonfrail versus 56% in frail patients ($P < .001$). Lengths of stay were longer and readmissions were more common in frail patients in both surgical types.

ANESTHESIA AND THE FRAIL PATIENT

There is no single approach to frail geriatric patients; instead meticulous care of elderly patients is important. Frail patients are patients with limited physiologic

Box 4: Frailty tests

1. Timed Up and Go Normal less than 15 seconds. This test is a measure of the time in seconds from sitting and rising from a chair to a standing position and walking 3 m (10 feet) on a flat surface, returning to the chair, and sitting again.
2. Independence of activities by the Katz Score. ADLs: bathing, feeding, dressing, transferring, walking, and toileting. Abnormal score defined as dependence of 1 or more activity.
3. Cognition test using the Mini-Cog test, which includes the 3-paired item recall and clock drawing.
4. Comorbidity assessment using the Charlson Index. This index measures burden of disease using 19 categories of comorbidity.
5. Chronic disease anemia, defined as hematocrit level of less than 35%.
6. A low albumin of less than 3.4 g/dL, which is a measure of nutrition.
7. History of 1 or more falls in the last 6 months.

Patients are grouped by number of positive characteristics: 0–1, nonfrail; 2–3 positives, prefrail; 4–7 abnormalities, frail.

From Robinson TN, Wu DS, Pointer L, et al. Simple frailty score predicts postoperative complications across surgical specialties. Am J Surg 2013;206:544–50; with permission.

reserve, who are thus vulnerable to even the slightest insult; for example, through hypotension or hypovolemia. Frail patients undergoing surgery and anesthesia carry an increased risk from complications and poor outcomes, including delirium. The contribution of the intraoperative anesthetic to these adverse outcomes is not well understood. In adults, deep anesthesia, defined using the bispectral index (BIS), has been associated with increased mortality in patients, especially those with low blood pressure and hematocrit. From these studies it is unclear whether the low BIS in these patients was a marker of overall poor preoperative status or a reflection of the impact of anesthetic agents on the brain [52]. Several studies have recently assessed the relationship between the depth of anesthesia and the risk of developing cognitive dysfunction following surgery. Siebert and colleagues [53] randomized elderly patients having hip fracture repair under spinal anesthesia to 2 different levels of sedation. Both groups received sedation with propofol and/or midazolam. The incidence of delirium was 50% less in the light sedation group, in which a BIS greater than 50 was maintained, versus the deep sedation group, which had BIS less than 50. On follow-up the 1-year mortality was 50% higher in patients with multiple comorbidities in the deep sedation group versus the light sedation group [51]. In a series of other studies of general anesthesia with anesthetic gases, patients who are maintained with higher BIS levels (45 or more) have a faster emergence and less likelihood of short-term delirium or longer-term postoperative cognitive dysfunction. These studies have not been directed at frail patients but, given the known increased risk of delirium and the reduction in reserve function, it is intuitive that these

Box 5: Elements of prehabilitation programs

1. Walking 15 to 20 minutes 3 times per week
2. Strength exercises: upper arm and shoulder; lower limbs including hamstring curls, ankle pronation
3. Abdominal breathing exercises

Data from Lee DH, Buth KJ, Martin BJ, et al. Frail patients are at increased risk for mortality and prolonged institutional care after cardiac surgery. Circulation 2010;121:973–8; and Kortebein P, Ferrando A, Lombeida J, et al. Effect of 10 days of bed rest on skeletal muscle in healthy older adults. JAMA 2007;297:1772–4.

patients will require less anesthesia. It is well known that the minimum alveolar concentration (MAC) of anesthesia is less in older patients, and these studies suggest there are advantages to monitoring the depth of anesthesia in very old and frail patients.

PREHABILITATION AND ENHANCED RECOVERY AFTER SURGERY PROGRAMS

Physical deconditioning (ie, a history of early exhaustion, diminished grip strength, weight loss, and generalized poor nutrition) is central in the identification of frail patients. Frail patients, especially those with sarcopenia, are at high risk of rapid deconditioning after any period of immobility [6]. Prehabilitation refers to a concentrated exercise program for patients before surgery, in contrast with the traditional rehabilitative physiotherapy and interventions offered after surgery (Box 5). It is known that resistance training in older frail community patients can lead to improvements in physical function [54,55]. This approach has also been tried in frail orthopedic patients. Some studies have shown benefit for patients undergoing elective knee surgery who underwent strength and endurance training for several weeks before elective surgery [56]. However, the feasibility and cost of prehabilitation for general surgery patients have yet to be established. It might be that, in selected surgeries, a period of prehabilitation can improve functional outcomes. ERAS refers to the enhanced recovery after surgery [6,41,57] programs. These clinical pathways guide preoperative and postsurgical care of patients, and improved outcomes have been shown for surgeries such as joint replacement, although most are not specific to frail patients [10].

SUMMARY

Frailty is an important syndrome in the geriatric population. The occurrence of frailty has important prognostic implications for patients in general and in particular at the time of surgery. Anesthesiologists should be able to recognize and diagnose frailty in older patients and understand the implications for outcomes. Measuring frailty may contribute to decision-making capability for patients and their families, as well as anesthesiologists and surgeons. Future research should be directed toward strategies to reverse frailty and reduce complications and readmissions in frail patients undergoing surgery.

References

[1] Hubbard RE, Story DA. Patient frailty: the elephant in the operating room. Anaesthesia 2014;69(Suppl 1):26–34.
[2] Amrock LG, Deiner S. The implication of frailty on preoperative risk assessment. Curr Opin Anaesthesiol 2014;27:330–5.
[3] Partridge JS, Harari D, Dhesi JK. Frailty in the older surgical patient: a review. Age Ageing 2012;41(2):142–7.
[4] Joseph B, Pandit V, Sadoun M, et al. Frailty in surgery. J Trauma Acute Care Surg 2014;76(4):1151–6.
[5] Peden CJ, Grocot MP. National Research Strategies: what outcomes are important in peri-operative elderly care? Anaesthesia 2014;69(Suppl 1):61–9.
[6] Robinson TN, Wu DS, Pointer L, et al. Simple frailty score predicts postoperative complications across surgical specialties. Am J Surg 2013;206:544–50.
[7] Robinson TN, Eiseman B, Wallace JI, et al. Redefining geriatric preoperative assessment using frailty, disability and co-morbidity. Ann Surg 2009;250:449–55.
[8] Bakker FC, Robben SH, Olde Rikkert MG. Effects of hospital-wide interventions to improve care for frail older inpatients: a systematic review. BMJ Qual Saf 2011;20:680–91.
[9] Chin A, Paw MJ, Dekker JM, et al. How to select a frail elderly population? A comparison of three working definitions. J Clin Epidemiol 1999;52:1015.
[10] Carli F, Brown R, Kennepohl S. Prehabilitation to enhance postoperative recovery for an octogenarian following robotic-assisted hysterectomy with endometrial cancer. Can J Anaesth 2012;59:779–84.
[11] Fedarko NS. The biology of aging and frailty. Clin Geriatr Med 2011;27:27–37.
[12] Fulop T, Larbi A, Witkowski JM, et al. Aging, frailty and age-related diseases. Biogerontology 2010;11:547–63.
[13] Walston J, McBurnie MA, Newman A, et al. Frailty and activation of the inflammation and coagulation systems with and without clinical comorbidities: results from the Cardiovascular Health Study. Arch Intern Med 2002;162:2333–41.
[14] Abellan van Kan G, Rolland Y, Bergman H, et al. The I.A.N.A task force on frailty assessment of older people in clinical practice. J Nutr Health Aging 2008;12:29–37.
[15] Bergman H, Ferrucci L, Guralnik J, et al. Frailty: an emerging research and clinical paradigm–issues and controversies. J Gerontol A Biol Sci Med Sci 2007;62:731–7.
[16] Shamliyan T, Talley KM, Ramakrishnan R, et al. Association of frailty with survival: a systematic literature review. Ageing Res Rev 2012;12:719–36.
[17] Chikwe J, Adams DH. Frailty: the missing element in predicting operative mortality. Semin Thorac Cardiovasc Surg 2010;22:109–10.
[18] Fried LP, Ferrucci L, Darer J, et al. Untangling the concepts of disability, frailty, and comorbidity: implications for improved targeting and care. J Gerontol A Biol Sci Med Sci 2004;59:255–63.
[19] Revenig LM, Canter DJ, Taylor MD, et al. Too frail for surgery? Initial results of a large multidisciplinary prospective study examining preoperative variables predictive of poor surgical outcomes. J Am Coll Surg 2013;217:665–70.
[20] Collard RM, Boter H, Schoevers RA, et al. Prevalence of frailty in community-dwelling older persons: a systematic review. J Am Geriatr Soc 2012;60:1487–92.
[21] Khan H, Kalogeropoulos AP, Georgiopoulou VV, et al. Frailty and risk for heart failure in older adults: the Health, Aging, and Body Composition Study. Am Heart J 2013;166:887–94.
[22] Afilalo J, Alexander KP, Mack MJ, et al. Frailty assessment in the cardiovascular care of older adults. J Am Coll Cardiol 2014;63(8):747–62.

[23] Sündermann S, Dademasch A, Praetorius J, et al. Comprehensive assessment of frailty for elderly high-risk patients undergoing cardiac surgery. Eur J Cardiothorac Surg 2011;39:33–7.
[24] Sündermann S, Dademasch A, Rastan A, et al. One-year follow-up of patients undergoing elective cardiac surgery assessed with the comprehensive assessment of frailty test and its simplified form. Interact Cardiovasc Thorac Surg 2011;13:119–23.
[25] Stortecky S, Schoenenberger AW, Moser A, et al. Evaluation of multidimensional geriatric assessment as a predictor of mortality and cardiovascular events after transcatheter aortic valve implantation. JACC Cardiovasc Interv 2012;5:489–96.
[26] Klein BE, Klein R, Knudtson MD, et al. Frailty, morbidity and survival. Arch Gerontol Geriatr 2005;41:141–9.
[27] Woods NF, Lacroix AZ, Gray SL, et al. Frailty: emergence and consequences in women aged 65 and older in the Women's Health Initiative Observational Study. J Am Geriatr Soc 2005;53:1321–30.
[28] Baylis D, Bartlett DB, Syddall HE, et al. Immune-endocrine bio-markers as predictors of frailty and mortality: a 10-year longitudinal study in community-dwelling older people. Age (Dordr) 2013;35:963–71.
[29] Barzilay JI, Blaum C, Moore T, et al. Insulin resistance and inflammation as precursors of frailty: the cardiovascular health study. Arch Intern Med 2007;167:635–41.
[30] Rockwood K, Mitnitski A. Frailty defined by deficit accumulation and geriatric medicine defined by frailty. Clin Geriatr Med 2011;27:17–26.
[31] Volpato S, Cavalieri M, Sioulis F, et al. Predictive value of the short physical performance battery following hospitalization in older patients. J Gerontol A Biol Sci Med Sci 2011;66: 89–96.
[32] Fried LP, Tangen CM, Walston J, et al. Frailty in older adults: evidence for a phenotype. J Gerontol A Biol Sci Med Sci 2001;56:M146–56.
[33] Bandeen-Roche K, Xue QL, Ferrucci L, et al. Phenotype of frailty: characterization in the women's health and aging studies. J Gerontol A Biol Sci Med Sci 2006;61:262–6.
[34] Guralnik JM, Simonsick EM, Ferrucci L, et al. A short physical performance battery assessing lower extremity function: association with self-reported disability and prediction of mortality and nursing home admission. J Gerontol 1994;49:M85–94.
[35] Ling CH, Taekema D, de Craen AJ, et al. Handgrip strength and mortality in the oldest old population: the Leiden 85-Plus study. CMAJ 2010;182:429–35.
[36] de Vries NM, Staal JB, van Ravensberg CD, et al. Outcome instruments to measure frailty: a systematic review. Ageing Res Rev 2011;10:104–14.
[37] Lasithiotakis K, Petrakis J, Venianaki M, et al. Frailty predicts outcome of elective laparoscopic cholecystectomy in geriatric patients. Surg Endosc 2013;27(4):1144–50.
[38] Adams P, Ghanem T, Stachler R, et al. Frailty as a predictor of morbidity and mortality in inpatient head and neck surgery. JAMA Otolaryngol Head Neck Surg 2013;139(8): 783–9.
[39] Keller DS, Bankwitz B, Nobel T, et al. Using frailty to predict who will fail early discharge after laparoscopic colorectal surgery with an established recovery pathway. Dis Colon Rectum 2014;57:337–42.
[40] Afilalo J, Karunananthan S, Eisenberg MJ, et al. Role of frailty in patients with cardiovascular disease. Am J Cardiol 2009;103:1616–21.
[41] Perera S, Mody SH, Woodman RC, et al. Meaningful change and responsiveness in common physical performance measures in older adults. J Am Geriatr Soc 2006;54:743–9.
[42] Afilalo J, Eisenberg MJ, Morin JF, et al. Gait speed as an incremental predictor of mortality and major morbidity in elderly patients undergoing cardiac surgery. J Am Coll Cardiol 2010;56:1668–76.
[43] Suh DH, Kim JW, Kim SH, et al. Pre-and intra-operative variables associated with surgical complications in elderly patients with gynecologic cancer: the clinical value of comprehensive geriatric assessment. J Geriatr Oncol 2014;5(3):315–22.

[44] Kim K, Park KH, Koo KH, et al. Comprehensive geriatric assessment can predict postoperative morbidity and mortality in elderly patients undergoing elective surgery. Arch Gerontol Geriatr 2013;56:507–12.
[45] Lee DH, Buth KJ, Martin BJ, et al. Frail patients are at increased risk for mortality and prolonged institutional care after cardiac surgery. Circulation 2010;121:973–8.
[46] Kortebein P, Ferrando A, Lombeida J, et al. Effect of 10 days of bed rest on skeletal muscle in healthy older adults. JAMA 2007;297:1772–4.
[47] Wall BT, Dirks ML, van Loon LJ. Skeletal muscle atrophy during short-term disuse: implications for age-related sarcopenia. Ageing Res Rev 2013;12:898–906.
[48] Newman AB, Gottdiener JS, Mcburnie MA, et al. Associations of subclinical cardiovascular disease with frailty. J Gerontol A Biol Sci Med Sci 2001;56:M158–66.
[49] Cacciatore F, Abete P, Mazzella F, et al. Frailty predicts long-term mortality in elderly subjects with chronic heart failure. Eur J Clin Invest 2005;35:723–30.
[50] Rozzini R, Sabatini T, Frisoni GB, et al. Frailty is a strong modulator of heart failure-associated mortality. Arch Intern Med 2003;163:737–8.
[51] Radtke FM, Franck M, Lendner JL, et al. Monitoring depth of anaesthesia in a randomized trial decreases the rate of postoperative delirium but not postoperative cognitive dysfunction. Br J Anaesth 2013;110(S1):i98–105.
[52] Sieber Fe, Zakriya KJ, Gottschalk A, et al. Sedation depth during spinal anesthesia and the development of postoperative delirium in elderly patients undergoing hip fracture repair. Mayo Clin Proc 2010;85:18–26.
[53] Brown CH, Azman AS, Gottschalk A, et al. Sedation depth during spinal anesthesia and survival in elderly patient undergoing hip fracture repair. Anesth Analg 2014;118:977–80.
[54] Latham NK, Bennett DA, Stretton CM, et al. Systematic review of progressive resistance strength training in older adults. J Gerontol A Biol Sci Med Sci 2004;59:48–61.
[55] Gill TM, Baker DI, Gottschalk M, et al. A program to prevent functional decline in physically frail, elderly persons who live at home. N Engl J Med 2002;347:1068–74.
[56] Huang SW, Chen PH, Chou YH. Effects of a preoperative simplified home rehabilitation education program on length of stay of total knee arthroplasty patients. Orthop Traumatol Surg Res 2012;98(3):259–64.
[57] Zhuang CL, Ye XZ, Zhang XD, et al. Enhanced recovery after surgery programs versus traditional care for colorectal surgery: a meta-analysis of randomized controlled trials. Dis Colon Rectum 2013;56:667–78.

Advances in Anesthesia 32 (2014) 133–147

ADVANCES IN ANESTHESIA

Liposomal Bupivacaine

Its Role in Regional Anesthesia and Postoperative Analgesia

Brian M. Ilfeld, MD, MS (Clinical Investigation)

Division of Regional Anesthesia and Acute Pain Medicine, Department of Anesthesiology, University of California San Diego, 200 West Arbor Drive, MC 8770, San Diego, CA 92103-8770, USA

Keywords

• Analgesia • Epidural • Liposome bupivacaine • Peripheral nerve block • Postoperative analgesia • Regional anesthesia • Long-acting local anesthetic

Key points

- Postsurgical pain duration is usually greater than the duration of analgesia provided by a single administration of traditional formulations of local anesthetics.
- Liposomes may be used to encase local anesthetics, which then release the active medication gradually over a period of multiple days, thus increasing the duration of a single-injection block.
- The United States Food and Drug Administration recently approved a liposomal bupivacaine formulation (Exparel) for use exclusively in wound infiltration.
- Exparel might soon be approved for use in epidural analgesia and peripheral nerve blocks. Initial clinical trials suggest a possible duration of more than 96 hours when administered in a femoral nerve block.
- At the time of this writing, there is no liposome bupivacaine formulation approved within the United States for use in either epidural or peripheral nerve blocks.

INTRODUCTION

Postsurgical pain usually outlasts the duration of analgesia provided by a single administration of traditional formulations of local anesthetics, whether introduced by infiltrating directly into a wound, into the epidural space, or as part of a peripheral nerve block. Bupivacaine hydrochloride (HCl) is currently the longest-acting local anesthetic approved by the United States Food and

Industry Relationships: The author has received funding for clinical research trials from Pacira Pharmaceuticals, Inc, manufacturer of a liposome bupivacaine formulation.

E-mail address: bilfeld@ucsd.edu

0737-6146/14/$ – see front matter
http://dx.doi.org/10.1016/j.aan.2014.08.004

Drug Administration (US FDA), with an analgesic duration of up to 18 to 24 hours when administered in some peripheral nerve blocks. Although multiple analgesic adjuvants such as epinephrine and clonidine have been reported, currently there is no US FDA–approved medication that reliably extends the effective analgesic duration of single-injection epidural or peripheral nerve blocks beyond 24 hours [1,2].

LIPOSOMES

Liposomes consist of a hydrophilic head and 2 hydrophobic tails and were first proposed as a medication carrier in 1965 (Fig. 1) [3]. They can be characterized structurally as unilamellar vesicles with a single outer lipid bilayer (Fig. 2), multilamellar vesicles with concentric lipid bilayers (see Fig. 2), or multivesicular liposomes with nonconcentric lipid bilayers (Fig. 3) [4]. Multivesicular liposomes with nonconcentric lipid bilayers facilitate medication drug loading because of their large size. These multivesicular liposomes create a medication depot gradually releasing local anesthetic, which potentially leads to an extended duration of analgesia [5]. Multiple medications have been encapsulated with multivesicular liposomes, including morphine, fentanyl, chemotherapeutics, ibuprofen, neostigmine, and local anesthetics [4]. There are several routes of administration [4–14]:

- Topical
- Subcutaneous
- Intramuscular
- Intravenous
- Intraperitoneal
- Subconjunctival
- Intravitreal
- Intra-articular
- Intrathecal
- Perineural
- Epidural

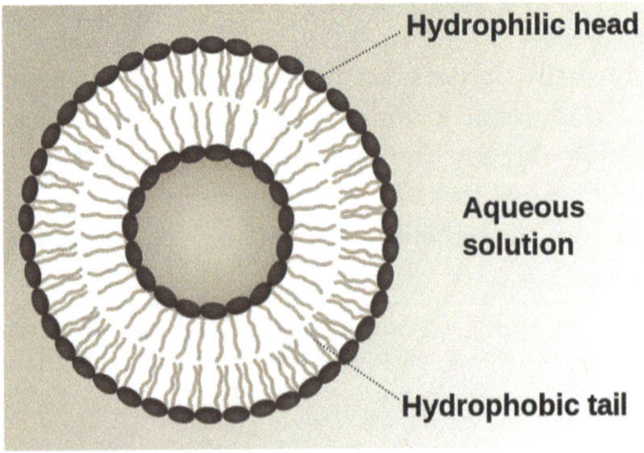

Fig. 1. Liposomes consisting of a hydrophilic head and 2 hydrophobic tails.

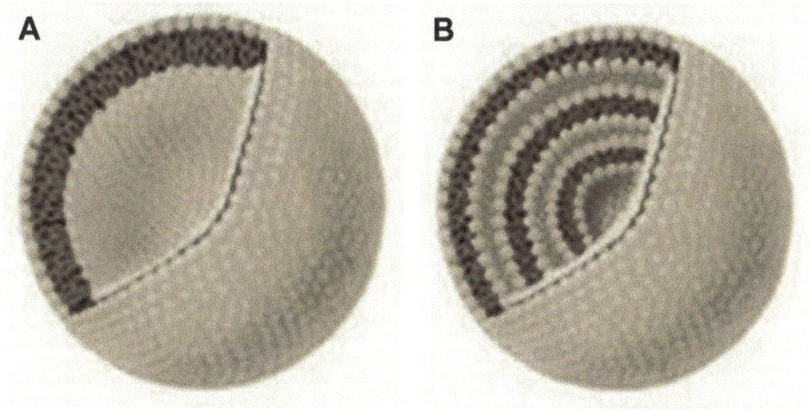

Fig. 2. Liposome in 2 forms: (*A*) unilamellar vesicle, and (*B*) multilamellar vesicles.

In 2004, liposome morphine (DepoDur, Pacira Pharmaceuticals, Parsippany, NJ) became the first liposome-encased medication to be approved for postoperative analgesia by the US FDA [15–18].

LIPOSOME LOCAL ANESTHETIC

Adding local anesthetic (lidocaine) to liposomes was first proposed in 1979 [11], and was soon followed by the first in vivo use in 1980 with dibucaine in guinea pigs [19]; the first use in humans involved topical tetracaine in 1988 [7]. The first report of liposome local anesthetic being used for postoperative analgesia

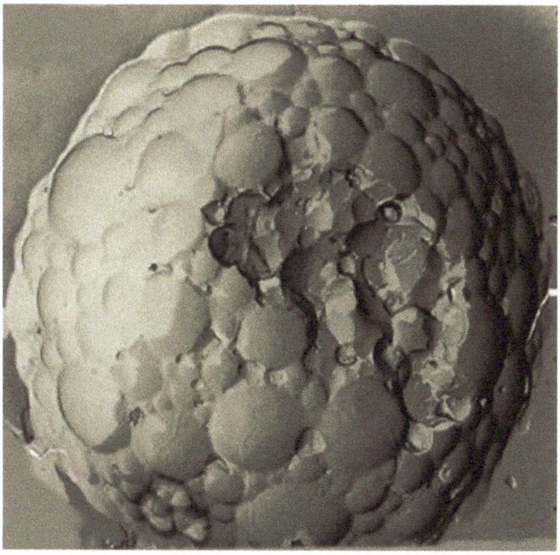

Fig. 3. Scanning electron microscope image of a multivesicular liposome with nonconcentric bilayers.

occurred in 1994: subjects undergoing major thoracic, abdominal, or major lower extremity orthopedic surgery were given a single epidural administration of either bupivacaine HCl 0.5% or liposome bupivacaine 0.5% (nonrandomized, but subject and observer masked) [9]. Subjects receiving standard bupivacaine experienced a mean (standard deviation) duration of analgesia of 3.2 hours (0.4 hours) versus 6.3 hours (1.1 hours) for those receiving liposome bupivacaine ($P<.05$). Such promising results helped to encourage future research involving animals and human volunteers [12,20,21], including use in peripheral nerve blocks [22]. Without exception, a plethora of studies conclusively showed that local anesthetic action is dramatically prolonged when the anesthetic is encapsulated in liposomes.

POTENTIAL TOXICITY

Preclinical research reports no myotoxicity on histologic examination in animals [23,24], and roughly twice as much liposome bupivacaine infused intravenously in rabbits to induce seizures, ventricular tachycardia, and asystole compared with bupivacaine HCl [25]. In humans, there have been 3 suspected intravenous injections of liposome bupivacaine, involving 150 mg, 450 mg, and 450 mg of injectate intended for wound infiltration following knee arthroplasty [26]. Other subjects within this study had mean bupivacaine plasma concentrations of 255 ng/mL (for the 150-mg group) and 520 ng/mL (450-mg group). In contrast, the 3 subjects with unintended intravascular injections had concentrations of 8290 to 34,331 ng/mL. However, none showed symptoms or signs of local anesthetic systemic toxicity, including no electrocardiogram or corrected QT interval changes from baseline [26].

EXPAREL

For the first time, in 2011 the US FDA approved a liposome-encapsulated bupivacaine (Exparel, Pacira Pharmaceuticals, Parsippany, NJ) with specific indications and parameters [27]:

- Administration (infiltration) solely into the surgical site
- Exclusively for postoperative analgesia
- Only for use in adult patients
- Each 20-mL ampule contains 266 mg of Exparel (13.3 mg/mL or 1.33%)
- Each ampule contains a small amount (<3%) of unencapsulated bupivacaine HCl
- Maximum approved dose is 266 mg
- May dilute 20 mL up to 280 mL (1:14) with normal saline
- Administer with a needle no smaller than 25 gauge
- Must use the vial within 4 hours of opening

Note that doses of Exparel are expressed as the free base, so 266 mg of Exparel is equivalent to 300 mg of bupivacaine HCl. If a local anesthetic other than bupivacaine HCl is to be administered at the same site following Exparel, 20 minutes must pass before introduction because the unencapsulated local anesthetic may displace the bupivacaine within the multivesicular liposomes, greatly altering the pharmacokinetics and pharmacodynamics of the Exparel. However, bupivacaine HCl may be introduced at the same or a different anatomic site without a time delay: the maximum recommended additional dose is 133 mg (approximately 50 mL of 0.25% bupivacaine HCl).

PHARMACOKINETICS

When infiltrated directly into the surgical site, Exparel shows a biphasic plasma peak concentration (Fig. 4) [28]. The initial peak occurring within 1 to 2 hours is caused by the extraliposome bupivacaine HCl (<3%) included in every ampule of Exparel. The initial peak is followed by a second plasma peak caused by the slow release of bupivacaine HCl from the liposomes at nearly twice the plasma concentration 24 to 48 hours following administration. Note that after 96 hours bupivacaine is still detectable within the plasma.

PHARMACODYNAMICS: WOUND INFILTRATION

There are multiple publications involving the infiltration of Exparel directly into a surgical wound [27]. The highest quality data may be derived from 10 randomized controlled trials involving a combined total of 823 subjects. Exparel was superior to placebo in providing postoperative analgesia for both bunionectomy [29] and hemorrhoidectomy [30]. In contrast, when Exparel was compared with bupivacaine HCl, only 1 study involving hemorrhoidectomy showed a statistically significant difference between the two treatments for the primary analgesic end point [31]. A similar clinical trial, also involving hemorrhoidectomy, was negative for its primary end point [32], as were trials

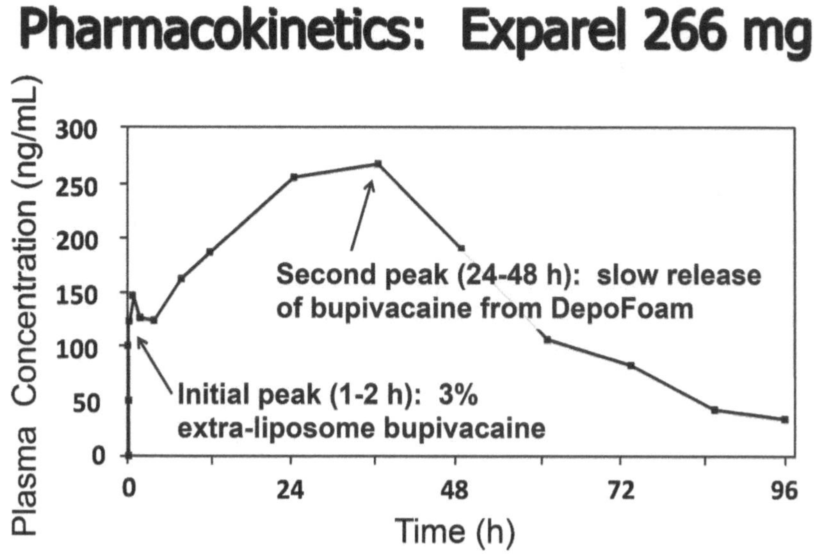

Fig. 4. Pharmacokinetics of a single 266-mg dose of Exparel infiltrated directly into tissue.

involving inguinal hernia repair [32], breast augmentation [32,33], and total knee arthroplasty [32,34].

Many of these trials were dose-response studies, not designed to be a defining test of efficacy. In addition, many trials did detect some benefits of Exparel compared with bupivacaine HCl in secondary end points, such as decreased opioid use (minimal differences) [35]. A systematic review of the efficacy of these 10 randomized controlled trials of wound infiltration found Exparel (doses, 66–532 mg) to be associated with a significantly longer time to first use of opioid analgesics following surgery (median, 9.3 hours vs 3.6 hours; $P<.0001$) [32]. Another analysis focused on pooled data from study subjects receiving liposome bupivacaine at doses up to and including the highest approved dose (266 mg) compared with bupivacaine HCl [35]. In this analysis, the mean cumulative area under the curve (AUC) pain intensity score in patients receiving liposome bupivacaine was 283 compared with 329 in those receiving bupivacaine HCl ($P=.039$). Administration of liposome bupivacaine was also associated with longer median time to first administration of postsurgical opioid rescue (9.9 hours) and a lower total amount of opioids consumed after surgery (12.2 mg) versus bupivacaine HCl (2.7 hours and 19.0 mg, respectively; $P<.0001$ for both comparisons).

However, with any newly introduced medication, it is incumbent on the manufacturer and scientific community to provide conclusive evidence of efficacy before widespread adoption in every everyday clinical practice, especially when the new medication is approximately 100 times the cost of the one it is proposed to replace. Although there is limited evidence from secondary end points suggesting that there may be some benefits to infiltrating Exparel into surgical wounds, at the present time there is only a single randomized controlled trial showing a statistically significant improvement in its primary endpoint for a single surgical procedure (hemorrhoidectomy) [31]. Health care providers should be cognizant of this dearth of conclusive evidence of benefits when making practice decisions.

ADVERSE EVENTS

On the positive side, the subjects exposed to Exparel within the 10 published randomized controlled trials noted previously (823 subjects total) experienced no more adverse events (AEs) than subjects receiving bupivacaine HCl (Table 1) [36]. Less than 1% of subjects receiving Exparel showed cardiac-related AEs, possibly related to treatment (none for subjects receiving placebo or bupivacaine HCl). None were deemed serious by investigators and none required an intervention. However, in a phase 1 study, a healthy volunteer with no history of seizures had a vasovagal episode before receiving any study medication [26]. This subject subsequently received subcutaneous injections of bupivacaine HCl 2.5 mg and Exparel 15 mg in the right and left forearms, respectively. Immediately after a 5-mm incision was made in the right forearm, he complained of nausea, seemed to have a vasovagal reaction, lowered his head between his knees, and then had what the principal investigator described

Table 1
AEs experienced by 823 subjects of 10 randomized controlled trials comparing Exparel with either bupivacaine HCl or placebo

	AEs (%)	Serious AEs (%)
Placebo	43	1
Bupivacaine HCl	75	5
Exparel	62	3

as a 15-second tonic-clonic seizure with micturition. He was subsequently lethargic for approximately 3 minutes. Although it was described by the principal investigator as a seizure, the investigators deemed the event unlikely to be related to the study drug. Considering the subject's preexposure vasovagal reaction, the extremely small subcutaneous injection of active medications, and the 3 subjects from a different study with extraordinarily high plasma levels of bupivacaine following suspected accidental intravascular injection of Exparel up to 450 mg without any neurologic or cardiovascular signs or symptoms of systemic toxicity [26], it is extremely unlikely that this healthy subject experienced a true seizure, as opposed to a second vasovagal reaction.

EPIDURAL ADMINISTRATION

In preclinical studies, Exparel showed no toxicity when administered in the epidural space of both rats and dogs [27]. In a phase 1 trial with healthy volunteers, subjects (n = 6) received epidural (via a catheter at L_{3-4}) bupivacaine HCl 50 mg (20 mL of 0.25%), or 1 of 3 doses of Exparel: 89, 155, or 266 mg in saline producing 20 mL of injectate (n = 8 for each dose) [37]. Subjects were observed for 96 hours following the single-bolus administration. Bupivacaine plasma concentrations were dose dependent, with a lower peak at all Exparel doses relative to the bupivacaine HCl controls. The 3 Exparel doses resulted in peak concentrations at approximately the same time (within 30 minutes) as the bupivacaine HCl controls; however, unlike the controls in whom plasma levels decreased precipitously almost immediately, the 3 Exparel doses resulted in stable plasma levels until they began to decrease after roughly 24 hours, and were still detectable within the plasma after 84 to 96 hours. Exparel had a significantly greater ($P < .001$) area under the plasma bupivacaine concentration–time curve from baseline to either last plasma sample or infinity compared with bupivacaine HCl. The elimination half-life of Exparel was approximately 3 times longer than that of bupivacaine HCl.

Because of the small number of subjects in each treatment group of this phase 1 study, no statistics were applied to the collected data. However, the results of this pilot study strongly suggest a dramatic increase in analgesia duration: median time until recovery of pinprick sensation was 11 hours for standard bupivacaine HCl, compared with 35 hours for Exparel (all doses combined) [37]. In contrast, subjects receiving bupivacaine HCl had a more intense motor block for a longer duration (Table 2). These results suggest an excellent sensory/motor block ratio with Exparel having a dramatic advantage compared bupivacaine HCl. Both epidural Exparel and bupivacaine HCl were well tolerated. The most common AEs were headache (21% with Exparel, 0% with bupivacaine HCl) and injection-site pain (83% with either treatment). All AEs were mild to moderate, and no study discontinuations resulted from AEs. It is emphasized that Exparel is not currently approved for use in the epidural space, and must be considered experimental at this time.

PERIPHERAL NERVE BLOCKS

Preclinical toxicology in rabbits and dogs showed similar findings for Exparel and bupivacaine HCl: mild granulomatous inflammation of adipose tissue considered a normal foreign body response [38]. No histologic evidence of peripheral (brachial plexus) nerve injury was observed. In a phase 1 study, 36 healthy volunteers were randomized to receive either bupivacaine HCl 75 mg or Exparel 66 to 155 mg as an infiltration peripheral nerve block at the ankle (including the saphenous, deep peroneal, and superficial peroneal nerves) [27]. Both medications were well tolerated, and the Exparel doses of 66 to 133 mg were roughly equivalent to the doses of bupivacaine HCl. However, the highest Exparel dose of 155 mg resulted in decreased sensation for more than 72 hours.

A subsequent phase 2 multicenter trial involving patients undergoing bunionectomy (n = 58) randomized subjects undergoing ankle blocks to either bupivacaine 125 mg or Exparel 155 to 310 mg [27]. Subjects who received Exparel reported higher pain scores within the first 12 hours compared with those who had received bupivacaine HCl, suggesting that Exparel in these doses produces a peripheral nerve block of lower potency (Fig. 5). From 24 to 96 hours, there were no statistically significant differences among treatments, although there was a trend of improved analgesia with Exparel (see Fig. 5). No statistically significant differences in opioid consumption were detected.

TRANSVERSUS ABDOMINIS PLANE BLOCKS

Although 2 phase 2 cohort studies of Exparel using blocks within the transversus abdominis plane (TAP) have been reported in abstract form [39,40], effectiveness cannot be determined because neither was randomized or controlled [27]. The first involved robotic prostatectomy, and subjects received TAP with Exparel 266 mg in 20 mL (n = 12) or 40 mL (n = 12) of diluent

Table 2
Epidural Exparel (n = 18) versus bupivacaine HCl (n = 6)

	Bupivacaine HCl	Exparel
Median time until pinprick sensation recovery (h)	11	35
Experiencing some degree of motor block (%)	100	57
Unable to ambulate after 4 h (%)	80	27
Median time for complete motor block resolution (h)	3	1

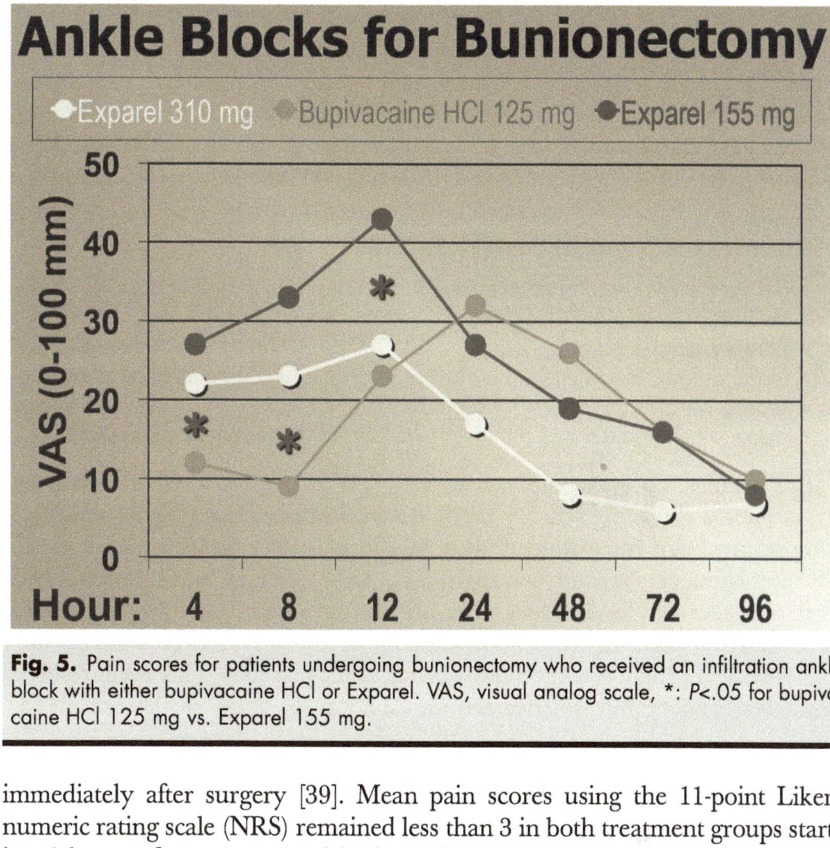

Fig. 5. Pain scores for patients undergoing bunionectomy who received an infiltration ankle block with either bupivacaine HCl or Exparel. VAS, visual analog scale, *: $P<.05$ for bupivacaine HCl 125 mg vs. Exparel 155 mg.

immediately after surgery [39]. Mean pain scores using the 11-point Likert numeric rating scale (NRS) remained less than 3 in both treatment groups starting 6 hours after surgery and lasting 96 hours. In the second study, a TAP block with 266 mg of Exparel 266 mg in 20 mL was administered in 13 subjects undergoing umbilical hernia repair. Average pain scores remained less than 3 on an NRS for at least 120 hours following surgery; the TAP infiltration failed in 1 subject who had a pain intensity score of 10 at 4 hours and was admitted to a hospital overnight for pain control.

FEMORAL NERVE BLOCKS

One volunteer dose-response study using Exparel in femoral nerve blocks has been published [41]. Subjects (n = 14) received Exparel 0 to 80 mg in 1 ultrasonography-guided single-injection femoral nerve block, with the contralateral side receiving a different dose of 0 to 80 mg. Sensory effects were measured with tolerance to transcutaneous electrical stimulation, whereas motor effects were assessed by measuring the maximum voluntary isometric contraction (MVIC) of the quadriceps femoris muscle. There was a wide variation in interindividual response, and paradoxically there was an inverse dose-related effect on sensory and motor function: the higher the dose, the lower the observed effect. With each milligram increase in bupivacaine, MVIC increased by a mean of

0.09% (standard error [SE], 0.03; 95% confidence interval [CI], 0.04–0.14; $P=$ .002) and tolerance to cutaneous current decreased by 0.03 mA (SE, 0.01; 95% CI, −0.04 to −0.02; $P<$.001). It is noteworthy that 2 subjects with anomalous dose-response profiles may have either experienced a placebo effect or intentionally falsified responses; with exclusion of these 2 individuals, the correlation between dose and sensory block was not significant and the correlation between dose and motor blockade reversed to the expected direction. The effects of the higher doses (40–80 mg) show sensory and motor deficits lasting 24 to 99 hours:

- Sensory block duration (doses 40–80 mg) was more than 24 hours in 100% of subjects
- Sensory block peaked in 2 subjects more than 80 hours after administration
- MVIC did not consistently return to within 20% of baseline until after 24 hours (doses 40–80 mg) in 90% of subjects
- Motor block peaked in 1 subject more than 40 hours after administration

In summary, liposome bupivacaine generally resulted in a partial quadriceps motor block; regarding sensory block, subjects who received higher doses had a more consistent response pattern of requiring greater transcutaneous electrical stimulation current to reach slight discomfort (sensory block) than did subjects who received lower doses. The only reported AE was transient pruritus and erythema at the injection site during the first few days after administration in 1 participant (on a side receiving normal saline placebo). This event resolved without treatment and was deemed unrelated to the study medication.

SURGICAL SUBJECTS

In 1 unpublished phase 2 dose-ranging study involving patients undergoing total knee arthroplasty, subjects (n = 100) received a preoperative 20-mL single-injection femoral nerve block with either normal saline (placebo, n = 24) or 1 of 3 possible doses of Exparel: 67, 133, or 266 mg (E. Onel, Pacira Pharmaceuticals, Inc; written communication; April 3, 2014). A complete (including statistical) analysis of the resulting data is not available at the time of this writing, but preliminary data suggest that the pain scores at rest were lower for the 2 higher doses of Exparel, and similar between the lower dose and placebo (Table 3). Data on motor strength and ambulation are currently unavailable.

Table 3
Preliminary results from a phase 2 dose-ranging study involving patients undergoing total knee arthroplasty (n = 100) who received a single-injection femoral nerve block with either normal saline or 1 of 3 possible doses of Exparel

	AUC_{0-24} NRS at rest	AUC_{0-24} NRS with flexion
Placebo (n = 24)	179	196
Exparel 67 mg (n = 22)	180	194
Exparel 133 mg (n = 24)	160	174
Exparel 266 mg (n = 24)	154	171

Abbreviations: AUC_{0-24}, AUC 0 to 24 postoperative hours; NRS, Numeric Rating Score (0–10).

This dose-response study was used to plan a subsequent phase 3 multicenter clinical trial, also involving patients undergoing total knee arthroplasty, which randomized subjects (n = 184) in a double-masked fashion to a 20-mL single-injection femoral nerve block with either 266 mg of Exparel or normal saline (E. Onel, Pacira Pharmaceuticals, Inc; written communication; April 3, 2014). All subjects received a femoral perineural catheter immediately following study solution injection to be used with a bupivacaine HCl infusion should 2 other opioid-based rescue medications prove insufficient. Again, currently available results are both preliminary and limited in scope, but, importantly, the prospectively designated primary end point of AUC for pain scores in the first 72 postoperative hours was positive ($P < .0001$). Although these results comparing an active medication with saline are not surprising, they are important for 2 reasons:

1. The manufacturer is using the results of this phase 3 study to petition the US FDA to grant approval for use of Exparel in peripheral nerve blocks. Should this petition be granted, a liposome bupivacaine formulation approved for use in peripheral nerve blocks would, after decades of study, be available to health care providers.
2. The AUC for pain scores was not only improved for the Exparel group in the first 24 hours (Fig. 6) but, in the periods of 24 to 48 hours and 48 to 72 hours as well

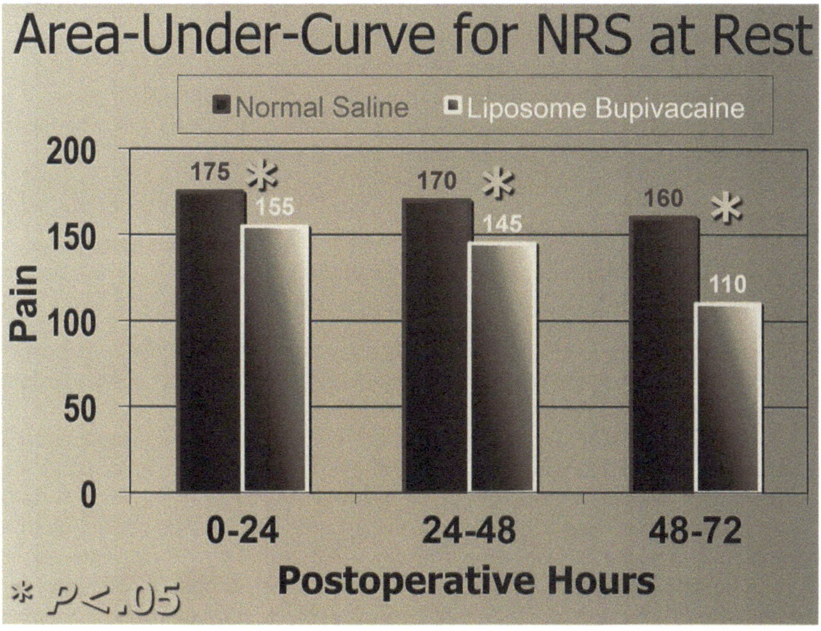

Fig. 6. AUC for pain scores at rest for subjects who underwent total knee arthroplasty with a preoperative single-injection femoral nerve block randomized to either Exparel (266 mg) or normal saline (placebo).

($P<.05$). This finding shows that Exparel provides postoperative analgesia in both of these additional time periods, and dramatically prolongs postoperative analgesia compared with unencapsulated bupivacaine HCl.

POTENTIAL IMPLICATIONS

At present, health care providers must insert a perineural catheter and provide a continuous perineural local anesthetic infusion to prolong the effects of a peripheral nerve block beyond the current 24-hour duration of unencapsulated bupivacaine HCl [42]. However, if Exparel (1) is approved for use in peripheral nerve blocks, and (2) is shown in well-controlled randomized trials to be at least noninferior in providing postoperative analgesia compared specifically with continuous peripheral nerve blocks, there are several important potential advantages of a single injection of liposomal bupivacaine rather than an infusion:

- No infusion pump, catheter, or large volume of local anesthetic (reservoir)
- Decreased costs
- Decreased provider time for block placement (without the need for catheter insertion)
- Decreased provider time for infusion management
- Decreased inconvenience to patients without having to carry a portable infusion pump and large reservoir of local anesthetic as well as having to remove a perineural catheter
- No potential for catheter leakage and dislodgement
- Decreased necessity for provider training (for catheter insertion)
- Decreased infection risk (without a perineural catheter left in situ)
- Possible decreased hemorrhage/hematoma formation risk without a perineural catheter (and possible use with potent anticoagulants)

POTENTIAL DISADVANTAGES

There are also potential disadvantages to using a long-acting single injection of local anesthetic rather than a continuous peripheral nerve block:

- Unclear whether surgical anesthesia is attainable with any dose of Exparel.
- Potentially inferior short-term analgesia (during the duration of unencapsulated bupivacaine HCl) if Exparel proves less potent.
- Inability to titrate down: too dense a sensory block may be disconcerting to patients or even increase the risk of limb injury; too dense a motor block may decrease physical therapy ability or increase the risk of falling; and a dense proprioception deficit might increase the risk of falling. In addition, a prolonged phrenic nerve block (with above-the-clavicle brachial plexus approaches) has the potential to result in prolonged symptomatic hemidiaphragmatic paresis.
- Inability to titrate up: inadequate sensory block may provide inadequate analgesia, and an inadequate duration of analgesia cannot be prolonged without a perineural infusion.
- Inability to administer bolus doses: inability to provide additional analgesia when sporadically needed (eg, physical therapy or dressing changes).

KNOWLEDGE GAPS AND FUTURE RESEARCH

Exparel used for wound infiltration for various surgical procedures must be validated against unencapsulated bupivacaine HCl with randomized controlled phase 4 clinical trials. Use of Exparel within the epidural space is at the very early stages of exploration, and multiple phase 2 and 3 studies are required before approval is sought from regulatory bodies. In addition, if the US FDA approves the use of Exparel in peripheral nerve blocks, an enormous amount of research is required:

- Exparel must be compared with single-injection bupivacaine HCl for various surgical procedures
- Exparel must be compared with continuous peripheral nerve blocks for various surgical procedures
- The optimal dose, concentration, and volume of Exparel must be determined for various peripheral nerve blocks and surgical procedures
- The appropriate surgical procedures to which Exparel may be applied must be determined
- Long-term cohort studies of Exparel used in single-injection peripheral nerve blocks must be conducted to identify the incidence of rare risks/complications

SUMMARY

- Postsurgical pain duration is usually greater than the duration of analgesia following a single administration of traditional formulations of local anesthetics.
- Liposomes may be used to encase local anesthetics, which then release the active medication gradually over a period of multiple days, thus increasing the duration of action of a single-injection block.
- The US FDA has recently approved a liposome bupivacaine formulation, Exparel, for use exclusively in wound infiltration.
- However, it might soon be approved for use in epidural analgesia and peripheral nerve blocks. Initial clinical trials suggest a possible duration of more than 96 hours when administered in a femoral nerve block.
- It is emphasized that, at the time of this writing, there is no liposome bupivacaine formulation approved within the United States for use in epidural or peripheral nerve blocks.

References

[1] Murphy DB, McCartney CJ, Chan VW. Novel analgesic adjuncts for brachial plexus block: a systematic review. Anesth Analg 2000;90:1122–8.

[2] McCartney CJ, Duggan E, Apatu E. Should we add clonidine to local anesthetic for peripheral nerve blockade? A qualitative systematic review of the literature. Reg Anesth Pain Med 2007;32:330–8.

[3] Bangham AD, Standish MM, Miller N. Cation permeability of phospholipid model membranes: effect of narcotics. Nature 1965;208:1295–7.

[4] Viscusi ER. Liposomal drug delivery for postoperative pain management. Reg Anesth Pain Med 2005;30:491–6.

[5] Howell SB. Clinical applications of a novel sustained-release injectable drug delivery system: DepoFoam technology. Cancer J 2001;7:219–27.

[6] Hung OR, Comeau L, Riley MR, et al. Comparative topical anaesthesia of EMLA and liposome-encapsulated tetracaine. Can J Anaesth 1997;44:707–11.

[7] Gesztes A, Mezei M. Topical anesthesia of the skin by liposome-encapsulated tetracaine. Anesth Analg 1988;67:1079–81.
[8] Kopacz DJ, Bernards CM, Allen HW, et al. A model to evaluate the pharmacokinetic and pharmacodynamic variables of extended-release products using in vivo tissue microdialysis in humans: bupivacaine-loaded microcapsules. Anesth Analg 2003;97:124–31.
[9] Boogaerts JG, Lafont ND, Declercq AG, et al. Epidural administration of liposome-associated bupivacaine for the management of postsurgical pain: a first study. J Clin Anesth 1994;6:315–20.
[10] Eichenfield LF, Funk A, Fallon-Friedlander S, et al. A clinical study to evaluate the efficacy of ELA-Max (4% liposomal lidocaine) as compared with eutectic mixture of local anesthetics cream for pain reduction of venipuncture in children. Pediatrics 2002;109:1093–9.
[11] Grant GJ, Bansinath M. Liposomal delivery systems for local anesthetics. Reg Anesth Pain Med 2001;26:61–3.
[12] Holte K, Werner MU, Lacouture PG, et al. Dexamethasone prolongs local analgesia after subcutaneous infiltration of bupivacaine microcapsules in human volunteers. Anesthesiology 2002;96:1331–5.
[13] Pedersen JL, Lilleso J, Hammer NA, et al. Bupivacaine in microcapsules prolongs analgesia after subcutaneous infiltration in humans: a dose-finding study. Anesth Analg 2004;99: 912–8.
[14] Lafont ND, Legros FJ, Boogaerts JG. Use of liposome-associated bupivacaine in a cancer pain syndrome. Anaesthesia 1996;51:578–9.
[15] Viscusi ER, Kopacz D, Hartrick C, et al. Single-dose extended-release epidural morphine for pain following hip arthroplasty. Am J Ther 2006;13:423–31.
[16] Viscusi ER, Martin G, Hartrick CT, et al. Forty-eight hours of postoperative pain relief after total hip arthroplasty with a novel, extended-release epidural morphine formulation. Anesthesiology 2005;102:1014–22.
[17] Gambling D, Hughes T, Martin G, et al. A comparison of Depodur, a novel, single-dose extended-release epidural morphine, with standard epidural morphine for pain relief after lower abdominal surgery. Anesth Analg 2005;100:1065–74.
[18] Carvalho B, Riley E, Cohen SE, et al. Single-dose, sustained-release epidural morphine in the management of postoperative pain after elective cesarean delivery: results of a multicenter randomized controlled study. Anesth Analg 2005;100:1150–8.
[19] Okano T, Haga M, Watanabe Y, et al. Duration of the local anesthetic action of dibucaine by liposomes and its mechanism (author's transl). Yakugaku Zasshi 1980;100:1097–103 [In Japanese].
[20] Ohri R, Blaskovich P, Wang JC, et al. Prolonged nerve block by microencapsulated bupivacaine prevents acute postoperative pain in rats. Reg Anesth Pain Med 2012;37: 607–15.
[21] Ohri R, Wang JC, Blaskovich PD, et al. Inhibition by local bupivacaine-releasing microspheres of acute postoperative pain from hairy skin incision. Anesth Analg 2013;117: 717–30.
[22] Estebe JP, Le Corre P, Du PL, et al. The pharmacokinetics and pharmacodynamics of bupivacaine-loaded microspheres on a brachial plexus block model in sheep. Anesth Analg 2001;93:447–55.
[23] McAlvin JB, Reznor G, Shankarappa SA, et al. Local toxicity from local anesthetic polymeric microparticles. Anesth Analg 2013;116:794–803.
[24] McAlvin JB, Padera RF, Shankarappa SA, et al. Multivesicular liposomal bupivacaine at the sciatic nerve. Biomaterials 2014;35:4557–64.
[25] Boogaerts J, Declercq A, Lafont N, et al. Toxicity of bupivacaine encapsulated into liposomes and injected intravenously: comparison with plain solutions. Anesth Analg 1993;76:553–5.
[26] Bergese SD, Onel E, Morren M, et al. Bupivacaine extended-release liposome injection exhibits a favorable cardiac safety profile. Reg Anesth Pain Med 2012;37:145–51.

[27] Ilfeld BM. Liposome bupivacaine in peripheral nerve blocks and epidural injections to manage postoperative pain. Expert Opin Pharmacother 2013;14:2421–31.
[28] Hu D, Onel E, Singla N, et al. Pharmacokinetic profile of liposome bupivacaine injection following a single administration at the surgical site. Clin Drug Investig 2013;33:109–15.
[29] Golf M, Daniels SE, Onel E. A phase 3, randomized, placebo-controlled trial of DepoFoam(R) bupivacaine (extended-release bupivacaine local analgesic) in bunionectomy. Adv Ther 2011;28:776–88.
[30] Gorfine SR, Onel E, Patou G, et al. Bupivacaine extended-release liposome injection for prolonged postsurgical analgesia in patients undergoing hemorrhoidectomy: a multicenter, randomized, double-blind, placebo-controlled trial. Dis Colon Rectum 2011;54:1552–9.
[31] Haas E, Onel E, Miller H, et al. A double-blind, randomized, active-controlled study for post-hemorrhoidectomy pain management with liposome bupivacaine, a novel local analgesic formulation. Am Surg 2012;78:574–81.
[32] Bergese SD, Ramamoorthy S, Patou G, et al. Efficacy profile of liposome bupivacaine, a novel formulation of bupivacaine for postsurgical analgesia. J Pain Res 2012;5:107–16.
[33] Smoot JD, Bergese SD, Onel E, et al. The efficacy and safety of DepoFoam bupivacaine in patients undergoing bilateral, cosmetic, submuscular augmentation mammaplasty: a randomized, double-blind, active-control study. Aesthet Surg J 2012;32:69–76.
[34] Bramlett K, Onel E, Viscusi ER, et al. A randomized, double-blind, dose-ranging study comparing wound infiltration of DepoFoam bupivacaine, an extended-release liposomal bupivacaine, to bupivacaine HCl for postsurgical analgesia in total knee arthroplasty. Knee 2012;19:530–6.
[35] Dasta J, Ramamoorthy S, Patou G, et al. Bupivacaine liposome injectable suspension compared with bupivacaine HCl for the reduction of opioid burden in the postsurgical setting. Curr Med Res Opin 2012;28:1609–15.
[36] Viscusi ER, Sinatra R, Onel E, et al. The safety of liposome bupivacaine, a novel local analgesic formulation. Clin J Pain 2014;30:102–10.
[37] Viscusi ER, Candiotti KA, Onel E, et al. The pharmacokinetics and pharmacodynamics of liposome bupivacaine administered via a single epidural injection to healthy volunteers. Reg Anesth Pain Med 2012;37:616–22.
[38] Richard BM, Newton P, Ott LR, et al. The safety of EXPAREL ® (bupivacaine liposome injectable suspension) administered by peripheral nerve block in rabbits and dogs. J Drug Deliv 2012;2012:962101.
[39] Sternlicht A, Shapiro M, Robelen G, et al. Initial findings using Exparel (bupivacaine liposome injectable suspension) via infiltration into the transversus abdominis plane for postsurgical analgesia in robotic prostatectomy, abstracted (A124). Presented at: Annual Fall Pain Meeting and Workshops of the American Society of Regional Anesthesia and Pain Medicine, November 15–18, 2012; Miami Beach, FL.
[40] Feierman DE, Kronenfeld M, Gupta PM, et al. Evaluation of Exparel use via infiltration into the transversus abdominis plane for prolonged postoperative analgesia in subjects undergoing open abdominal hernia repair, abstracted (S338). Presented at: Annual Meeting of the International Anesthesia Research Society, May 4–7, 2013; San Diego, CA.
[41] Ilfeld BM, Malhotra N, Furnish TJ, et al. Liposomal bupivacaine as a single-injection peripheral nerve block: a dose-response study. Anesth Analg 2013;117:1248–56.
[42] Ilfeld BM. Continuous peripheral nerve blocks: a review of the published evidence. Anesth Analg 2011;113:904–25.

Advances in Anesthesia 32 (2014) 149–169

ADVANCES IN ANESTHESIA

Ultrasound Guidance for Central Neuraxial Anesthesia and Analgesia

James Edward Johnson, MBBS, FANZCA,
Anahi Perlas, MD, FRCPC,
Ki Jinn Chin, MBBS, MMed, FANZCA, FRCPC*

Department of Anesthesia, Toronto Western Hospital, University of Toronto, 399 Bathurst Street, McL 2-405, Toronto, Ontario M5T 2S8, Canada

Keywords

• Neuraxial blockade • Spinal anesthesia • Epidural analgesia • Ultrasound

Key points

- Detailed knowledge of the bony contours of spine is essential for interpretation of neuraxial ultrasound scan.
- Preprocedural ultrasound imaging can reduce the technical difficulty of neuraxial blockade by identifying the presence and location of interlaminar and interspinous soft-tissue windows.
- Both transverse midline and parasagittal oblique ultrasound views should be obtained, as they provide complementary information.
- Ultrasound-guided neuraxial blockade is an advanced technique that is of particular value in patients whose surface anatomic landmarks are obscured, altered, or absent; however, we recommend that practitioners accumulate experience with the technique in normal individuals.

INTRODUCTION

The primary technical challenge in neuraxial blockade is accurate identification of a soft-tissue window into the vertebral canal. This is usually inferred from palpation of the spinous processes and tactile feedback from the needle as it is inserted. However, difficulty can be encountered if surface landmarks are obscured, altered, or absent or if the interlaminar or interspinous spaces are

Disclosures: None of the authors have any material conflicts of interest to report.

*Corresponding author. *E-mail address:* gasgenie@gmail.com

0737-6146/14/$ – see front matter
http://dx.doi.org/10.1016/j.aan.2014.08.002

narrowed by age-related changes. Technical difficulty and multiple needle insertion attempts are not only associated with patient discomfort but also with serious complications including spinal hematoma and neurologic injury [1–3]. Ultrasound guidance assists with identification of anatomy and target structures, which permits more accurate planning of needle insertion, trajectory, and depth and, in turn, improves technical ease of performance.

Ultrasound guidance in this context generally refers to the performance of a preprocedural scan that delineates the spinal anatomy, following which spinal or epidural needle insertion occurs in the usual manner. Real-time ultrasound-guided neuraxial blockade, however, refers to needle insertion under direct ultrasonographic visualization.

ANATOMY AND SONOANATOMY OF THE LUMBAR SPINE

Knowledge of the gross bony anatomy of the spine is essential for interpretation of neuraxial ultrasound scan. It is particularly important to appreciate the contours of the posterior bony surfaces of the spine (Fig. 1), as these are responsible for the characteristic shapes of the acoustic dropout shadows seen on ultrasound scan, which, in turn, are key to recognition of anatomic structures.

A curvilinear low-frequency ultrasound probe (transducer) with its wider field of view and better beam penetration is recommended for use in all adult patients. Two imaging planes and probe orientations are commonly used to image the spine (Fig. 2), transverse (or axial) and parasagittal (or longitudinal).

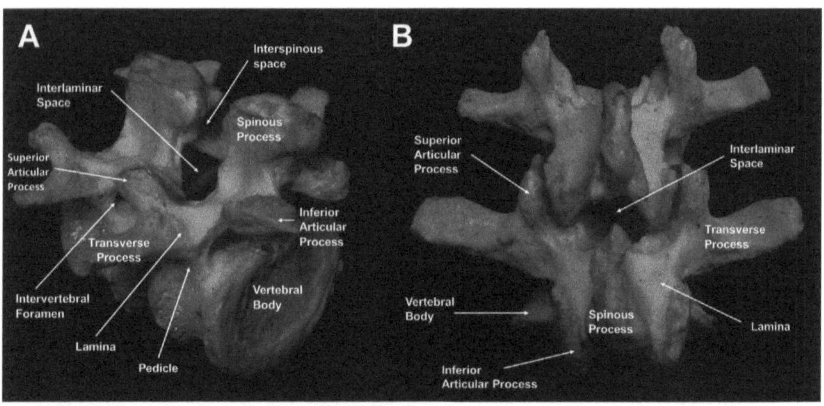

Fig. 1. Three-quarter oblique view (*A*) and posterior view (*B*) of adjacent lumbar vertebrae. The interlaminar space is located posteriorly and is bounded by the bases of the spinous processes, the laminae, and the inferior articular processes. It is roofed over by the ligamentum flavum. The interspinous space lies in the midline and is filled by the supraspinous and interspinous ligaments. The intervertebral foramina are located laterally and are bounded by the pedicles, the vertebral body, the laminae, and the superior and inferior articular processes and contain the spinal nerve roots and their accompanying blood vessels. (*Courtesy of* www.usra.ca; with permission.)

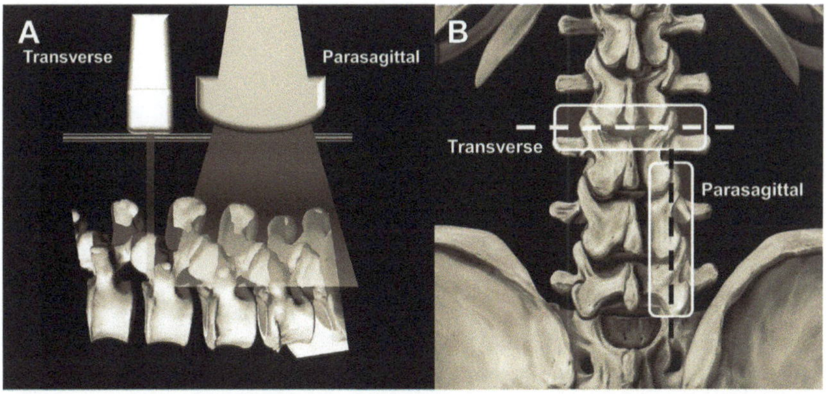

Fig. 2. The ultrasound probe may be placed in 2 basic orientations: transverse or parasagittal, which determines the cut of the spine that will be visualized. Figure *A* is a lateral view, and Figure *B* is a posterior view, of the surface placement of the transducer over the lumbar spine in the 2 basic orientations. (*Courtesy of* www.usra.ca; with permission.)

The transverse plane is most useful to determine an appropriate needle insertion point for a midline approach; however, the parasagittal plane provides valuable additional information on the location and identity of interlaminar spaces, particularly in the patient with more difficult anatomy. The ultrasound examination should, therefore, always use both probe orientations. Five typical ultrasonographic views of the lumbar spine can be obtained: 3 in the parasagittal plane and 2 in the transverse plane.

1. Parasagittal oblique view
2. Parasagittal transverse process view
3. Parasagittal articular process view
4. Transverse midline interlaminar view
5. Transverse midline spinous process view

The parasagittal oblique (PSO) and transverse midline (TM) interlaminar views are the 2 most important views to obtain.

Parasagittal oblique view

To obtain the PSO view, the ultrasound probe is placed in a longitudinal parasagittal orientation and angled toward the midline to direct the beam through the paramedian interlaminar spaces. The beam transects the sloping laminae of the lumbar vertebrae, producing a characteristic "sawtooth" pattern of acoustic shadows (Fig. 3). Two hyperechoic linear structures are seen in the interlaminar gap between the sawteeth. The more superficial one that adjoins the bases of adjacent sawteeth is the posterior complex and represents the ligamentum flavum, epidural space, and posterior dura. The deeper hyperechoic structure is the anterior complex and represents the anterior dura, posterior longitudinal ligament, and posterior aspect of the vertebral body and intervertebral disc, which together make up the anterior wall of the vertebral canal. The

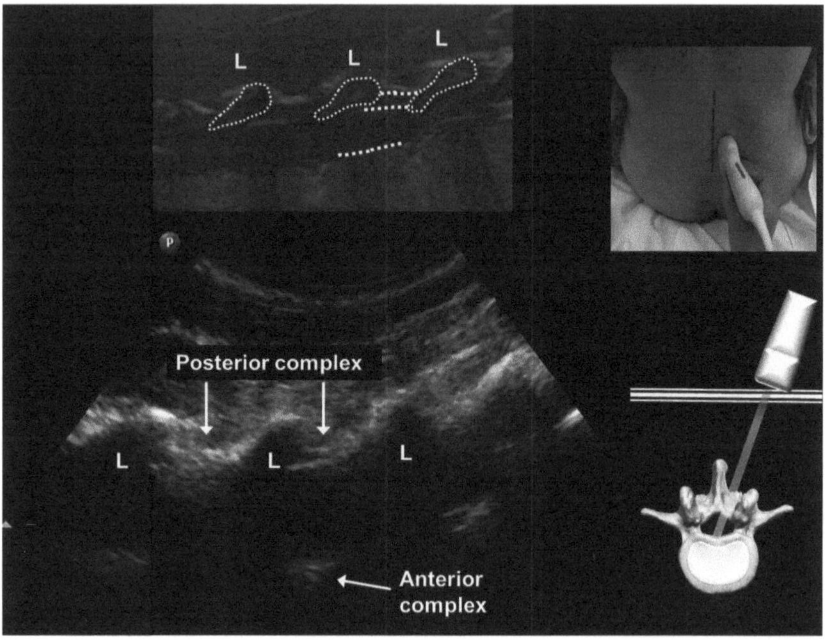

Fig. 3. PSO view of the lumbar spine with corresponding magnetic resonance image (*above*). The laminae (L) are visible in cross-section as sloping hyperechoic lines with acoustic shadowing beneath and form a sawtooth pattern. The hyperechoic posterior complex, consisting of ligamentum flavum, posterior epidural space, and posterior dura, is visible between laminae; these structures cannot always be distinguished from one another. The deeper hyperechoic linear structure is the anterior complex, consisting of anterior dura, anterior epidural space, posterior longitudinal ligament, and the posterior aspect of the vertebral body and intervertebral disc. (*Courtesy of* www.usra.ca; with permission.)

intervening hypoechoic area is the intrathecal space. The conus medullaris has the same echogenicity as cerebrospinal fluid and cannot be distinguished in the adult patient. Pulsatile hyperechoic streaks may occasionally be seen within the intrathecal space and most likely represent elements of the cauda equina.

Parasagittal views of the articular processes and transverse processes

If the ultrasound probe is positioned more laterally in the parasagittal plane or is insufficiently angled toward the midline, an image of the articular processes or transverse processes may be obtained instead. The overlapping superior and inferior articular processes can be recognized as a continuous, wavy hyperechoic line with a dense acoustic shadow beneath (Fig. 4).

The transverse processes, however, cast characteristic fingerlike acoustic shadows with the psoas major muscle visible in the acoustic window between the transverse processes (Fig. 5). Recognition of these 2 views guide the operator as to the appropriate manipulation of the probe required to obtain the PSO view.

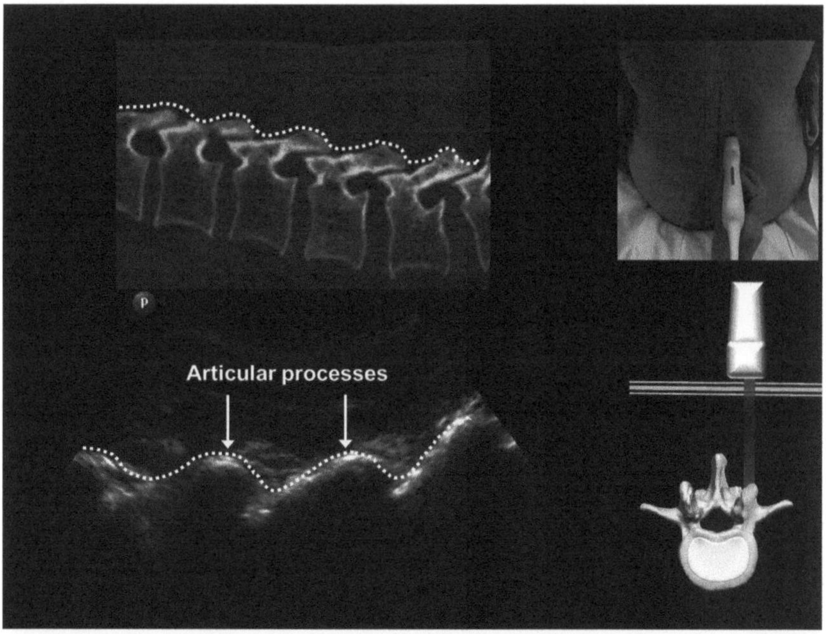

Fig. 4. Parasagittal articular process view of the lumbar spine and corresponding computed tomography image (*above*). The overlapping bony superior and inferior articular processes are seen as a continuous hyperechoic line of humps with acoustic shadowing beneath. (*Courtesy of* www.usra.ca; with permission.)

Transverse midline interlaminar view

The most important characteristic of the TM interlaminar view is visualization of the hyperechoic anterior complex, which signifies that the ultrasound beam has penetrated the vertebral canal through the interspinous and interlaminar spaces (Fig. 6). The posterior complex is usually visible as well but is generally less distinct compared with the PSO view. The articular processes and transverse processes lie in the same transverse plane, and their bony contours are usually visible lateral to the posterior and anterior complexes.

Transverse midline spinous process view

The TM spinous process view is easily recognized by the hyperechoic appearance of the tip of the spinous process and adjacent lamina and the dense acoustic dropout shadow that they cast (Fig. 7). This view is a cue to manipulate the ultrasound probe cephalad or caudad to obtain the TM interlaminar view.

RECOMMENDED PREPROCEDURAL SCANNING TECHNIQUE IN THE LUMBAR SPINE

The operator stands or sits behind the patient, who may be placed in the sitting or lateral decubitus position. The ultrasound machine is ideally placed on the opposite side of the bed from the operator.

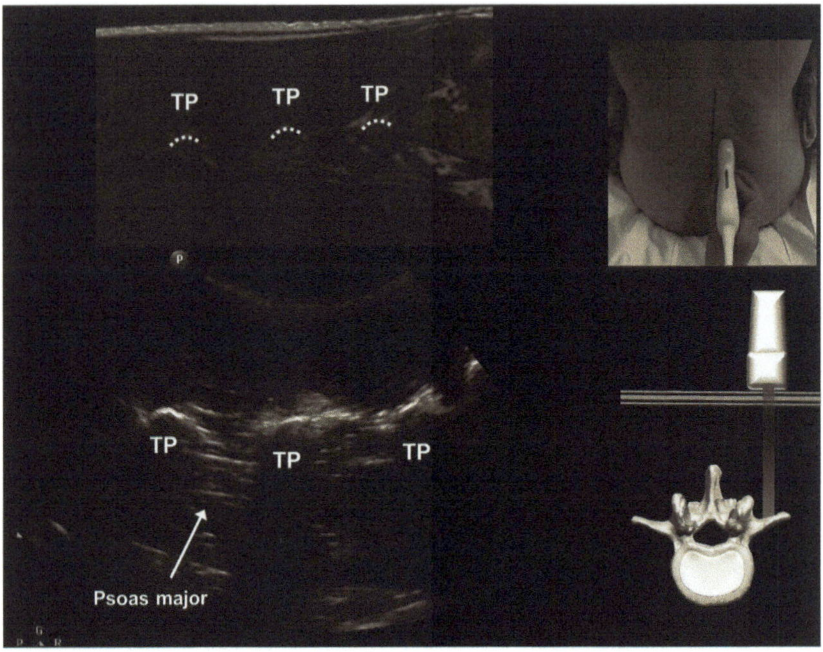

Fig. 5. Parasagittal transverse process view of the lumbar spine and corresponding magnetic resonance image (*above*). The probe is placed over the tips of the transverse processes (TP), which appear as hyperechoic curvilinear structures with fingerlike acoustic shadowing beneath. The erector spinae muscle and the psoas muscle lie superficial and deep to the transverse processes, respectively. (*Courtesy of* www.usra.ca; with permission.)

The probe is first placed in a parasagittal orientation over the sacrum of the patient. The sacrum is easily recognizable as a continuous hyperechoic line with acoustic shadowing beneath (Fig. 8). The probe is slid in a cephalad direction and angled toward the midline to obtain a PSO view of the L5–S1 interlaminar space. Successive interlaminar spaces are identified by continuing to slide the probe in a cephalad direction. Each interlaminar space should be centered on the ultrasound screen and a corresponding mark made on the patient's skin in the middle of the long edge of the probe (Fig. 9). These marks serve to confirm the identity of the intervertebral level being imaged when scanning in the transverse plane. In the event an adequate TM interlaminar view cannot be obtained, these marks indicate the approximate location of the interlaminar space and can thus guide needle insertion.

The probe is then rotated into the transverse plane and manipulated to obtain the TM interlaminar views at the relevant interspaces. Slight cephalad tilting of the probe may be required to optimize image quality in patients with limited spine flexion. When the appropriate view is obtained, skin marks made at the midpoints of the long and short edges of the probe will indicate the locations of the neuraxial midline and interlaminar space, respectively (Fig. 10).

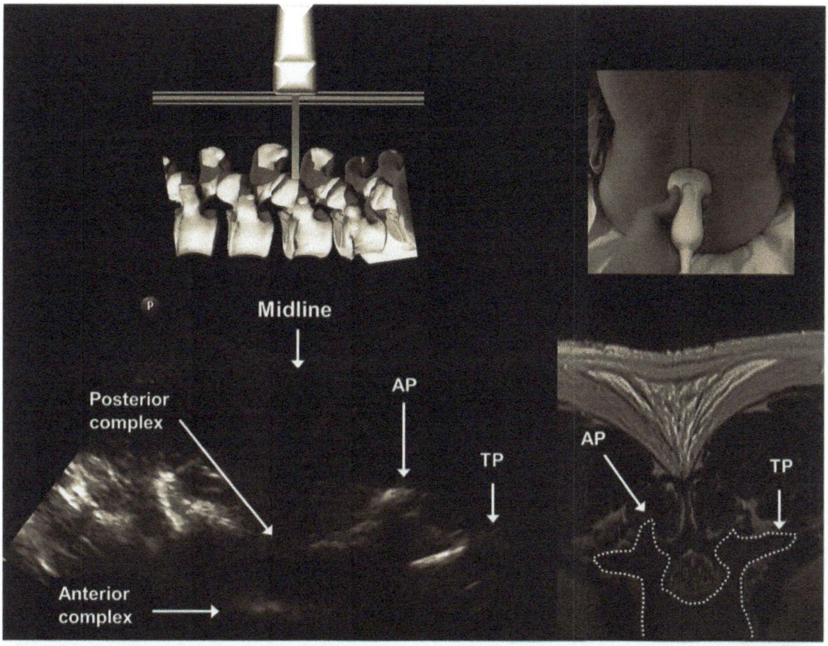

Fig. 6. Transverse midline interlaminar view of the lumbar spine and corresponding magnetic resonance imaging scan (*right*). The intrathecal space is a dark hypoechoic band sandwiched between the hyperechoic posterior and anterior complex. The transverse processes and articular processes lie in the same transverse plane and are usually visible. The ligamentum flavum, posterior epidural space, and dura usually cannot be distinguished from one another in the transverse view. The midline is indicated by the dark vertical stripe of the interspinous ligament. (*Courtesy of* www.usra.ca; with permission.)

The intersection of these 2 marks is an appropriate needle insertion point for a midline approach to the vertebral canal.

The depth to the deep aspect of the posterior complex may be measured in either the PSO or TM interlaminar view, and either correlates well with actual needle depth to the epidural and intrathecal space. The actual depth to the central neuraxial space is slightly deeper, as a slight amount of pressure is required to maintain contact between the ultrasound probe and skin surface.

Strategies in subjects with poor-quality views

Good-quality images can be difficult to obtain in certain populations, particularly the morbidly obese and elderly. In the obese patient, image quality may be improved by adjustments in gain and focus and reducing frequency to enhance penetration. Firm probe pressure may also help by enhancing skin probe contact and reducing the effective depth to the structures of interest. Experience in scanning and image interpretation will also facilitate recognition of more subtle appearances of the characteristic patterns described previously (Fig. 11).

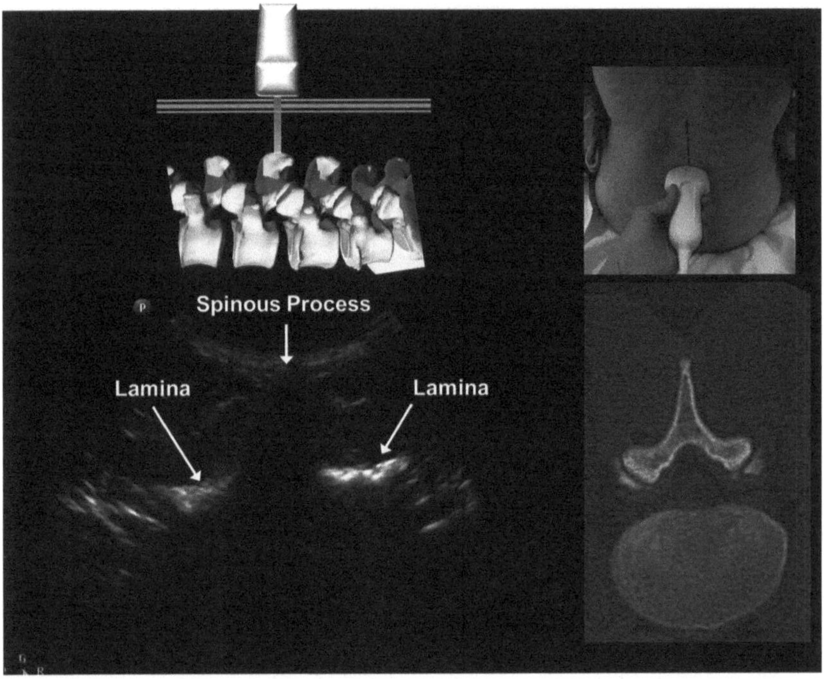

Fig. 7. Transverse midline spinous process view of the lumbar spine and corresponding computed tomography image (*right*). The tip of the spinous process and the lamina are brightly hyperechoic on ultrasound scan with pronounced acoustic shadowing that obscures all deeper structures. (*Courtesy of* www.usra.ca; with permission.)

Elderly patients may present a challenge because of narrowing of the interspinous and interlaminar spaces associated with age-related degenerative changes. Prominent spinous processes in a thinner elderly patient may hinder adequate skin probe contact and contribute to poor visualization of neuraxial structures. In such patients, a TM interlaminar view may be physically difficult or impossible to obtain, and the PSO view may be a better alternative. Contact may also be improved by using a probe with a smaller footprint.

ANATOMY AND SONOANATOMY OF THE THORACIC SPINE

There are significant differences in the morphology of the thoracic spine relative to the lumbar spine (Fig. 12). In the midthoracic spine (T5–8), the spinous processes angle steeply in a caudad direction such that the inferior border of the spinous process overlies the midpoint of the lamina below. The thoracic laminae also lie closer together, and the interlaminar spaces are, therefore, much narrower. The lower 4 thoracic vertebrae (T9–12) are similar to lumbar vertebrae in that their spinous processes are broad, flat, and only slightly angled.

A curvilinear low-frequency probe is generally recommended; however, in slimmer individuals, a linear high-frequency probe may also produce adequate

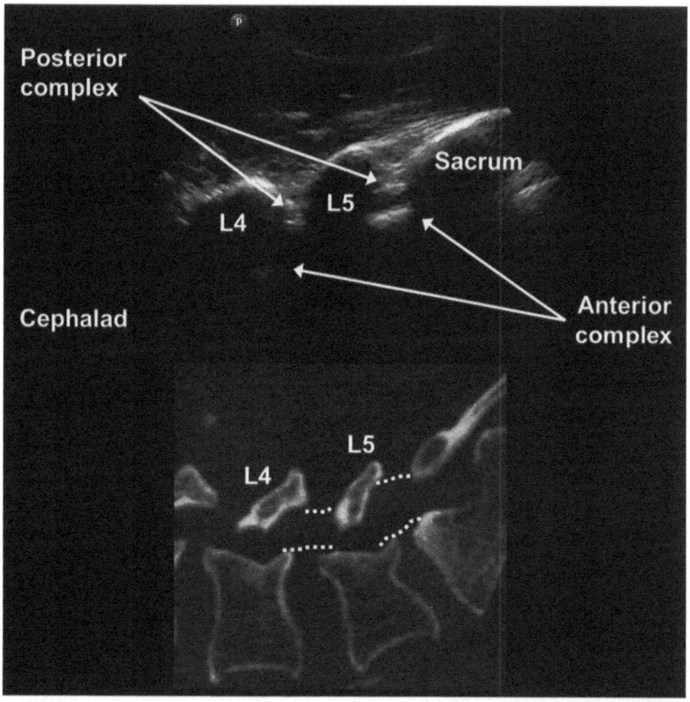

Fig. 8. Parasagittal oblique view of the L5–S1 junction and corresponding computed tomography image (*below*). The sacrum is recognizable as a horizontal hyperechoic linear structure, and the L5 lamina has the typical sawtooth appearance. The posterior and anterior complexes are visible through the intervening gap. (*Courtesy of* www.usra.ca; with permission.)

images. As in the lumbar spine, the 2 most important views are the PSO and TM interlaminar views. In the lower thoracic spine, these views are similar to those of the lumbar spine except that the interlaminar spaces tend to be narrower. The midthoracic views are quite different, however.

Parasagittal oblique view of the midthoracic spine

The midthoracic laminae appear as almost horizontal hyperechoic linear structures separated by narrow gaps, which represent the paramedian interlaminar spaces (Fig. 13). Because of the narrow interlaminar spaces, the posterior complex and anterior complex are only sometimes visible and are usually smaller and fainter than in the lumbar spine [4].

Transverse midline view of the midthoracic spine

The overlapping spinous processes in the midthoracic spine make it impossible to obtain a TM interlaminar view of posterior and anterior complexes. The visible structures are the hyperechoic bony contours of the spinous process, lamina, and transverse processes and, more laterally, the ribs and pleura (Fig. 14).

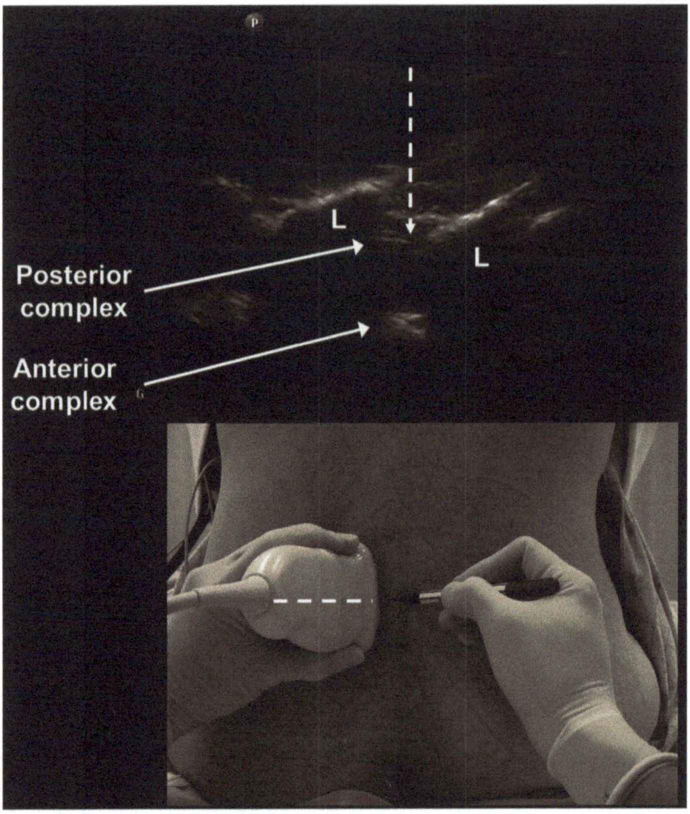

Fig. 9. In the parasagittal oblique view, each interlaminar space is centered in turn on the ultrasound screen. A corresponding skin mark is made at the midpoint of the probe's long edge to mark its position. (*Courtesy of* www.usra.ca; with permission.)

RECOMMENDED PREPROCEDURAL SCANNING TECHNIQUE IN THE THORACIC SPINE

The patient is placed in the position in which the block is to be performed, generally lateral decubitus or sitting. The interlaminar spaces are identified and marked using the PSO view in a process similar to that described for the lumbar spine. The depth to the lamina or posterior complex is measured to estimate needle depth to the epidural space. The TM view is used mainly to map and mark out the location of the neuraxial midline, particularly if it cannot be palpated or if it is distorted, for example, by scoliosis. With this additional information, the needle approach to the thoracic epidural space can be triangulated more accurately.

Identification of intervertebral level can be achieved by counting upwards from the L5–S1 junction. Alternatively, the spaces can also be counted down from T1 or up from T12, having first identified the articulation of the first rib with T1 or the 12th rib with T12, respectively.

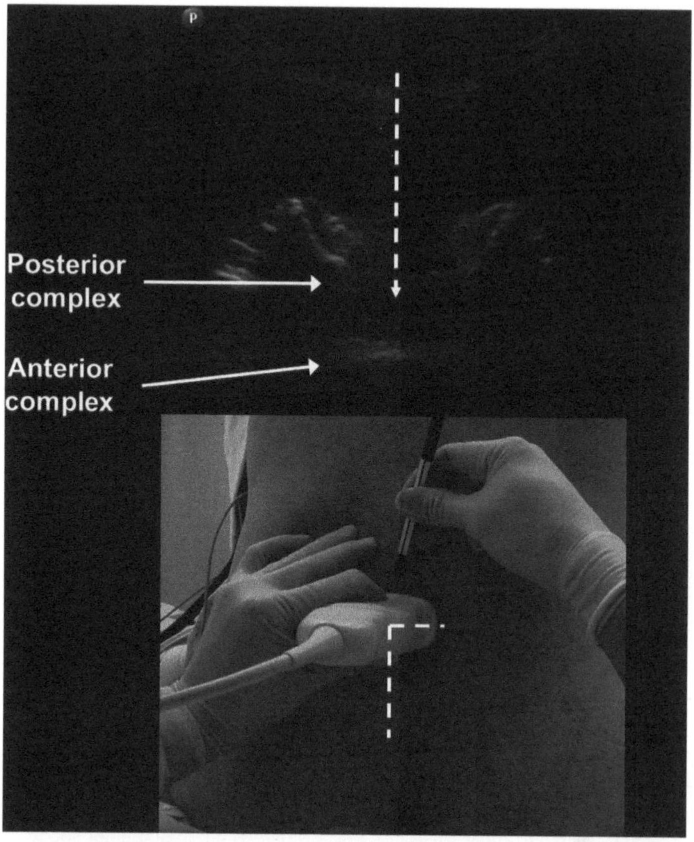

Fig. 10. In the transverse midline interlaminar view, the midline is centered on the ultrasound screen, and skin marks are made at the midpoint of the probe's long and short edges. The intersection of these 2 marks provides an appropriate needle insertion point for a midline approach to the epidural or intrathecal space at that level. (*Courtesy of* www.usra.ca; with permission.)

THE CLINICAL APPLICATION OF NEURAXIAL ULTRASOUND SCAN

Identification of specific intervertebral levels

Accurate identification of intervertebral levels is desirable in neuraxial anesthesia for reasons of efficacy (eg, ensuring congruency of epidural needle and catheter tip placement with the surgical incision) and safety (eg, avoiding conus medullaris injury in spinal anesthesia).

Lumbar spine

In the lumbar spine, clinical assessment using Tuffier's line identifies the correct intervertebral level in as few as 29% of patients compared with magnetic resonance imaging [5]. In contrast, ultrasound scan appears to be much more accurate. In a 2002 study comparing clinical assessment, ultrasound scan, and lateral spine x-ray examination [6], ultrasound scan correctly identified the

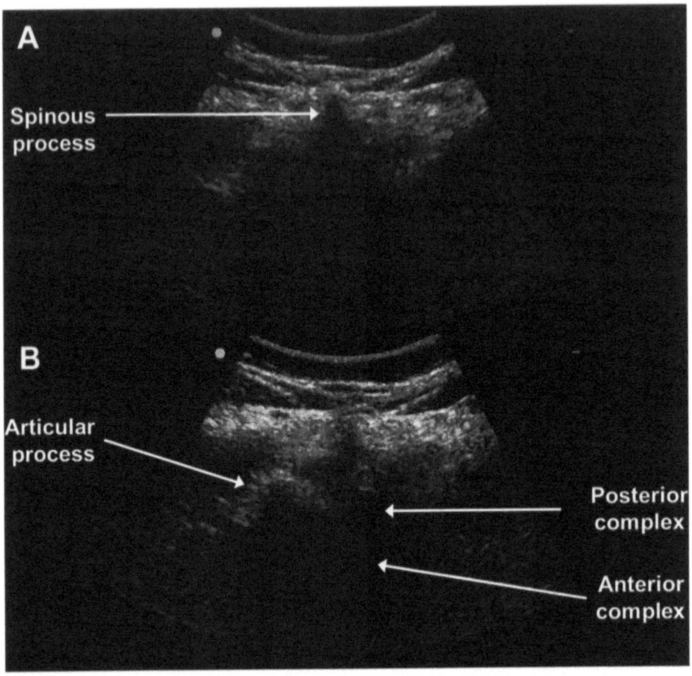

Fig. 11. An example of poor-quality transverse midline spinous process (*A*) and interlaminar (*B*) views in one individual. In the interlaminar view (*B*), the posterior and anterior complexes are only faintly hyperechoic, but nevertheless are visible, especially when contrasted with the dense acoustic shadow cast by the spinous process and lamina in (*A*). The other visual cue that (*B*) is an interlaminar view as opposed to a spinous process view is the contour of the tip of the articular process which lies in the same transverse plane as the interlaminar space. (*Courtesy of* www.usra.ca; with permission.)

L2–3 interspace or immediately adjacent spinous processes in 84% of cases compared with only 37% of the time when surface landmarks were used. The margin of error with ultrasound scan was at most either 1 space above (9%) or below (7%).

Other studies have consistently found a discrepancy between ultrasound-guided and clinical assessments of lumbar intervertebral level in 28% to 63% of patients [7–10]. More concerning is that in most cases (72%–93%) in which discrepancy was observed, the clinically identified level was 1 to 2 interspaces higher than that identified by ultrasound scan [8–10].

Thoracic spine

Surface anatomic landmark-based methods of identifying thoracic intervertebral levels have also been found to be inaccurate when referenced to the gold standard of magnetic resonance imaging or x-ray imaging [11–13]. A similar discrepancy between ultrasound identification of thoracic intervertebral level (using a counting-up method from the sacrum and 12th rib) and surface

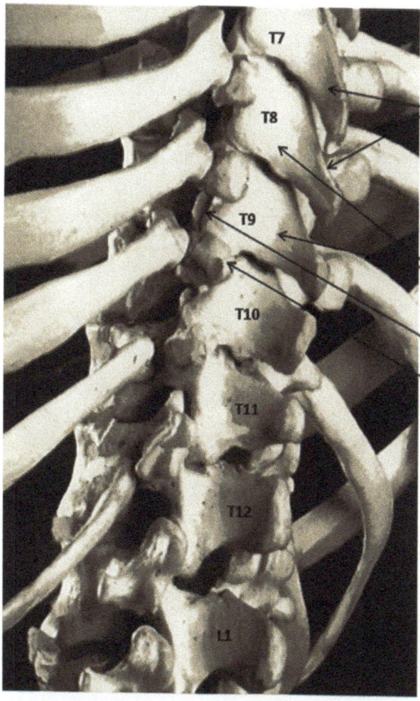

Fig. 12. The lower thoracic vertebrae (T10–T12) are similar in morphology and ultrasonographic appearance to lumbar vertebrae. The middle thoracic vertebrae have steeply sloping spinous processes that make it impossible to obtain a transverse interlaminar view. The interlaminar spaces are also small, and the paramedian sagittal oblique view into the vertebral canal is limited as a result. (*Courtesy of* www.usra.ca; with permission.)

anatomic landmarks (vertebral prominens for C7 and inferior angle of the scapula for T7) has been shown [14]. Ultrasound scan is likely to be more accurate than surface landmarks; however; this has not been verified against a gold standard imaging technique.

Measuring depth to the epidural or intrathecal space

Lumbar spine

Excellent correlation between ultrasound-measured depth and actual needle insertion depth to the epidural and intrathecal space has been found in numerous studies, regardless of whether the measurements were made using sagittal, PSO, or TM views [7,15–20]. In addition, the difference between measured and actual depth in most studies is small (approximately 0.5 cm), with ultrasound scan usually underestimating needle depth because of the slightly varying amounts of pressure applied to the probe to main adequate skin surface contact.

Thoracic spine

Two studies compared ultrasound-measured depth in the PSO view with actual needle insertion depth during thoracic epidural anesthesia [21,22]. Good

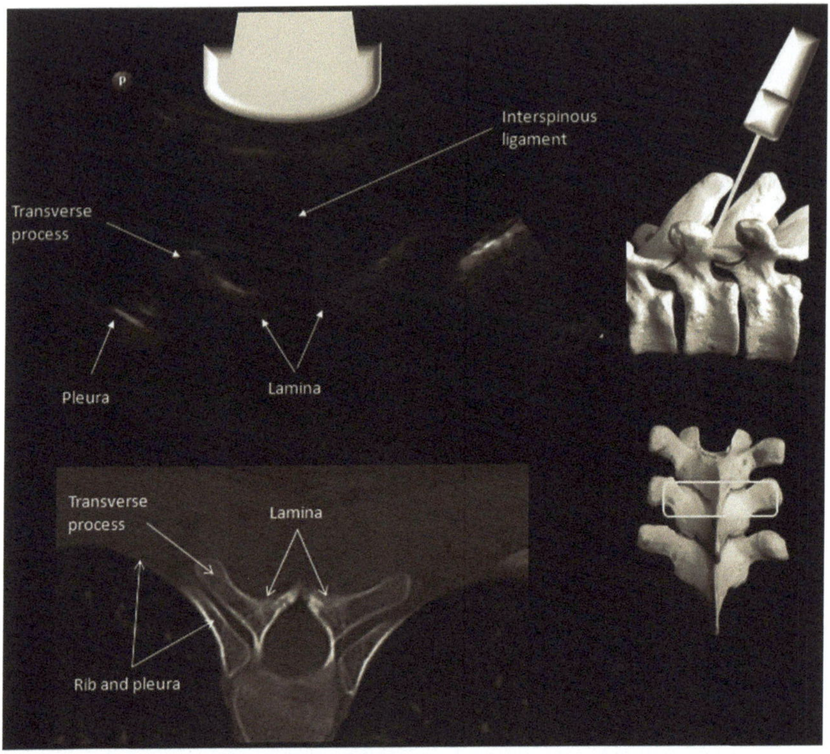

Fig. 13. Transverse view of the midthoracic spine and corresponding computed tomography image. An interlaminar view into the vertebral canal cannot be obtained because of the steeply sloping spinous processes and overlapping laminae. (*Courtesy of* www.usra.ca; with permission.)

correlation was observed in both studies with ultrasound scan tending to underestimate actual depth by only 0.5 to 0.7 cm.

Improving the clinical efficacy of neuraxial blockade

Three randomized, controlled trials (RCTs) suggest that ultrasound improves the clinical efficacy of obstetric epidural analgesia compared with surface landmark-guided neuraxial techniques [15,16,23]. In 2 of the studies, in which a single experienced operator performed both the scan and the block, there was a decrease in postblock pain scores in the ultrasound-guided groups, which may be partly explained by reductions in asymmetric and patchy blocks [15,23]. There was also a significant reduction in the rate of incomplete analgesia (2% vs 8%) in one study [23] and epidural failure (0% vs 5.6%) in the other [15]. More recently, Vallejo and colleagues [16] randomly assigned 15 first-year anesthesia trainees to perform 370 labor epidurals with or without the assistance of a preprocedural ultrasound scan performed by a single experienced operator. The epidural failure rate in this study was again significantly lower in the ultrasound-guided patient group (1.6% vs 5.5%).

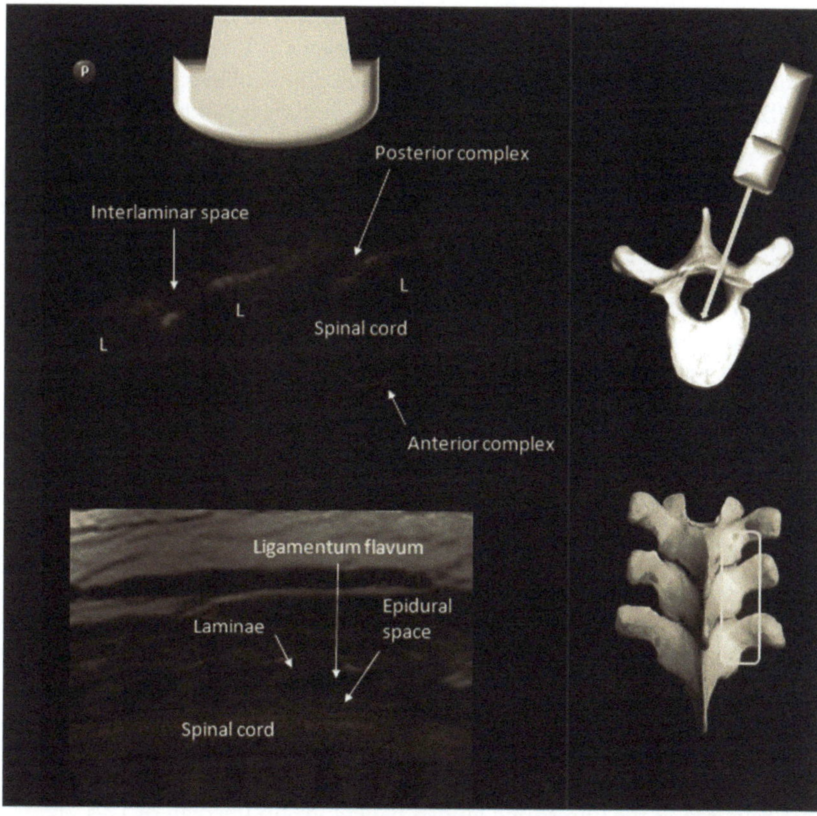

Fig. 14. Paramedian sagittal oblique view of the midthoracic spine and corresponding magnetic resonance image. Despite the narrow interlaminar space, it is possible to visualize the posterior and anterior complex at one or more levels. At a minimum, the location of the interlaminar space can be determined by the dip or gap between successive laminae (L). Note that the spinal cord is hypoechoic and cannot be distinguished from the surrounding cerebrospinal fluid. (*Courtesy of* www.usra.ca; with permission.)

A recent systematic review and meta-analysis also suggest that ultrasound guidance results in greater block success. Shaikh and colleagues [24] identified 14 publications involving 1334 patients that compared ultrasound-guided and non–ultrasound-guided neuraxial procedures, including diagnostic lumbar punctures and epidural and spinal anesthetics. Overall, ultrasound guidance reduced the risk of procedure failure by 79%, with a number needed to treat to avoid 1 failure of 16. Subgroup analysis confirmed that this effect was equally strong for both intrathecal (relative risk, 0.19) and epidural (relative risk, 0.23) procedures.

Improving technical performance of neuraxial blockade

Lumbar spine

Numerous case reports show that ultrasound scan facilitates neuraxial blockade in patients with difficult spinal anatomy, including marked obesity [25,26], previous spinal surgery [27–29], and spinal deformity [30]. In addition, 3 RCTs support its use in this context. Grau and colleagues [15] randomly assigned 72 parturients with a history of difficult epidural, kyphoscoliosis, or body mass index (BMI) greater than 33 kg/m^2 to surface landmark-guided or ultrasound-guided epidural placement by a single experienced operator. Successful epidural needle placement in the surface landmark-guided group required significantly more puncture attempts compared with the ultrasound-guided group (2.6 vs 1.5). Chin and colleagues [31] studied an older population of 120 orthopedic patients with BMI greater than 35 kg/m^2, scoliosis, or previous lumbar surgery, and randomly assigned them to either surface landmark-guided or ultrasound-guided spinal anesthesia by one of several experienced operators. Use of ultrasound scan halved the median number of needle insertions from 2 to 1 and significantly reduced the need for additional needle passes (6 vs 13). Most recently, Sahin and colleagues [32] studied a population of 100 parturients undergoing elective cesarean section, dividing them into nonobese (BMI $<$30 kg/m^2) and obese (BMI $\geq$30 kg/m^2) subgroups and randomly assigning them to surface landmark-guided or ultrasound-guided spinal anesthesia. There was a higher incidence of block success within 2 needle passes when ultrasound scan was used in both subgroups (obese, 88% vs 52%; nonobese, 80% vs 52%).

Ultrasound guidance may improve the technical performance of obstetric epidural anesthesia even in patients without predictors of technical difficulty. In an RCT of 300 parturients, Grau and colleagues [23] reported that the mean number of needle passes was significantly lower with the use of ultrasound compared with surface landmarks alone (1.3 vs 2.2). Vallejo and colleagues [16], in their afore-mentioned study, similarly found that fewer insertion attempts were required in the ultrasound-guided patient group (median of 1 vs 2).

The benefit in spinal anesthesia is less clear, however. In 150 parturients undergoing elective cesarean section, all of whom had easily palpable landmarks and BMI less than 35 kg/m^2, spinal anesthesia was performed by 3 experienced anesthesiologists using either the surface landmark or ultrasound-guided technique [33]. There were no significant differences in needle passes (mean 2.0 vs 1.7) or block performance time (52.5 vs 41.4 seconds). This is in contrast to the findings of Sahin and colleagues [32], who found significant benefits of ultrasound scan in their nonobese subgroup of patients.

Thoracic spine

Ultrasound scan is expected to have a similar benefit in improving technical performance of thoracic epidurals; however, currently, there is limited evidence to support this finding. In a case series of mid-to-lower thoracic epidural insertion in 35 healthy adult patients, the PSO view on ultrasound scan was used to determine the optimal needle insertion point for a paramedian approach [22]. Successful insertion was achieved with 1 skin puncture on average and within 2 or fewer redirections in 88% of cases. Other case reports indicate that ultrasound scan is useful in evaluating the abnormal anatomy and in determining the optimal needle insertion site and trajectory in scoliosis patients [34,35].

Predicting the ease of performance of neuraxial blockade

Ultrasound scan may also be used as an evaluation tool to guide preanesthetic planning [30]. The premise is that the quality of ultrasonographic views should correspond to ease of needle insertion, as both rely on the presence of a suitable soft tissue window. Weed and colleagues [36] performed ultrasound scans using the PSO view in 60 orthopedic patients undergoing spinal anesthesia. Anesthesiologists performing the block were blinded to the ultrasound scan. The positive predictive value of a poor-quality image in the PSO view for difficult spinal anesthesia was 82.3%, and the negative predictive value 67.4%.

In a similar study, Chin and colleagues [37] attempted to predict ease of spinal anesthesia in 100 orthopedic patients using both the PSO and TM views. Anesthesiologists performing the spinal anesthetic were blinded to the ultrasound scan. If both posterior and anterior complexes were visible (a good-quality view) in the TM view, the positive predictive value for absence of technical difficulty at that level was 85%. The PSO view was a less useful predictor, which may reflect the use of a midline as opposed to paramedian needle approach. In some patients, spinal anesthesia was challenging despite a good-quality TM view. The authors hypothesized that this could have been avoided if the information from the ultrasound scan had been used to guide the spinal procedure, as would be the case in the clinical setting.

Reducing the risk of adverse outcomes

Ultrasound scan may reduce adverse effects related to epidural analgesia, including postpartum headache and backache [23]. The ability to measure depth to the epidural space may also reduce the risk of inadvertent dural puncture.

Neurologic injury and spinal hematoma are rare but dreaded complications of neuraxial blockade. Because of the low baseline incidence (<0.001%), it is not surprising that strong evidence for a reduction in risk with ultrasound scan is lacking. Nevertheless, there are sound reasons why ultrasound guidance might increase safety. Both spinal hematoma and permanent neurologic sequelae have been associated with difficult block performance [1–3]. The recent meta-analysis by Shaikh and colleagues [24] reported a 73% reduction in the risk of traumatic procedures with ultrasound guidance, which further supports a potential safety advantage. Conus medullaris injury during spinal anesthesia is another rare but devastating complication of spinal anesthesia [38,39] that could be prevented by the improved accuracy of intervertebral level identification with ultrasound scan.

ACQUIRING COMPETENCY IN NEURAXIAL ULTRASOUND SCAN

The learning curve in neuraxial ultrasound scan

Neuraxial ultrasound scan can be challenging because of to the relatively complex sonoanatomy of the spine, and significant training and experience may be required for its benefits to be fully realized.

Two studies using cumulative-sum analysis examined the learning curve of anesthesiologists with no prior experience in neuraxial ultrasound scan [40,41].

In the first, 2 anesthesiologists attempted to identify a specific lumbar spinous process, which was then verified by computed tomography [40]. The first subject required 36 procedures to achieve the predetermined accuracy level of 90% successful identifications, whereas the second subject required 22 procedures. In the second study, 18 anesthesiologists were provided with comprehensive didactic and hands-on training [41]. The subjects were evaluated several days later on 3 tasks: identification of a specific intervertebral level, marking an optimal needle insertion point, and measuring depth to the epidural space. Participants were allowed a maximum of 20 trials of each task, and only 27% of candidates achieved competence in intervertebral-level identification. No candidate achieved competence in the other 2 tasks. It should be noted, however, that only 61% of subjects completed 20 trials. The authors also remarked that most of the errors stemmed from imprecision in skin marking and depth measurement and could have been avoided with greater attention to detail.

These small studies suggest that each component of the neuraxial ultrasound scan skillset may have a different learning curve and that the number of attempts to achieve competency is likely to vary widely between individuals. Although the optimal number is unclear, it would seem that experience of at least 40 cases may be required.

Training strategies in neuraxial ultrasound scan

Familiarization with the gross anatomy and sonoanatomy of the spine is essential before performing the ultrasound-guided neuraxial blockade in clinical practice. This can be done by reviewing didactic material [42–44], attending educational workshops, and repetitive practice on a water-based spine phantom or human volunteers.

An additional educational resource is an interactive 3-dimensional digital spine model available online at http://www.usra.ca/vspine.php. When combined with a multimodal educational strategy that included didactic lectures, cadaveric dissections, and hands-on scanning of volunteers, exposure to this model improved the ability of junior residents to perform a preprocedural ultrasound scan [45]. More work is needed to confirm persistence of the learning effect and if this multimodal approach translates into effective clinical performance.

REAL-TIME ULTRASOUND-GUIDED NEURAXIAL BLOCK

Real-time ultrasound-guided spinal or epidural anesthesia has been reported in a small number of case series [46–50]. Most descriptions involve a single operator, freehand technique which requires expertise in probe and needle handling. The largest series, using an in-plane needle approach and modified PSO view, reported a success rate of 97% and a mean block performance time of 8 minutes [50]. It is uncertain if this more complex approach has advantages over preprocedural ultrasound imaging or the surface landmark-guided technique.

More recently, the application of a needle tracking ultrasound system to real-time ultrasound-guided spinal anesthesia has been explored [51–54]. Displaying an overlay of needle position and trajectory on the ultrasound screen removes some of the challenges of the freehand technique. Nevertheless, it remains a cumbersome technique with limitations, including accuracy of the overlay and the need to use a large (17G) proprietary introducer needle.

SUMMARY

Preprocedural ultrasound imaging can clearly reduce the technical difficulty of lumbar neuraxial blockade, particularly in patients with challenging anatomy, and may also improve clinical efficacy. Evidence for its utility in thoracic epidurals is more limited, but ultrasound scan has been found to reliably estimate depth to the epidural space and to accurately determine the correct intervertebral level in both the lumbar and thoracic spine.

Currently, the efficacy of the conventional surface landmark-guided technique in most patients means that ultrasound-guided neuraxial blockade is unlikely to become routine. A pilot survey of anesthesiologists from selected international centers reported that neuraxial ultrasound scan is most commonly used to facilitate training and learning in selected cases in which difficulty is anticipated and when difficult insertion is encountered [55]. In this respect, it is analogous to advanced airway management techniques such as videolaryngoscopy or fiberoptic intubation. As with any advanced technique, however, competency in ultrasound-guided neuraxial blockade should ideally be acquired by accumulating experience in normal patients before encountering a clinically difficult scenario.

References

[1] Drug safety communications: updated recommendations to decrease risk of spinal column bleeding and paralysis in patients on low molecular weight heparins (Safety Announcement). c2013. [Internet]. Available at: http://www.fda.gov/downloads/Drugs/DrugSafety/UCM373735.pdf. Accessed May 1, 2014.

[2] Vandermeulen EP, Van Aken H, Vermylen J. Anticoagulants and spinal-epidural anesthesia. Anesth Analg 1994;79:1165–77.

[3] de Sèze M, Sztark F, Janvier G, et al. Severe and long-lasting complications of the nerve root and spinal cord after central neuraxial blockade. Anesth Analg 2007;104:975–9.

[4] Avramescu S, Arzola C, Tharmaratnam U, et al. Sonoanatomy of the thoracic spine in adult volunteers. Reg Anesth Pain Med 2012;37:349–53.

[5] Broadbent CR, Maxwell WB, Ferrie R, et al. Ability of anaesthetists to identify a marked lumbar interspace. Anaesthesia 2000;55:1122–6.

[6] Furness G, Reilly MP, Kuchi S. An evaluation of ultrasound imaging for identification of lumbar intervertebral level. Anaesthesia 2002;57:277–80.

[7] Chin KJ, Perlas A, Singh M, et al. An ultrasound-assisted approach facilitates spinal anesthesia for total joint arthroplasty. Can J Anaesth 2009;56:643–50.

[8] Locks Gde F, Almeida MC, Pereira AA. Use of the ultrasound to determine the level of lumbar puncture in pregnant women. Rev Bras Anestesiol 2010;60:13–9.

[9] Schlotterbeck H, Schaeffer R, Dow WA, et al. Ultrasonographic control of the puncture level for lumbar neuraxial block in obstetric anaesthesia. Br J Anaesth 2008;100:230–4.

[10] Whitty R, Moore M, Macarthur A. Identification of the lumbar interspinous spaces: palpation versus ultrasound. Anesth Analg 2008;106:538–40.

[11] Teoh DA, Santosham KL, Lydell CC, et al. Surface anatomy as a guide to vertebral level for thoracic epidural placement. Anesth Analg 2009;108:1705–7.

[12] Holmaas G, Frederiksen D, Ulvik A, et al. Identification of thoracic intervertebral spaces by means of surface anatomy: a magnetic resonance imaging study. Acta Anaesthesiol Scand 2006;50:368–73.

[13] Stonelake PS, Burwell RG, Webb JK. Variation in vertebral levels of the vertebra prominens and sacral dimples in subjects with scoliosis. J Anat 1988;159:165–72.

[14] Arzola C, Avramescu S, Tharmaratnam U, et al. Identification of cervicothoracic intervertebral spaces by landmarks and ultrasound. Can J Anaesth 2011;58:1069–74.

[15] Grau T, Leipold RW, Conradi R, et al. Ultrasound control for presumed difficult epidural puncture. Acta Anaesthesiol Scand 2001;45:766–71.

[16] Vallejo MC, Phelps AL, Singh S, et al. Ultrasound decreases the failed labor epidural rate in resident trainees. Int J Obstet Anesth 2010;19:373–8.

[17] Arzola C, Davies S, Rofaeel A, et al. Ultrasound using the transverse approach to the lumbar spine provides reliable landmarks for labor epidurals. Anesth Analg 2007;104:1188–92.

[18] Balki M, Lee Y, Halpern S, et al. Ultrasound imaging of the lumbar spine in the transverse plane: the correlation between estimated and actual depth to the epidural space in obese parturients. Anesth Analg 2009;108:1876–81.

[19] Tran D, Kamani AA, Lessoway VA, et al. Preinsertion paramedian ultrasound guidance for epidural anesthesia. Anesth Analg 2009;109:661–7.

[20] Sahota JS, Carvalho JC, Balki M, et al. Ultrasound estimates for midline epidural punctures in the obese parturient: paramedian sagittal oblique is comparable to transverse median plane. Anesth Analg 2013;116:829–35.

[21] Rasoulian A, Lohser J, Najafi M, et al. Utility of prepuncture ultrasound for localization of the thoracic epidural space. Can J Anaesth 2011;58:815–23.

[22] Salman A, Arzola C, Tharmaratnam U, et al. Ultrasound imaging of the thoracic spine in paramedian sagittal oblique plane. Reg Anesth Pain Med 2011;36:542–7.

[23] Grau T, Leipold RW, Conradi R, et al. Efficacy of ultrasound imaging in obstetric epidural anesthesia. J Clin Anesth 2002;14:169–75.

[24] Shaikh F, Brzezinsi J, Alexander S, et al. Ultrasound imaging for lumbar punctures and epidural catheterisations: systematic review and meta-analysis. BMJ 2013;346:f1720–31.

[25] O'Donnell D, Prasad A, Perlas A. Ultrasound-assisted spinal anesthesia in obese patients. Can J Anaesth 2009;56:982–3.

[26] Whitty RJ, Maxwell CV, Carvalho JC. Complications of neuraxial anesthesia in an extreme morbidly obese patient for Cesarean section. Int J Obstet Anesth 2007;16:139–44.

[27] Costello JF, Balki M. Cesarean delivery under ultrasound-guided spinal anesthesia in a parturient with poliomyelitis and Harrington instrumentation. Can J Anaesth 2008;55:606–11.

[28] Prasad GA, Tumber PS, Lupu CM. Ultrasound guided spinal anesthesia. Can J Anaesth 2008;55:716–7.

[29] Chin KJ, Macfarlane AJ, Chan V, et al. The use of ultrasound to facilitate spinal anesthesia in a patient with previous lumbar laminectomy and fusion: a case report. J Clin Ultrasound 2009;37:482–5.

[30] Chin KJ, Chan V. Ultrasonography as a preoperative assessment tool: predicting the feasibility of central neuraxial blockade. Anesth Analg 2010;110:252–3.

[31] Chin KJ, Perlas A, Chan V, et al. Ultrasound imaging facilitates spinal anesthesia in adults with difficult surface anatomic landmarks. Anesthesiology 2011;115:94–101.

[32] Sahin T, Balaban O, Sahin L. A randomized controlled comparison of presinsertion ultrasound guidance for spinal anesthesia in pregnancy; outcomes among obese and lean parturients. J Anesth 2014;28(3):413–9.

[33] Ansari T, Yousef A, El Gamassy A, et al. Ultrasound-guided spinal anesthesia in obstetrics: is there an advantage over the landmark technique in patients with easily palpable spines? Int J Obstet Anesth 2014;23(3):213–6.

[34] McLeod A, Roche A, Fennelly M. Case series: ultrasonography may assist epidural insertion in scoliosis patients. Can J Anaesth 2005;52:717–20.
[35] Pandin P, Haentjens L, Salengros JC, et al. Combined ultrasound and nerve stimulation-guided thoracic epidural catheter placement for analgesia following anterior spine fusion in scoliosis. Pain Pract 2009;9:230–4.
[36] Weed JT, Taenzer AH, Finkel KJ, et al. Evaluation of pre-procedure ultrasound examination as a screening tool for difficult spinal anaesthesia. Anaesthesia 2011;66:925–30.
[37] Chin KJ, Ramlogan R, Arzola C, et al. The utility of ultrasound imaging in predicting ease of performance of spinal anesthesia in an orthopedic patient population. Reg Anesth Pain Med 2013;38:34–8.
[38] Hamandi K, Mottershead J, Lewis T, et al. Irreversible damage to the spinal cord following spinal anesthesia. Neurology 2002;59:624–66.
[39] Reynolds F. Damage to the conus medullaris following spinal anaesthesia. Anaesthesia 2001;56:235–47.
[40] Halpern SH, Banerjee A, Stocche R, et al. The use of ultrasound for lumbar spinous process identification: a pilot study. Can J Anaesth 2010;57:817–22.
[41] Margarido CB, Arzola C, Balki M, et al. Anesthesiologists' learning curves for ultrasound assessment of the lumbar spine. Can J Anaesth 2010;57:120–6.
[42] Chin KJ, Karmakar MK, Peng P. Ultrasonography of the adult thoracic and lumbar spine for central neuraxial blockade. Anesthesiology 2011;114:1459–85.
[43] Balki M. Locating the epidural space in obstetric patients-ultrasound a useful tool: continuing professional development. Can J Anaesth 2011;57:1111–26.
[44] Karmakar MK, Li X, Kwok WH, et al. Sonoanatomy relevant for ultrasound-guided central neuraxial blocks via the paramedian approach in the lumbar region. Br J Radiol 2012;85: e262–9.
[45] Niazi AU, Tait G, Carvalho JCA, et al. The use of an online three-dimensional model improves performance in ultrasound scanning of the spine: a randomized trial. Can J Anaesth 2013;60:458–64.
[46] Karmakar MK, Li X, Ho AM, et al. Real-time ultrasound-guided paramedian epidural access: evaluation of a novel in-plane technique. Br J Anaesth 2009;102:845–54.
[47] Chin KJ, Chan VW, Ramlogan R, et al. Real-time ultrasound-guided spinal anesthesia in patients with challenging spinal anatomy: two case reports. Acta Anaesthesiol Scand 2010;54:252–5.
[48] Tran D, Kamani AA, Al-Attas E, et al. Single-operator real-time ultrasound-guidance to aim and insert a lumbar epidural needle. Can J Anaesth 2010;57:313–21.
[49] Lee PJ, Tang R, Sawka A, et al. Brief report: real-time ultrasound-guided spinal anesthesia using Taylor's approach. Anesth Analg 2011;112:1236–8.
[50] Conroy PH, Luyet C, McCartney CJ, et al. Real-time ultrasound-guided spinal anaesthesia: a prospective observational study of a new approach. Anesthesiol Res Pract 2013;2013: 525818.
[51] Brinkmann S, Tang R, Vaghadia H, et al. Assessment of a real-time ultrasound-guided spinal technique using SonixGPS in human cadavers. Can J Anaesth 2012;59:1156–7.
[52] Wong SW, Niazi AU, Chin KJ, et al. Real-time ultrasound-guided spinal anesthesia using the SonixGPS. Can J Anaesth 2013;60:50.
[53] Brinkmann S, Tang R, Sawka A, et al. Single-operator real-time ultrasound-guided spinal injection using SonixGPS: a case series. Can J Anaesth 2013;60:896–901.
[54] Niazi AU, Chin KJ, Jin R, et al. Real-time ultrasound-guided spinal anesthesia using the SonixGPS ultrasound guidance system: a feasibility study. Acta Anaesthesiol Scand 2014;58(7):875–81.
[55] Paech MJ, Hillyard SG. New techniques and technologies for obstetric anaesthesia. Int J Obstet Anesth 2012;21:101–2.

Advances in Anesthesia 32 (2014) 171–190

ADVANCES IN ANESTHESIA

Perioperative Management of the Patient with Diabetes

Timothy B. Curry, MD, PhD[a,b,*], Daniel R. Brown, MD, PhD[a,c]

[a]Department of Anesthesiology, Mayo Clinic, 200 First Street Southwest, Rochester, MN 55905, USA; [b]Department of Physiology and Biomedical Engineering, Mayo Clinic, 200 First Street Southwest, Rochester, MN 55905, USA; [c]Division of Anesthesiology Critical Care, Mayo Clinic, 200 First Street Southwest, Rochester, MN 55905, USA

Keywords

• Diabetes • Glycemic control • Insulin • Hypoglycemia • Hyperglycemia

Key points

- Diabetes is common in patients undergoing surgical procedures and is an important risk factor for adverse perioperative outcomes.
- Patients with type 1 diabetes must be provided with a continuous source of insulin at all times.
- For most patients with diabetes, glucose lower than 180 mg/dL (10 mmol/L) is a reasonable target.
- Insulin therapy resulting in hypoglycemia is associated with worse outcomes.
- Any efforts to prevent or treat hyperglycemia must include strategies to prevent, monitor for, and treat hypoglycemia.
- A multidisciplinary perioperative glycemic control program can result in safe and effective care.

INTRODUCTION

Background

The term "diabetes" describes several diseases of abnormal carbohydrate metabolism that are characterized by hyperglycemia, along with a relative or an absolute impairment of insulin secretion and varying degrees of peripheral resistance to the metabolic effects of insulin. According to the Centers for Disease Control and Prevention, the prevalence of diabetes in the United States among individuals 20 years or older is now approximately 8.3% and rates among those older than 65 years is greater than 25%. The economic burden

*Corresponding author. Department of Anesthesiology, Mayo Clinic, 200 First Street Southwest, Rochester, MN 55905. *E-mail address*: Curry.Timothy@mayo.edu

0737-6146/14/$ – see front matter
http://dx.doi.org/10.1016/j.aan.2014.08.001

of diabetes has been estimated at $245 billion in the United States alone, with $176 billion being direct medical costs, an increase of 41% compared with 2007 estimates [1]. The impact of diabetes on health systems is expected to grow, as rates of obesity and prediabetes, major risk factors for the development of diabetes, increase.

Diabetes is overrepresented in patients undergoing anesthesia compared with the general population. Approximately 14% of noncardiac surgical patients carry the diagnosis of diabetes. In patients undergoing cardiac surgery, some reports suggest more than 30% have diabetes [2]. Additionally, a significant number of patients who require surgery are diabetic, but have not been formally diagnosed [2–5]. Diabetes is an independent risk factor for adverse outcomes after surgery [6–8], and diabetes and prediabetes are risk factors for perioperative hyperglycemia and hypoglycemia [9–11]. Thus, the perioperative management of patients with diabetes is a modifiable risk factor and is of significant importance to patients and health care systems. This importance has contributed to perioperative glycemic management being identified as a quality metric by multiple patient advocacy groups, as well as payers. This review describes current classifications and treatments of diabetes, discusses the anesthetic implications of diabetes and the current literature addressing perioperative glycemic control and outcomes, and provides recommendations for developing a perioperative glycemic management program.

Classification of diabetes

Diabetes is classified into 4 clinical categories with a range of insulin requirements and sensitivities (Fig. 1) [12].

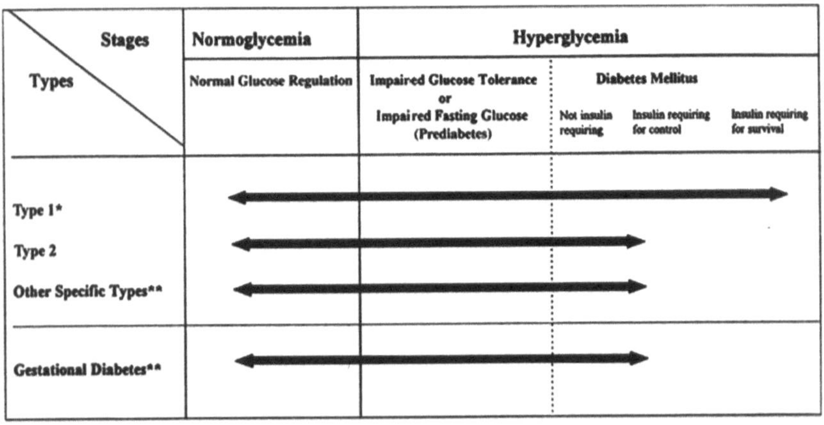

Fig. 1. Disorders of glycemia: etiologic types and stages. *Even after presenting in ketoacidosis, these patients can briefly return to normoglycemia without requiring continuous therapy (ie, "honeymoon" remission); **in rare instances, patients in these categories (eg, Vacor toxicity, type 1 diabetes presenting in pregnancy) may require insulin for survival. (*From* American Diabetes Association. Diagnosis and classification of diabetes mellitus. Diabetes Care 2013;36(Suppl 1):S68; with permission.)

Type 1 diabetes

Type 1 diabetes accounts for 5% to 10% of patients with diabetes and is usually due to autoimmune-mediated destruction of pancreatic β-cells, leading to an absolute insulin deficiency and requirement for exogenous insulin for survival. The disease is often diagnosed during childhood, although a minority of patients present as adults and are considered to have adult-onset type 1 diabetes. The presenting symptom of type 1 diabetes may be ketoacidosis but in other patients fasting, hyperglycemia occurs first, with ketoacidosis only occurring during times of stress.

Type 2 diabetes

Type 2 diabetes is the most common type of diabetes, accounting for more than 90% of patients with diabetes [12]. The prevalence of type 2 diabetes has tripled in the United States since 1980 [13]. It is characterized by varying degrees of a combination of insulin deficiency and resistance of tissues to the actions of insulin. Type 2 diabetes is closely associated with aging and obesity and is often accompanied by a cluster of risk factors for cardiovascular disease known as the metabolic syndrome [14]. Previous terms for type 2 diabetes have included non–insulin-dependent diabetes mellitus and adult-onset diabetes. However, it is now recognized that patients with type 2 diabetes may require insulin for glycemic control, can present with ketoacidosis during periods of stress, and the prevalence of type 2 diabetes in children is a growing public health problem, making these terms obsolete [15].

Gestational diabetes

Diabetes diagnosed during pregnancy that is clearly not overt diabetes is referred to as gestational diabetes. Gestational diabetes is due to an inadequate increase in insulin secretion to compensate for the decrease in insulin sensitivity that accompanies pregnancy. Although 90% of diabetes during pregnancy is gestational, the number of pregnant women with type 2 diabetes who become pregnant is increasing rapidly [16]. Differentiating between the 2 types of diabetes may be difficult, but diagnostic criteria for gestational diabetes versus overt diabetes during pregnancy have been developed [12].

Other forms of diabetes

Genetic defects in insulin action, pancreatic disease (eg, cystic fibrosis, pancreatitis, pancreatectomy), other endocrinopathies (Cushing syndrome), and drugs or chemicals (corticosteroids) may also cause diabetes. Although these causes may have other important implications for anesthesia and perioperative management, the treatment of these forms of diabetes still centers on supplementing deficient insulin states and controlling hyperglycemia, as in diabetes mellitus types 1 and 2.

Prediabetes

Impaired fasting glucose (IFG) and impaired glucose tolerance (IGT) are risks factors for both the development of diabetes and cardiovascular disease and are sometimes referred to as prediabetes (Table 1). Additionally, A1C levels below

Table 1
Diagnostic criteria for prediabetes and diabetes

	A1C (%)	FPG	OGTT	RPG
Normal	<5.7	<100 mg/dL (5.6 mmol/L)	<140 mg/dL (7.8 mmol/L)	
Prediabetes[a]	5.7–6.4	100–125 mg/dL (5.6–6.9 mmol/L)	140–199 mg/dL (7.8–11 mmol/L)	
Diabetes	≥6.5	≥126 mg/dL (7 mmol/L)	≥200 mg/dL (11.1 mmol/L)	≥200 mg/dL (11.1 mmol/L)
Gestational diabetes		92–125 mg/dL (5.1–6.9 mmol/L)	153–199 mg/dL (8.5–11 mmol/L)	

Abbreviations: A1C, glycosylated hemoglobin; FPG, fasting plasma glucose; OGTT, 2-hour oral glucose (75 g) tolerance test; RPG, random plasma glucose.

[a]Impaired fasting glucose, glucose intolerance, or at-risk for diabetes may also be used, depending on criteria.

Data from American Diabetes Association. Standards of medical care in diabetes–2014. Diabetes Care 2014;37 Suppl 1:S17.

the cutoff for diabetes but above normal levels is also a risk factor for developing diabetes and cardiovascular disease. This information may be useful for risk stratification and is used to identify patients in whom preventative strategies should be initiated.

Diagnosis

The prevalence of undiagnosed diabetes in surgical patients is considerable [2–5]. Thus, the perioperative period represents an important opportunity for making the diagnosis of diabetes. This is important, as proper management of diabetes improves long-term patient outcomes, such as renal and cardiovascular morbidity. Traditionally, the diagnosis of diabetes has been based on plasma glucose criteria, both fasting or during an oral glucose tolerance test. More recently, glycosylated hemoglobin (as defined by the hemoglobin A1C percentage) has been advocated for both the diagnosis of diabetes and monitoring the effectiveness of disease management, as this value reflects the past several months of glucose control (see Table 1) [12]. Patients with prediabetes (see Table 1) are also at increased risk for hyperglycemia in the perioperative period compared with nondiabetic patients and should be included in any comprehensive strategies for perioperative management of patients with diabetes.

Treatment of diabetes

Many different drugs are used in the treatment of diabetes and they have different mechanisms of action, pharmacokinetics, pharmacodynamics, and risk profiles. The type of treatment influences preoperative patient education and management, as well as intraoperative therapy, and it is important that all perioperative providers are familiar with principles of diabetes management, even if they do not chronically manage diabetes medications. Details of the types of drugs used to treat diabetes along with algorithms and strategies for the medical management of diabetes can be found elsewhere [17–19]. Briefly, patients with type 1 diabetes must be provided exogenous insulin and most likely will be treated with a combination of long-acting and short-acting insulin preparations or a continuous subcutaneous insulin infusion via an ambulatory pump. Some patients with type 2 diabetes and prediabetes may attempt to control their diabetes with lifestyle modifications, such as diet and exercise, but most will eventually be treated with a variety of oral medications with or without insulin. The treatment of diabetes during pregnancy centers on insulin as a first-line therapy, because of its effectiveness and safety profile, and women with type 2 diabetes who are planning on becoming pregnant are often switched from oral diabetes drugs to insulin [20].

PERIOPERATIVE MANAGEMENT GOALS

The challenge of caring for a patient with diabetes during the perioperative period is related to a number of separate but related issues, including (1) identification and optimal blood glucose management, (2) management of end-organ complications and chronic diseases associated with diabetes, (3) prevention and management of hyperglycemia and hypoglycemia, and (4) postprocedure follow-up and management. Although a number of guidelines for the care of the hospitalized patient with diabetes exist, there are few guidelines that encompass the entire perioperative period. The Society for Ambulatory Anesthesia has produced a consensus statement that does include guidance on adjustment of medications and glycemic targets, but these are tailored to ambulatory surgery [21]. The British and Australian Diabetes Societies have developed more comprehensive guidelines [22,23], yet development of a perioperative strategy for patients with diabetes is highly institution-specific due to differing resources, infrastructures, and patient populations. A multidisciplinary approach encompassing the entire procedural episode of care that uses an ongoing quality improvement process is likely to be most successful.

Prehospital evaluation, management and education

Diabetes is associated with a large number of long-term medical consequences, including retinopathy, nephropathy, neuropathy (sensory and autonomic), coronary heart disease, cerebrovascular disease, peripheral vascular disease, sleep apnea, and dental disease. Many of these comorbid diseases increase the risk of major perioperative morbidity, such as cardiac events, kidney injury, and infection. Additionally, diabetes is associated with problems of particular importance to anesthesiologists, such as limiting neck range of motion due to glycosylation of connecting tissues. Therefore, the perioperative evaluation of patients with diabetes by a medical provider, anesthesiologist, or preoperative clinic is recommended so that proper risk assessment and testing and medical optimization can be performed before surgery (Box 1).

Preoperative evaluation of glycemic control

Patients with a known diagnosis of diabetes, including those who are attempting to control their diabetes with lifestyle interventions, should have their

Box 1: Components of a targeted preoperative diabetes evaluation

Medical history

Age and characteristics of onset of diabetes (eg, ketoacidosis, laboratory finding)

Eating patterns, physical activity habits, nutritional status, and weight history; growth and development in children and adolescents

Diabetes education

Previous and current treatment of diabetes, including medications, medication adherence, meal plan, physical activity patterns, results of glucose monitoring, response to therapy (A1C records)

DKA frequency, severity, and causes

Hypoglycemic episodes, including frequency, cause, and hypoglycemia awareness

Diabetes-related complications

Physical examination

Height, weight, body mass index, blood pressure (including orthostatic measurements)

Airway, especially neck range of motion, mouth opening and dentition

Cardiovascular examination

Sleep apnea risk assessment

Targeted musculoskeletal and neurologic examinations

Skin/foot examination (skin breakdown/chronic infection)

Laboratory evaluation

A1C, if results not available within past 2–3 months

If not performed/available within past year, consider

- Fasting lipid profile, including total, LDL, and HDL cholesterol and triglycerides
- Liver function tests
- Test for urine albumin excretion with spot urine albumin-to-creatinine ratio
- Serum creatinine and calculated glomerular filtration rate
- Thyroid-stimulating hormone (type 1 diabetes, dyslipidemia, women older than 50 years)

Abbreviations: A1C, glycosylated hemoglobin; DKA, diabetic ketoacidosis; HDL, high-density lipoprotein; LDL, low-density lipoprotein.

Modified from American Diabetes Association. Standards of medical care in diabetes–2014. Diabetes Care 2014;37 Suppl 1:S21; with permission.

glycemic control tested. Hemoglobin A1C testing provides information regarding long-term (approximately 3 months) glycemic control and does not require the patient be fasting (Table 2). Although the relationship between elevated A1C and perioperative outcomes is still not completely clear [24],

Table 2
Relationship between A1C and estimated average daily glucose (eAG)

A1C, %	eAG, mg/dL (mmol/L)
6	126 (7.0)
7	154 (8.6)
8	183 (10.2)
9	212 (11.8)
10	240 (13.3)
11	269 (14.9)
12	298 (16.6)

Modified from American Diabetes Association. Standards of medical care in diabetes–2014. Diabetes Care 2014;37 Suppl 1:S23; with permission.

there is growing evidence that elevated A1C is associated with worse outcomes after surgery [6,25–27]. Additionally, greater A1C is associated with increased risks of hyperglycemia and variability in perioperative plasma glucose concentrations. Both of these have been associated with increased adverse outcomes [28–31]. Although cutoffs for the delay or cancellation of elective surgery have been proposed, there are few data to suggest that correcting A1C before surgery improves outcomes, and normalization of A1C is likely to be an unrealistic goal for some patients [32]. Additionally, it has been shown in some settings that intensive therapy to lower A1C in patients with diabetic retinopathy or cardiovascular risk factors is associated with worse outcomes [33,34]. Therefore, although it seems reasonable for patients with markedly abnormal A1C (eg, <4% or >8%) to be referred for optimization of medical therapy before elective surgery, A1C may be best used to identify patients with diabetes, to identify patients at greatest risk of perioperative hyperglycemia, and to identify patients who may benefit from specialized care pathways.

Many patients who present for surgery have not had regular medical care, and for some, the surgical episode of care may be their first entry into the health care system. Additionally, surgery has been shown to be an important opportunity for initiation of plans for lifestyle modifications: a "teachable moment" [35]. Therefore, patients with risk factors for diabetes (eg, age, obesity, other components of the metabolic syndrome) who have not been previously diagnosed might benefit from evaluation for diabetes or prediabetes in the perioperative period. Not only would this allow for proper risk identification and institution of plans for optimization and perioperative management, but it may have important long-term public health implications.

Preoperative evaluation of complications of diabetes

Cardiovascular disease. Patients with diabetes are 2 to 4 times more likely to die of heart disease than individuals without diabetes. Diabetes is a risk factor for hypertension, coronary artery disease, diastolic dysfunction, congestive heart failure, peripheral vascular disease, and cerebrovascular disease. Myocardial infarction and sudden death occur more often in patients with diabetes who are asymptomatic [36], and approximately 30% of patients with diabetes have significant coronary disease [37]. Current preoperative guidelines for perioperative cardiovascular evaluation list diabetes, along with a history of ischemic heart disease, compensated or previous heart failure, cerebrovascular disease, and renal insufficiency as clinical risk factors to be considered when determining which patients are candidates for preoperative cardiac testing [38].

Renal disease. Renal dysfunction commonly develops in diabetic patients, and diabetes is the leading cause of renal failure requiring renal replacement therapy. Diabetes is also a risk factor for perioperative acute kidney injury and contrast-induced nephropathy [39,40]. Evaluation of renal function is warranted in patients with diabetes and should be considered in selecting and dosing renally cleared drugs to avoid nephrotoxic and drug toxicity.

Other complications of diabetes. Peripheral and autonomic neuropathies are common in diabetic patients and preexisting neurologic deficits should be noted before procedures. Although the prevalence of diabetes and the potential benefits of regional anesthesia and analgesia lead many to continue to use regional techniques in patients with diabetes, the increased risk of neurologic complications in patients with diabetes and/or diabetic neuropathy should be considered [41,42]. Cardiovascular autonomic neuropathy predisposes patients to hemodynamic lability and the need for vasopressor support [43], and may reduce hypoxic ventilatory drive [44]. Autonomic neuropathy also can cause gastroparesis, predisposing diabetic patients to pulmonary aspiration.

Chronic hyperglycemia may result in decreased joint mobility, making positioning difficult, and decreased mobility in the temporomandibular and cervical spine joints makes diabetes a known risk factor for difficult intubation [45,46]. Some, but not all, studies have found that diabetes is a risk factor for postoperative visual loss after spine surgery [47,48]. Finally, as obesity and type 2 diabetes often coexist, the myriad of anesthetic implications related to obesity also must be evaluated and managed.

Preoperative medication management

Patients with type 1 diabetes have an absolute requirement for exogenous insulin administration and, therefore, require special attention in the perioperative period. Expert consultation by endocrinologists or diabetes specialists should be considered. Patients should continue to use their long-acting insulin with modifications to dose made depending on the type of insulin used and the timing of their surgery and anticipated resumption of oral intake (Table 3). There is a growing prevalence of the use of ambulatory insulin infusion pumps that provide a continuous subcutaneous insulin infusion, and patients should continue to use their insulin pumps the day of their procedure until a more definitive plan, dictated by the nature of the procedure and patient-specific factors, is initiated. Most pumps provide for lower infusion rates during periods of sleep or illness.

Patients with type 2 diabetes are usually treated with one or more oral drugs and also may be using subcutaneous insulin. It is recommended that patients

Table 3
Diabetic medication for fasting guidelines

Medications	Instructions
Oral medications or noninsulin injectables: sulfonylureas (chlorpropamide, glipizide, glyburide, glimepiride), biguanides (metformin), meglitinides (repaglinide, nateglinide), thiazolidinediones (rosiglitazone, pioglitazone), dipeptidyl peptidase 4 inhibitors (sitagliptin, saxagliptin, linagliptin, alogliptin), sodium-glucose cotransporter 2 inhibitors (canagliflozin and dapagliflozin), alpha-glucosidase inhibitors (acarbose, meglitol), noninsulin injectables (exenatide, pramlintide, larglutide)	Hold dose while fasting
Long-acting insulin (glargine, detemir)	If morning procedure, usual morning dose. If later procedure, 50%–75% of usual morning dose or on arrival to hospital. Reduce evening dose if history of hypoglycemia.
Intermediate-acting insulin (NPH, zinc insulin)	50%–75% of usual morning dose or on arrival to hospital. Reduce evening dose if history of hypoglycemia.
Short/rapid-acting insulin (regular, lispro, aspart, glulisine)	Hold while fasting
Premixed insulin (70/30 NPH regular, 50/50 NPH/regular, 70/30 aspart protamine/aspart, 75/25 lispro protamine/lispro, 50/50 lispro protamine/lispro)	Do not use premixed; use 50%–75% of usual dose of intermediate-acting insulin only (use NPH for lispro-protamine mixtures) or on arrival to hospital. Reduce evening dose if history of hypoglycemia.
Continuous subcutaneous insulin infusion (ambulatory insulin infusion pump)	Continue basal insulin; "sick" or "sleep" rates may be used. Hold bolus doses while fasting.

Suggested management of diabetes medications on the day of surgery to account for usual fasting guidelines (based on the literature [21,77] and expert recommendations). Insulin doses should be reduced in patients with a history of hypoglycemia or hypoglycemia unawareness who are fasting.

Abbreviation: NPH, neutral protamine Hagedorn (insulin).

discontinue oral drugs when they begin fasting and should not take any drug on the day of surgery, even if they continue to consume clear liquids, until their normal diet is resumed (see Table 3). The growing number of patients with type 2 diabetes using insulin (including ambulatory subcutaneous insulin infusion pumps) requires that their insulin dosing also be adjusted perioperatively.

Perioperative glycemic control strategies for patients with diabetes

The goals of a glycemic control program should be to prevent and/or treat hyperglycemia while monitoring for and minimizing hypoglycemia. This requires a coordinated, multidisciplinary approach throughout the surgical episode, building off of the preoperative evaluation and management (Table 4).

Evidence for benefit of glycemic control

There are a growing number of studies that suggest that hyperglycemia, particular in patients with diabetes, is associated with worse outcomes [8,10,49–53]. It appears that blood glucose variability, not just mean glucose, is also important [30,31,54], but the optimal balance between target blood glucose and glucose variability is unknown [55]. Given the evidence that diabetes and hyperglycemia are predictors of worse outcomes, the question of whether treatment of hyperglycemia results in better outcomes has been a topic of considerable interest and controversy. A comprehensive review of the literature is beyond the scope of the current work; however, there are a few key concepts that are worthwhile to discuss in the context of the current interpretation of the literature.

Table 4
Multidisciplinary perioperative glycemic control program for patients with diabetes

Admission	Documentation of glucose, recent diabetes medication use
	Medication reconciliation
	Initiation of glycemic control plan
	  Glucose monitoring
	  Expert consultation vs protocol-based management
	  Long-acting basal insulin for overall control
	  Short-acting correction insulin for immediate control

Preoperative area Procedural area Postanesthesia care area Postsurgical care areas	Glucose monitoring Short-acting insulin or insulin infusions Effective transfers of care between providers Glucose monitoring Continuation of perioperative glycemic control plan, protocol-based or expert management, modified to individual patient response

Discharge	Patient education
	  Diet
	  Diabetic medication regimen
	  Blood glucose testing
	Updated medication lists
	Recommendations for follow-up

A surge of interest in glycemic control occurred in the early 2000s after the publication of prospective, randomized trials in critically ill adult patients who demonstrated significant reductions in mortality with intensive insulin therapy when compared with usual care [56,57]. These trials prompted a number of follow-up studies that had differing conclusions and concerns about the safety and effectiveness of intensive glycemic control in hospitalized patients with and without diabetes [58,59]. The adverse outcomes associated with intensive glycemic management may be related to greater rates of hypoglycemia [60]. Although there are limited prospective data comparing intensive intraoperative insulin therapy to conventional intraoperative glucose management, at least one study found greater numbers of deaths and strokes with intensive intraoperative therapy [61]. Despite the variable outcomes reported and the potential risks of intensive glucose control, most would suggest that avoiding extremes in glucose, high or low, is associated with better outcomes [9,10,62–66].

Glucose targets for patients with diabetes

Although certain subpopulations may benefit from stricter glycemic control, most guidelines on the care of patients with diabetes now recommend that insulin should be administered when glucose reaches 140 to 150 mg/dL (7.8–8.3 mmol/L) with the goal of preventing glucose levels of greater than 180 mg/dL (10 mmol/L) (Table 5). Individual insulin sensitivity, a history of hypoglycemia and/or hypoglycemia unawareness, and the duration of surgery and recovery, and time to resumption of oral intake should all be factored into the decision to administer insulin. In some instances, such as short outpatient procedures with a low risk of complications, higher glucose targets may be acceptable [21].

Methods of glycemic control in patients with diabetes

Expert guidelines recommended that insulin be the drug used to treat hyperglycemia in the hospitalized patient [17]. However, for noncritically ill patients or

Table 5
Recommendations of select professional societies for target plasma glucose in hospitalized and/or perioperative patients with diabetes

American Society of Clinical Endocrinologists [18]	Random glucose <180 mg/dL (10 mmol/L), fasting glucose <140 mg/dL (7.8 mmol/L)
American Diabetes Association [17]	Random glucose <180 mg/dL (10 mmol/L), fasting glucose <140 mg/dL (7.8 mmol/L)
Society for Ambulatory Anesthesiology [21]	Intraoperative glucose <180 mg/dL (10 mmol/L)
Society of Critical Care Medicine [71]	Blood glucose most <150 mg/dL (8.3 mmol/L), absolutely <180 mg/dL (10 mmol/L), initiate at ≥150 mg/dL (8.3 mmol/L)
Joint British Diabetes Society/NHS Diabetes [23]	Target blood glucose should be 108–180 mg/dL (6–10 mmol/L), acceptable range 72–216 mg dL (4–12 mmol/L)
Australian Diabetes Society [22]	90–180 mg/dL (5–10 mmol/L)

outpatients with type 2 diabetes treated with oral agents and/or insulin, the subcutaneous insulin route may be preferred. The use of "sliding" scale insulin algorithms alone or intravenous bolus insulin leads to poor/variable control [67,68]; the use of long-acting subcutaneous basal insulin with correction scale therapy using rapid-acting subcutaneous insulin provides superior control throughout the perioperative period [69]. One approach is to provide long-acting basal insulin on admission to select patients who have not taken their oral medications and/or insulin. When this approach is used, it is imperative that procedures and protocols for blood glucose monitoring and treatment of hypoglycemia be in place. For shorter, less stressful procedures in stable patients or when patients will be resuming their normal diet and diabetic drug therapy soon after the procedure, treating elevated glucose levels with rapid-acting subcutaneous insulin may be all that is required throughout the procedure and recovery. Specific examples of insulin protocols have been published [61,70], but it is advisable that practices validate the safety and performance of glucose protocols on an ongoing basis to account for local differences in practices and patient populations. Support of this approach is within the Joint Commission expectations.

For longer procedures, unstable/critically ill patients, procedures associated with hemodynamic instability, or when subcutaneous administration is not feasible, guidelines suggest the use of intravenous insulin infusions [71]. Protocols that allow for changes in the relative dosing of insulin for a given glucose range should be used, as these allow for compensation for differences and changes in insulin sensitivity [61]. Procedures should be in place to ensure timely communication and appropriate follow-up when transferring patients between care areas when insulin infusions are used due to the potential for medication errors and delays in glucose monitoring. Transition to basal/bolus subcutaneous insulin should be initiated before discontinuing the insulin infusion to prevent hyperglycemia.

Patients with type 1 diabetes should have either long-acting basal insulin provided or have a continuous infusion of insulin throughout the perioperative period. Increasingly, patients with type 1 (and some with type 2) will be treated using ambulatory infusion pumps. The perioperative use of continuous subcutaneous insulin infusions is an evolving practice and some institutions permit the use of these pumps during surgical procedures when possible. When the infusion site is in a surgical field or during surgeries when skin perfusion may be altered due to temperature fluctuations or hemodynamic instability, discontinuation of the infusion may be most appropriate. When subcutaneous insulin pumps are removed from patients with type 1 diabetes, another source of exogenous insulin must be provided. This is often in the form of an intravenous insulin infusion, but long-acting subcutaneous insulin may be used if providers are familiar with use under these circumstances or expert consultation is available. In all cases, frequent monitoring for hypoglycemia and hyperglycemia should be provided due to a large variation in insulin sensitivity and the risk of diabetic ketoacidosis (DKA) in these patients. Finally, transitioning back to a subcutaneous insulin regimen may be challenging, as changes in oral intake or other physiologic effects of surgery will influence insulin needs or sensitivity.

Glucose monitoring

Regular, accurate measurement of glucose is the single most important component of the safe and effective perioperative management of a diabetic patient's blood glucose. When insulin infusions are initiated, blood glucose should be measured at least every hour; if subcutaneous insulin is used, blood glucose should be monitored at a minimum of every 2 hours and more frequently in patients with type 1 diabetes, those who exhibit a greater sensitivity to the effects of insulin, or those who have hypoglycemia unawareness. Once the patient has recovered from anesthesia and resumes nutritional intake, the frequency of monitoring may be able to be decreased and a nutritional insulin therapy component added.

Point-of-care glucose testing using glucose meters is often performed because of the speed of return of results and the lower associated per-test costs. However, studies have shown glucose measured using point-of-care devices, particularly during surgery, can vary significantly from laboratory-performed results and has the potential to adversely affect clinical outcomes [72–74]. The testing of capillary blood samples with glucose meters, although convenient, is not recommended when perfusion of the extremities may be altered due to tissue edema, altered tissue perfusion, or other factors that change the temporal or quantitative relationship between capillary and blood glucose values. For these reasons, capillary blood testing also is not recommended for use in critically ill patients [71]. The use of capillary blood for glucose testing in patients in surgery or under anesthesia needs further study. Plans for obtaining blood samples repeatedly during the surgical procedure are needed. Venous blood can be obtained from a peripheral vein, central venous catheters, or peripherally inserted central venous catheters. Placement of arterial catheters is a safe method for obtaining blood for repeated measurements of glucose and should be considered when venous access is anticipated to be limited [75]. When point-of-care glucose monitoring is used, training of providers in the use of glucose meters and strict quality control measures are needed. Experts from laboratory medicine should be involved in the development of programs when the frequent use of glucose meters is anticipated.

Development of a perioperative glycemic control program

As perioperative glycemic control becomes a common performance improvement metric, it is important that institutions, practice groups, and practitioners become familiar with the steps required to develop a program that focuses on the safe, effective treatment of patients with diabetes. The development of effective glycemic control programs faces a number of challenges and optimal practice requires multidisciplinary development and endorsement, including physicians, nurses, technicians, pharmacists, laboratories, and administrators [76,77]. Furthermore, development of comprehensive programs for perioperative management of diabetes may require significant resources in the form of personnel, information technology infrastructure, and equipment to fully accomplish their goals. However, significant cost savings can be realized through these diabetes management programs [78]. Additionally, several regulatory and patient advocacy organizations include glycemic control as a marker of quality of care [79], and it may be an important component of future reimbursement models.

Discharge and follow-up

Many patients who are found to be hyperglycemic during the perioperative period will not have been previously diagnosed with diabetes [2,5]. The diagnosis of diabetes during states of stress may be difficult, but patients with hyperglycemia should be referred for follow-up. Measurements of A1C in the perioperative period may be useful to make a presumptive diagnosis of diabetes; however, A1C during periods of acute stress has not been validated and there are a number of known confounders, including transfusion and hemolysis [80]. Still, recent data would suggest that resources expended in identifying patients with diabetes during the perioperative period may result in considerable benefit [81]. Proper follow-up is encouraged for all patients with diabetes, as the risk of adverse outcomes does not end at discharge and information regarding glycemic control and specific changes to diabetes management must be clearly communicated. This is especially important when rapid changes in oral intake or insulin sensitivity/production are anticipated, such as in otorhinological, thoracic, gastrointestinal, endocrine, or weight-loss surgery.

Special considerations

Treatment of diabetes during labor and delivery

Hyperglycemia during labor and delivery is a risk factor for fetal distress and neonatal hypoglycemia and, therefore, it is suggested that glucose be targeted between 72 and 126 mg/dL (4–7 mmol/L). Glucose monitoring and treatment of hyperglycemia of the parturient should be continued 24 to 72 hours postpartum [20]. Insulin infusions with frequent blood glucose monitoring may be the best way of treatment. Additionally, monitoring of the neonate for hypoglycemia is mandatory after birth in women who have diabetes during pregnancy.

Acute medical conditions associated with hyperglycemia

Hyperglycemia can result in metabolic alterations, such as DKA and a nonketotic hyperosmolar state (NKHS) [82]. In addition, surgical stress may alter glycometabolic regulation, contributing to disruption of glucose homeostasis. The response of glucose metabolism during stress and surgery is difficult to predict but, in general, the perioperative period is associated with relative insulin hyposecretion, increased insulin resistance, and subsequent hyperglycemia. Frequently, factors that precipitate these severe alterations in glucose regulation necessitate surgical intervention; therefore, it is important that perioperative care providers understand the pathophysiology and treatment of these disorders. Blood glucose should be checked in all patients before surgery, and a glucose greater than 300 mg/dL should prompt evaluation of blood or urine for ketones and nonemergent surgery delayed until hyperglycemia and/or ketosis is corrected.

Ketoacidosis is a life-threatening complication (reported mortality 5%–10%), seen predominantly in type 1 diabetic patients, that results from insulin deficiency and is characterized by hyperglycemia, dehydration, hyperosmolarity, and ketoacidosis. A precipitating event such as infection, surgical stress, trauma, or lack of insulin therapy may be identified. Management is focused on identifying and treating precipitating factors, intravenous insulin infusion, fluid resuscitation, electrolyte replacement, and frequent glucose monitoring. Patients are at risk for cerebral edema during treatment and careful monitoring of neurologic status is warranted. NKHS occurs predominantly in type 2 diabetic patients, often during periods of stress, such as infection or other illness. Compared with patients with DKA, patients in NKHS are typically more dehydrated, hyperosmolar, and hyperglycemic. Neurologic alterations are often present and may include confusion, coma, seizures, and/or focal neurologic deficits. Although patients with NKHS lack the acidemia that is caused by ketone production, severe dehydration may result in significant hypotension leading to lactic acidosis as well as predisposing to thrombotic events. Gradual fluid resuscitation over more than 24 hours guided by serial sodium measurements is the mainstay of treatment. A more gradual time frame for metabolic correction is advocated due to the greater degree of hyperosmolarity and concerns for cerebral edema with rapid correction of metabolic and electrolyte profiles.

Hypoglycemia

Hypoglycemia is commonly defined in adults as plasma glucose less than 70 mg/dL (3.9 mmol/L). Altered mental status, progressing to coma and death, along with the physiologic responses to increased catecholamines are the 2 major ways by which hypoglycemia is most commonly detected. In the perioperative environment, and to a greater extent in the setting of general anesthesia, the ability to recognize these signs and symptoms may be compromised. Clinicians need to have a high index of suspicion for hypoglycemia and, again, frequent determination of glucose should be a part of all care processes developed for the care of diabetic patients. Hypoglycemia may develop due to residual effects of long-acting drugs, overaggressive antidiabetic treatment, or decreased caloric intake. Treatment consists of dextrose administration and correction of the precipitating cause. Because the response to dextrose administration is quite variable, following an initial bolus (25–50 mL of 50% dextrose in adults), serial glucose determinations should be performed and a dextrose infusion considered based on the patient's response.

SUMMARY

1. Type 2 diabetes is common in patients undergoing surgical procedures and is an important risk factor for adverse perioperative outcomes.

2. Patients with type 1 diabetes benefit from a continuous source of insulin at all times.
3. For most patients with diabetes, glucose lower than 180 mg/dL (10 mmol/L) is a reasonable target. Insulin therapy should be initiated at 140 to 150 mg/dL (7.8–8.3 mmol/L).
4. Intensive insulin therapy with lower glucose targets is associated with hypoglycemia and worse outcomes.
5. Any efforts to prevent or treat hyperglycemia must include strategies to prevent, monitor for, and treat hypoglycemia.
6. To safely and effectively care for patients with diabetes, a perioperative glycemic control program should be developed using a multidisciplinary approach.

References

[1] American Diabetes Association. Economic costs of diabetes in the U.S. in 2012. Diabetes Care 2013;36:1033–46.

[2] Lauruschkat AH, Arnrich B, Albert AA, et al. Prevalence and risks of undiagnosed diabetes mellitus in patients undergoing coronary artery bypass grafting. Circulation 2005;112: 2397–402.

[3] Abdelmalak B, Abdelmalak JB, Knittel J, et al. The prevalence of undiagnosed diabetes in non-cardiac surgery patients, an observational study. Can J Anaesth 2010;57: 1058–64.

[4] Hudson CC, Welsby IJ, Phillips-Bute B, et al. Glycosylated hemoglobin levels and outcome in non-diabetic cardiac surgery patients. Can J Anaesth 2010;57:565–72.

[5] Levetan CS, Passaro M, Jablonski K, et al. Unrecognized diabetes among hospitalized patients. Diabetes Care 1998;21:246–9.

[6] Halkos ME, Puskas JD, Lattouf OM, et al. Elevated preoperative hemoglobin A1c level is predictive of adverse events after coronary artery bypass surgery. J Thorac Cardiovasc Surg 2008;136:631–40.

[7] Frisch A, Chandra P, Smiley D, et al. Prevalence and clinical outcome of hyperglycemia in the perioperative period in noncardiac surgery. Diabetes Care 2010;33:1783–8.

[8] Gandhi GY, Nuttall GA, Abel MD, et al. Intraoperative hyperglycemia and perioperative outcomes in cardiac surgery patients. Mayo Clin Proc 2005;80:862–6.

[9] Kwon S, Thompson R, Dellinger P, et al. Importance of perioperative glycemic control in general surgery: a report from the Surgical Care and Outcomes Assessment Program. Ann Surg 2013;257:8–14.

[10] King JT Jr, Goulet JL, Perkal MF, et al. Glycemic control and infections in patients with diabetes undergoing noncardiac surgery. Ann Surg 2011;253:158–65.

[11] Abdelmalak BB, Bonilla AM, Yang D, et al. The hyperglycemic response to major noncardiac surgery and the added effect of steroid administration in patients with and without diabetes. Anesth Analg 2013;116:1116–22.

[12] American Diabetes Association. Diagnosis and classification of diabetes mellitus. Diabetes Care 2013;36(Suppl 1):S67–74.

[13] Centers for Disease Control and Prevention. National Surveillance Data Diagnosed Diabetes. 2014. Available at: http://www.cdc.gov/diabetes/statistics/prevalence_national.htm. Accessed June 2, 2014.

[14] Alberti KG, Eckel RH, Grundy SM, et al. Harmonizing the Metabolic Syndrome: a Joint Interim Statement of the International Diabetes Federation Task Force on Epidemiology and Prevention; National Heart, Lung, and Blood Institute; American Heart Association; World Heart Federation; International Atherosclerosis Society; and International Association for the Study of Obesity. Circulation 2009;120:1640–5.

[15] Swinburn BA, Sacks G, Hall KD, et al. The global obesity pandemic: shaped by global drivers and local environments. Lancet 2011;378:804–14.

[16] Lawrence JM, Contreras R, Chen W, et al. Trends in the prevalence of preexisting diabetes and gestational diabetes mellitus among a racially/ethnically diverse population of pregnant women, 1999-2005. Diabetes Care 2008;31:899–904.
[17] American Diabetes Association. Standards of medical care in diabetes–2014. Diabetes Care 2014;37(Suppl 1):S14–80.
[18] Garber AJ, Abrahamson MJ, Barzilay JI, et al. AACE comprehensive diabetes management algorithm 2013. Endocr Pract 2013;19:327–36.
[19] American Diabetes Association. Executive summary: standards of medical care in diabetes–2014. Diabetes Care 2014;37:S5–13.
[20] Hartling L, Dryden DM, Guthrie A, et al. Benefits and harms of treating gestational diabetes mellitus: a systematic review and meta-analysis for the U.S. Preventive Services Task Force and the National Institutes of Health Office of Medical Applications of Research. Ann Intern Med 2013;159:123–9.
[21] Joshi GP, Chung F, Vann MA, et al. Society for Ambulatory Anesthesia consensus statement on perioperative blood glucose management in diabetic patients undergoing ambulatory surgery. Anesth Analg 2010;111:1378–87.
[22] Wong J, Zoungas S, Wright C, et al. Evidence-based guidelines for perioperative management of diabetes in cardiac and vascular surgery. World J Surg 2010;34:500–13.
[23] Dhatariya K, Levy N, Kilvert A, et al. NHS diabetes guideline for the perioperative management of the adult patient with diabetes. Diabet Med 2012;29:420–33.
[24] Acott AA, Theus SA, Kim LT. Long-term glucose control and risk of perioperative complications. Am J Surg 2009;198:596–9.
[25] Underwood P, Askari R, Hurwitz S, et al. Preoperative A1C and clinical outcomes in patients with diabetes undergoing major noncardiac surgical procedures. Diabetes Care 2014;37:611–6.
[26] Faritous Z, Ardeshiri M, Yazdanian F, et al. Hyperglycemia or high hemoglobin A1C: which one is more associated with morbidity and mortality after coronary artery bypass graft surgery? Ann Thorac Cardiovasc Surg 2014;20(3):223–8.
[27] Marchant MH Jr, Viens NA, Cook C, et al. The impact of glycemic control and diabetes mellitus on perioperative outcomes after total joint arthroplasty. J Bone Joint Surg Am 2009;91:1621–9.
[28] Koumpan Y, Vandenkerkhof E, van Vlymen J. An observational cohort study to assess glycosylated hemoglobin screening for elective surgical patients. Can J Anaesth 2014;61: 407–16.
[29] Subramaniam B, Lerner A, Novack V, et al. Increased glycemic variability in patients with elevated preoperative HbA1C predicts adverse outcomes following coronary artery bypass grafting surgery. Anesth Analg 2014;118:277–87.
[30] Jeon CY, Furuya EY, Berman MF, et al. The role of pre-operative and post-operative glucose control in surgical-site infections and mortality. PLoS One 2012;7:e45616.
[31] Egi M, Bellomo R, Stachowski E, et al. Variability of blood glucose concentration and short-term mortality in critically ill patients. Anesthesiology 2006;105:244–52.
[32] Giori NJ, Ellerbe LS, Bowe T, et al. Many diabetic total joint arthroplasty candidates are unable to achieve a preoperative hemoglobin a1c goal of 7% or less. J Bone Joint Surg Am 2014;96:500–4.
[33] Suto C, Hori S, Kato S, et al. Effect of perioperative glycemic control in progression of diabetic retinopathy and maculopathy. Arch Ophthalmol 2006;124:38–45.
[34] Gerstein HC, Miller ME, Byington RP, et al. Effects of intensive glucose lowering in type 2 diabetes. N Engl J Med 2008;358:2545–59.
[35] Shi Y, Warner DO. Surgery as a teachable moment for smoking cessation. Anesthesiology 2010;112:102–7.
[36] Young LH, Wackers FJ, Chyun DA, et al. Cardiac outcomes after screening for asymptomatic coronary artery disease in patients with type 2 diabetes: the DIAD study: a randomized controlled trial. JAMA 2009;301:1547–55.

[37] Park GM, Lee SW, Cho YR, et al. Coronary computed tomographic angiographic findings in asymptomatic patients with type 2 diabetes mellitus. Am J Cardiol 2014;113:765–71.
[38] Fleisher LA, Beckman JA, Brown KA, et al. ACC/AHA 2007 guidelines on perioperative cardiovascular evaluation and care for noncardiac surgery. J Am Coll Cardiol 2007;50:1707–32.
[39] McCullough PA, Wolyn R, Rocher LL, et al. Acute renal failure after coronary intervention: incidence, risk factors, and relationship to mortality. Am J Med 1997;103:368–75.
[40] Weingarten TN, Gurrieri C, McCaffrey JM, et al. Acute kidney injury following bariatric surgery. Obes Surg 2013;23:64–70.
[41] Hebl JR, Kopp SL, Schroeder DR, et al. Neurologic complications after neuraxial anesthesia or analgesia in patients with preexisting peripheral sensorimotor neuropathy or diabetic polyneuropathy. Anesth Analg 2006;103:1294–9.
[42] Lirk P, Rutten MV, Haller I, et al. Management of the patient with diabetic peripheral neuropathy presenting for peripheral regional anesthesia: a European survey and review of literature. Minerva Anestesiol 2013;79:1039–48.
[43] Burgos LG, Ebert TJ, Asiddao C, et al. Increased intraoperative cardiovascular morbidity in diabetics with autonomic neuropathy. Anesthesiology 1989;70:591–7.
[44] Sobotka PA, Liss HP, Vinik AI. Impaired hypoxic ventilatory drive in diabetic patients with autonomic neuropathy. J Clin Endocrinol Metab 1986;62:658–63.
[45] Mashour GA, Kheterpal S, Vanaharam V, et al. The extended Mallampati score and a diagnosis of diabetes mellitus are predictors of difficult laryngoscopy in the morbidly obese. Anesth Analg 2008;107:1919–23.
[46] Warner ME, Contreras MG, Warner MA, et al. Diabetes mellitus and difficult laryngoscopy in renal and pancreatic transplant patients. Anesth Analg 1998;86:516–9.
[47] Nandyala SV, Marquez-Lara A, Fineberg SJ, et al. Incidence and risk factors for perioperative visual loss after spinal fusion. Spine J 2014;14(9):1866–72.
[48] Postoperative Visual Loss Study Group. Risk factors associated with ischemic optic neuropathy after spinal fusion surgery. Anesthesiology 2012;116:15–24.
[49] Umpierrez GE, Isaacs SD, Bazargan N, et al. Hyperglycemia: an independent marker of in-hospital mortality in patients with undiagnosed diabetes. J Clin Endocrinol Metab 2002;87:978–82.
[50] Doenst T, Wijeysundera D, Karkouti K, et al. Hyperglycemia during cardiopulmonary bypass is an independent risk factor for mortality in patients undergoing cardiac surgery. J Thorac Cardiovasc Surg 2005;130:1144–50.
[51] Ouattara A, Lecomte P, Le Manach Y, et al. Poor intraoperative blood glucose control is associated with a worsened hospital outcome after cardiac surgery in diabetic patients. Anesthesiology 2005;103:687–94.
[52] McGirt MJ, Woodworth GF, Brooke BS, et al. Hyperglycemia independently increases the risk of perioperative stroke, myocardial infarction, and death after carotid endarterectomy. Neurosurgery 2006;58:1066–73.
[53] Malmstedt J, Wahlberg E, Jörneskog G, et al. Influence of perioperative blood glucose levels on outcome after infrainguinal bypass surgery in patients with diabetes. Br J Surg 2006;93:1360–7.
[54] Hirsch IB, Brownlee M. Should minimal blood glucose variability become the gold standard of glycemic control? J Diabetes Complications 2005;19:178–81.
[55] Eslami S, Taherzadeh Z, Schultz MJ, et al. Glucose variability measures and their effect on mortality: a systematic review. Intensive Care Med 2011;37:583–93.
[56] Van den Berghe G, Wilmer A, Hermans G, et al. Intensive insulin therapy in the medical ICU. N Engl J Med 2006;354:449–61.
[57] Van den Berghe G, Wouters P, Weekers F, et al. Intensive insulin therapy in critically ill patients. N Engl J Med 2001;345:1359–67.

[58] Kosiborod M, Inzucchi SE, Krumholz HM, et al. Glucometrics in patients hospitalized with acute myocardial infarction: defining the optimal outcomes-based measure of risk. Circulation 2008;117:1018–27.
[59] The NICE-SUGAR Study Investigators, Finfer S, Chittock DR, et al. Intensive versus conventional glucose control in critically ill patients. N Engl J Med 2009;360:1283–97.
[60] Hermanides J, Bosman RJ, Vriesendorp TM, et al. Hypoglycemia is associated with intensive care unit mortality. Crit Care Med 2010;38:1430–4.
[61] Gandhi GY, Nuttall GA, Abel MD, et al. Intensive intraoperative insulin therapy versus conventional glucose management during cardiac surgery a randomized trial. Ann Intern Med 2007;146:233–43.
[62] Furnary AP, Gao G, Grunkemeier GL, et al. Continuous insulin infusion reduces mortality in patients with diabetes undergoing coronary artery bypass grafting. J Thorac Cardiovasc Surg 2003;125:1007–21.
[63] D'Alessandro C, Leprince P, Golmard JL, et al. Strict glycemic control reduces EuroSCORE expected mortality in diabetic patients undergoing myocardial revascularization. J Thorac Cardiovasc Surg 2007;134:29–37.
[64] Schmeltz LR, DeSantis AJ, Thiyagarajan V, et al. Reduction of surgical mortality and morbidity in diabetic patients undergoing cardiac surgery with a combined intravenous and subcutaneous insulin glucose management strategy. Diabetes Care 2007;30:823–8.
[65] McConnell YJ, Johnson PM, Porter GA. Surgical site infections following colorectal surgery in patients with diabetes: association with postoperative hyperglycemia. J Gastrointest Surg 2009;13:508–15.
[66] Ramos M, Khalpey Z, Lipsitz S, et al. Relationship of perioperative hyperglycemia and postoperative infections in patients who undergo general and vascular surgery. Ann Surg 2008;248:585–91.
[67] Queale WS, Seidler AJ, Brancati FL. Glycemic control and sliding scale insulin use in medical inpatients with diabetes mellitus. Arch Intern Med 1997;157:545–52.
[68] Subramaniam B, Panzica PJ, Novack V, et al. Continuous perioperative insulin infusion decreases major cardiovascular events in patients undergoing vascular surgery: a prospective, randomized trial. Anesthesiology 2009;110:970–7.
[69] Umpierrez GE, Hor T, Smiley D, et al. Comparison of inpatient insulin regimens with detemir plus aspart versus neutral protamine hagedorn plus regular in medical patients with type 2 diabetes. J Clin Endocrinol Metab 2009;94:564–9.
[70] Umpierrez GE, Hellman R, Korytkowski MT, et al. Management of hyperglycemia in hospitalized patients in non-critical care setting: an endocrine society clinical practice guideline. J Clin Endocrinol Metab 2012;97:16–38.
[71] Jacobi J, Bircher N, Krinsley J, et al. Guidelines for the use of an insulin infusion for the management of hyperglycemia in critically ill patients. Crit Care Med 2012;40:3251–76.
[72] Mraovic B, Schwenk ES, Epstein RH. Intraoperative accuracy of a point-of-care glucose meter compared with simultaneous central laboratory measurements. J Diabetes Sci Technol 2012;6:541–6.
[73] Kanji S, Buffie J, Hutton B, et al. Reliability of point-of-care testing for glucose measurement in critically ill adults. Crit Care Med 2005;33:2778–85.
[74] Rice MJ, Pitkin AD, Coursin DB. Review article: glucose measurement in the operating room: more complicated than it seems. Anesth Analg 2010;110:1056–65.
[75] Raurell-Torreda M, Del Llano-Serrano C, Almirall-Solsona D, et al. Arterial catheter setup for glucose control in critically ill patients: a randomized controlled trial. Am J Crit Care 2014;23:150–9.
[76] Magee MF. Hospital protocols for targeted glycemic control: development, implementation, and models for cost justification. Am J Health Syst Pharm 2007;64:S15–20.
[77] Alexanian SM, McDonnell ME, Akhtar S. Creating a perioperative glycemic control program. Anesthesiol Res Pract 2011;2011:465974.

[78] Newton CA, Young S. Financial implications of glycemic control: results of an inpatient diabetes management program. Endocr Pract 2006;12:43–8.
[79] Centers for Medicare & Medicaid Services and The Joint Commission. Specifications Manual for National Hospital Inpatient Quality Measures Discharge Dates 01-01-14 (1Q14) through 09-30-14 (3Q14) v4.3a. Available at: http://www.jointcommission.org/specifications_manual_for_national_hospital_inpatient_quality_measures.aspx. Accessed June 2, 2014.
[80] Bonora E, Tuomilehto J. The pros and cons of diagnosing diabetes with A1C. Diabetes Care 2011;34:S184–90.
[81] DeFronzo RA, Abdul-Ghani M. Type 2 diabetes can be prevented with early pharmacological intervention. Diabetes Care 2011;34:S202–9.
[82] Kitabchi AE, Umpierrez GE, Miles JM, et al. Hyperglycemic crises in adult patients with diabetes. Diabetes Care 2009;32(7):1335–43.

Advances in Anesthesia 32 (2014) 191–203

ADVANCES IN ANESTHESIA

Anesthetic Care of Septic Patients

R. Eliot Fagley, MD

Virginia Mason Medical Center, 1100 Ninth Avenue, Seattle, WA 98111, USA

Keywords

• Anesthesia • Sepsis • Mortality • Infection

Key points

- Septic patients are often brought to the operating room emergently, with the hope of achieving source control, which is the definitive therapy for septic shock.
- Safe induction can be achieved in several ways, most of which require catecholamine supplementation.
- Adequate hemodynamic monitoring, often with an arterial line and a central venous catheter, can aid clinical decision making.
- Central venous access also provides a safe, reliable route for vasoactive infusions.
- It is important for the clinician to be constantly vigilant for changes in patients' hemodynamic and pulmonary functions.

INTRODUCTION

Sepsis is one of the leading causes of mortality worldwide. However, since the publication of the first surviving sepsis guidelines [1], the mortalities associated with the systemic inflammatory response syndrome, sepsis, severe sepsis, and septic shock have decreased remarkably. This decrease is a result of several factors: early recognition, early treatment with broad-spectrum antimicrobial therapy, source control, early goal-directed fluid and vasopressor therapy, improved ventilator management, and prevention of target organ injury [2–4].

Anesthesiologists are frequently called on to care for patients who are at various points on the spectrum of the inflammatory response. As such, it is advisable to approach the care of septic patients with a construct comprises a plan for monitoring, induction, and maintenance of anesthesia; hemodynamic

E-mail address: eliot.fagley@vmmc.org

0737-6146/14/$ – see front matter
http://dx.doi.org/10.1016/j.aan.2014.08.003

goals; ventilatory strategies to minimize lung injury; strategies to minimize end-organ injury; and determination of the prudence of postprocedural extubation. It is also important to have a frank discussion with patients or their surrogates specifically addressing the risks of complications, including the need for prolonged intubation and mechanical ventilation, ventilator-associated pneumonia, delirium, large-volume fluid resuscitation (including blood and blood products), and mortality.

PREOPERATIVE EVALUATION

As in every case, the preoperative evaluation of septic patients should be thorough. Particular attention should be paid to physical examination and laboratory values that indicate sufficient systemic perfusion. The physical examination allows the clinician to determine whether the patient is warm and well perfused versus cool and mottled. Acid-base status, ventilation and oxygenation, renal function, white blood cell count, blood cultures, antibiotic therapy and sensitivity, and coagulation status are of particular interest. However, perioperative care of septic patients often revolves around source control, which is the prime directive in the care of this population. As such, source control should not be delayed while waiting for the aforementioned tests.

The patient's preoperative acid-base status gives the clinician an indication of the severity and trajectory of the patient's illness. The patient's pH, $Pa{CO_2}$ and $Pa{O_2}$, as measured by arterial blood gas, help to establish the patient's ability to ventilate and oxygenate appropriately. Ventilation and oxygenation, in turn, provide insight into the development of acute respiratory distress syndrome (ARDS), which is often associated with sepsis [4]. Creatinine, blood urea nitrogen (BUN), and pH provide insight into the quality of systemic perfusion and renal function. Plasma acid-base status also may affect pharmacodynamics of endogenous and exogenous catecholamines, which can have adverse effects on vascular tone and myocardial contractility. The white blood cell count can be confirmatory when there is no obvious infection, and it may bring up concerns for conditions not previously in the differential diagnosis. For example, leukopenia is sometimes an indicator of fungal infection [5]. By contrast, profound leukocytosis out of proportion to the level of illness is sometimes an indicator of *Clostridium difficile* colitis or device infection, such as central line–associated blood stream infection or pacemaker lead infection [6,7]. Blood cultures and antimicrobial sensitivities allow the anesthesiologist to verify appropriate antimicrobial coverage of the pathogenic organisms under consideration [5]. In addition, hepatic enzymes and coagulation status should be checked in similar fashion to the BUN and creatinine. Derangements in both plasma concentrations of hepatic enzymes and in liver synthetic function, as measured by coagulation studies (prothrombin time, international normalized ratio, activated partial thromboplastin time), often indicate severe hepatic injury in sepsis.

It is reasonable for the anesthesiologist to establish a baseline set of surrogates for systemic perfusion and cardiac function in the preoperative period. These secondary parameters include lactate, central venous oxygen saturation

($ScvO_2$), B-type natriuretic peptide (BNP), and troponins. Lactate and $ScvO_2$ are particularly useful because they can be sampled intermittently throughout the intraoperative period and compared with the established baseline [2]. BNP is useful as an indicator of atrial stretch, which is a surrogate for volume overload or ventricular hypokinesis [8]. Again, it is important to stress that these are secondary parameters and should not delay the start of an urgent, source-control (open surgical or percutaneous) intervention.

The preoperative examination should be focused but detailed, with particular attention paid to indicators of volume status, renal function, cardiac pump function, and pulmonary function. Patients are often profoundly hypovolemic in early septic shock, with dry mucous membranes, skin tenting, low urine output, and flat jugular veins. With aggressive crystalloid resuscitation and the capillary leak of the inflammatory response, patients often develop significant hydrostatic edema, particularly in dependent regions. However, the hydrostatic edema belies their intravascular volume depletion.

The potentially contradictory physical examination findings pose the question of what is the optimal method to monitor septic patients in the operating room. This question has been the subject of much debate across generations of physicians. Transesophageal echocardiography (TEE) is the gold standard for intraoperative monitoring of cardiac function and adequacy of ventricular filling [9]. However, TEE is not always indicated or recommended, particularly for patients whose source of infection may necessitate exploration of the esophagus, stomach, duodenum, proximal jejunum, mediastinum, or oropharynx. Direct intra-arterial catheterization and continuous pressure monitoring allows beat-to-beat determination of blood pressure, and it provides a reliable route by which to sample arterial blood gases. Although controversial, many clinicians still consider the pulmonary artery catheter (PAC), particularly the continuous mixed venous O_2 type (SvO_2), to be useful. Although the device has never been shown to improve outcomes, it does increase the richness of data available to the anesthesiologist [10,11]. One step removed from the PAC is the central venous catheter (CVC) with central venous pressure (CVP) monitoring. As a point piece of data, the CVP is probably not useful [12,13]. However, if the waveform is interpreted and the pressure is followed over time, the CVP may be diagnostic of acute changes in right heart function. These acute changes include right heart failure and acute tricuspid valve regurgitation, both of which are common in septic shock [14].

A new class of less invasive monitors has emerged in the past 2 decades. It is beyond the scope of this article to examine each in the detail it deserves. However, it is increasingly important for anesthesiologists to familiarize themselves with transthoracic echocardiography (TTE), stroke volume variation analysis, esophageal Doppler probes, lithium-dilution cardiac output, noninvasive cardiac output monitors, and thoracic impedance-based cardiac output devices [15]. Adjunctive devices such as these may be used as the anesthesiologist sees fit, particularly if there are contraindications to the use of TEE, PAC, and CVP placement or monitoring.

All of these devices should be used after defining a clear set of hemodynamic goals before entering the operating theater. Those goals are set with consideration for the patient's chronic conditions, because those conditions may alter the patient's ability to autoregulate blood flow to various vascular beds, particularly the brain, heart, and kidneys. For patients who have no medical conditions before the onset of sepsis, a mean arterial pressure goal of 65 mm Hg is reasonable. That goal often needs to be higher in patients with chronic conditions that adversely affect the microvasculature, such as chronic hypertension and peripheral vascular disease [16].

INDUCTION OF ANESTHESIA

Induction of anesthesia is a particularly important time for septic patients. While awake, their sympathetic nervous systems compensate for the vasodilatation of sepsis by releasing large amounts of endogenous catecholamines. On induction, septic patients experience a sympathectomy with unantagonized vasodilatation. They can become profoundly hypotensive if induction is not performed in a careful manner, and a safe induction nearly always requires supplementation with exogenous catecholamines. The choice of induction agent, induction technique, and exogenous catecholamine support may be altered for each individual situation.

In addition to hypotension, many of the drugs used for induction of anesthesia have been associated with increased delirium in the postoperative period [17,18]. Delirium has been associated with increased mortality in hospitalized patients [19]. As such, choosing induction agents with regard to the avoidance of delirium has great potential benefits for septic patients.

Neuromuscular blockade with either a depolarizing muscle relaxant (eg, succinylcholine) or a nondepolarizing muscle relaxant (eg, cisatracurium, rocuronium) is frequently used to facilitate endotracheal intubation and optimize surgical conditions. These drugs may have unpredictable and prolonged effects in septic patients, particularly in the postoperative period.

Available induction agents include propofol, etomidate, ketamine, and a combination of benzodiazepines and opiates. Available neuromuscular blockers are numerous, comprising 3 classes: depolarizing, nondepolarizing curares, and nondepolarizing steroids.

Propofol is the most frequently used induction agent. It is a powerful gamma-aminobutyric acid (GABA)–ergic drug that is capable of inducing electroencephalographic isoelectricity in clinically relevant doses. It also causes a profound sympathectomy. Induction with propofol is rapid in onset (1 arm-to-brain circulation time), and rapid in its offset, relying on redistribution to organs other than the brain. The residual effects of propofol are few, with a very low incidence of delirium, dysphoria, nausea, vomiting, or constipation. When supplemented with exogenous catecholamines during a careful induction, propofol can be used safely and effectively to induce anesthesia in septic patients.

The use of etomidate in the critically ill, which septic patients often are, is controversial. Etomidate is an alternative induction agent. It is a steroid-based drug that crosses the blood-brain barrier and sensitizes neurons to the effects of GABA, thus depressing the reticular activating system, and inducing a state of hypnosis and anesthesia. It causes less of a sympathectomy and less muscle relaxation than propofol in clinically relevant doses. It seems to be a more appropriate agent for inducing medically unstable patients. However, there is debate in the literature about adrenal gland suppression by even a single dose of etomidate [20–22]. There seems to be an association between the use of etomidate and an increase in mortality in the critically ill [23]. Also, the use of etomidate is associated with increased nausea and vomiting, feelings of dysphoria, and delirium. With these considerations in mind, etomidate can be used safely and effectively to induce anesthesia in septic patients.

Ketamine is a novel drug that results in a dissociative anesthetic state by disrupting communication between the thalamus and the limbic system. Unlike all other anesthetic drugs, vascular sympathetic tone is maintained, responsiveness to CO_2 is maintained, and it provides excellent analgesia without requiring supplementation with other agents. Its side effect profile is the main reason that it falls into and out of favor in anesthesiology every few years. In addition to hypertension and myocardial depression, ketamine causes powerful and realistic visual and auditory hallucinations. It can also induce a profound dysphoria, with patients often reporting that they think they are going to die. The dysphoria can be managed with anxiolytic drugs before the administration of ketamine, but the hallucinations usually persist. However, at subanesthetic doses ketamine maintains its excellent analgesic properties, and it is increasingly used as an adjunct in septic and critically ill patients [24]. With these considerations in mind, ketamine can be used safely and effectively to induce anesthesia in septic patients [25].

Benzodiazepines, often in combination with opiates to provide analgesia, have been used for many years to induce a state of anesthesia. Compared with the previously discussed agents, they are significantly longer acting, and are more variable in their anxiolytic efficacy from patient to patient. Benzodiazepines may be administered as either bolus or infusion, and may be continued into the postoperative period if the patient's clinical status warrants long-term intubation and mechanical ventilation. However, there is an emerging body of evidence showing a strong association between benzodiazepines and delirium [18]. With a further association between episodes of delirium and in-hospital mortality, many clinicians are seeking to limit the use of benzodiazepines, particularly in the elderly [19]. With these considerations in mind, benzodiazepines may safely be used to induce anesthesia in septic patients, but caution should be exercised.

Neuromuscular blockade with either depolarizing agents or nondepolarizing agents is often used to facilitate endotracheal intubation. Similar to all of the other previously discussed agents, neuromuscular blockers carry increased risk in septic patients, and avoidance of neuromuscular blockers (NMBs) is recommended in septic patients without ARDS [26].

Succinylcholine, the only depolarizing neuromuscular blocker available on the market, causes an increase in plasma potassium (K). This increase can be particularly problematic in septic patients who have renal dysfunction, and may result in hyperkalemia, with resulting arrhythmias. As the K leaves the intracellular fraction for the plasma fraction, it brings hydrogen (H) ions along with it, resulting in worsening acidemia. This decrease in pH may exacerbate myocardial dysfunction and vasoplegia. As such, it is prudent to check a plasma K level before the use of succinylcholine in septic patients.

Steroid-based nondepolarizing NMBs, such as rocuronium and vecuronium, competitively inhibit the action of acetylcholine on the postsynaptic membrane of the neuromuscular junction. They do not carry the same risk of hyperkalemia as succinylcholine. Instead, the concerns surrounding steroid-based nondepolarizing NMBs are for unpredictability in onset, metabolism by the liver and kidneys, and most importantly for prolonged respiratory muscle weakness [27]. The prolonged respiratory muscle weakness can result in extended ventilator times, and seems to be most common when patients are in a proinflammatory state [28,29]. Perhaps the worst complication of prolonged steroid-based NMB administration is neuropathy and myopathy of critical illness. Neuropathy and myopathy of critical illness result in profound voluntary and respiratory muscle weakness that can persist for months, often necessitating prolonged mechanical ventilatory support and protracted physical rehabilitation [28].

Nondepolarizing curare-derived NMBs (eg, cisatracurium and atracurium) also act by competitive inhibition to the action of acetylcholine, but their metabolism and elimination are less organ dependent. Atracurium is metabolized by a combination of plasma esterases and Hofmann degradation (spontaneous degradation at physiologic temperature and pH). Its use is limited by its active metabolite, laudanosine, which may accumulate and prolong the neuromuscular blockade. Cisatracurium also undergoes Hofmann degradation, but it has no known active metabolite. This quality makes cisatracurium the NMB of choice for septic patients [29].

MONITORING AND MAINTENANCE OF ANESTHESIA

In septic patients, the maintenance period of anesthetic administration can be particularly dynamic with frequent dramatic changes in volume status, vascular tone (systemic vascular resistance [SVR]), and myocardial contractility. Significant instability may occur as source control is achieved and inflammatory mediators are released into the blood stream. Add the relative hypovolemia of septic patients, and maintaining an adequate mean arterial pressure (MAP) can become challenging. As such, it is often prudent to place an arterial line in either the preoperative period or immediately after induction to facilitate maintaining MAP goals and frequent blood sampling for laboratory tests [30].

Maintenance of an MAP that allows sufficient systemic perfusion is imperative, because it minimizes the likelihood of myocardial ischemia, cerebral ischemia, acute kidney injury, acute liver injury, and bowel ischemia. Achievement of the target MAP goal is best accomplished using a strategy that optimizes preload, SVR, and contractility.

Optimizing preload sounds simple, but it can be particularly challenging. The gold standard for intraoperative preload determination is left ventricular volumetric quantification via TEE [9]. However, not every anesthesiologist is trained in the use of TEE, and there are times when use of TEE is either contraindicated or not possible. Therefore, anesthesiologists must rely on surrogates for preload, such as CVP, pulmonary capillary wedge pressure (PCWP), pulmonary artery diastolic pressure (PAD), continuous venous oxygen saturation (Svo_2), and continuous $Scvo_2$.

Measurement of CVP requires placement of a CVC. With the increased use of ultrasonography for CVC placement, the incidence of CVC placement–related complications has decreased significantly [31]. However, the risk of bleeding, vascular injury, and line infection are important to keep in mind. Although not a perfect indicator of right atrial pressure, and therefore right ventricular pressure, the CVP followed as a trend over a protracted period of time has been used for decades in medicine, and many clinicians are very comfortable with it. A preload CVP goal of 8 to 12 mm Hg is reasonable in intubated, mechanically ventilated patients. If patients are mechanically ventilated, and they are hypotensive, and the CVP is less than 8 mm Hg, then a fluid challenge is warranted (30 mL/kg) [30]. If they are hypotensive and the CVP is normal, then a vasopressor (eg, norepinephrine) should be started. If the CVP is high, then an inotropic agent (eg, epinephrine) should be started [30]. Concentrated infusions of vasoactive agents often require administration via CVC into a large central vessel.

The $Scvo_2$ catheter uses a fiberoptic oximeter at its tip to determine the blood oxygen saturation in the vessel in which it is located. As preload increases, the ventricle moves to a more favorable position on the Starling curve, systemic perfusion improves, and the $Scvo_2$ increases. The $Scvo_2$ provides useful data when viewed as a trend, much like the CVP.

PCWP, PAD, and Svo_2 require placement of a PAC. In addition to the CVC placement risks mentioned earlier, the PAC carries the additional risk of causing arrhythmias and thrombosis, in addition to other, less common complications. Because of the potential complications, studies that have shown no improvement in outcomes with the use of PACs, and studies that have shown worse outcomes with the use of PACs, the device has fallen out of favor for the routine care of septic patients [11].

In the absence of either an arterial line or a central line, the only available continuous data for the determination of preload are physical examination and urine output. Physical examination is often not possible in the operating room because patients are under sterile drapes. Urine output is notoriously unreliable during the physiologic stress of surgery, particularly in septic patients with acute kidney injury. It is therefore prudent to place an arterial line, a CVC, or both.

When resuscitating septic patients, there has long been debate as to the right choice of fluid: crystalloid, colloid, red blood cells, blood products, or hydroxyethyl starch (HES). HES and other synthetic colloids are associated with a greater incidence of kidney injury and mortality, and they have fallen out of favor [32–34]. Blood products (eg, fresh frozen plasma) carry an unacceptably high risk of infection, lung injury, and immune suppression when used for the purposes of volume expansion without coagulopathy. In sepsis, blood products should be reserved for the treatment of factor deficiency–related coagulopathy with active bleeding [30]. Red blood cells carry a risk of infection, lung injury, and immune suppression, and are associated with poor wound healing. There are also good data that point to a dose-dependent increase in mortality associated with red blood cell transfusion [35]. The role of red blood cell transfusion should be limited to the treatment of symptomatic anemia, with transfusion triggers between 7 and 9 g/dL depending on the patient's comorbidities [36,37]. Large-volume blood product transfusions should be periodically supplemented with either calcium gluconate or calcium chloride to counteract the preservative citrate in each transfused product. The decision between crystalloid and colloid may be left to the clinician's discretion, and often a mixed strategy works well.

The clinician must expect that conditions will change frequently, and sometimes rapidly. In gaining source control, large quantities of inflammatory mediators are often released into the patient's systemic circulation, which may result in vasodilation necessitating vasopressor support. It may result in an acute decrease in plasma pH that depresses myocardial contractility. It may also cause acute kidney injury that further decreases the plasma pH because of hyperkalemia and an inability to secrete H ions into the urine. Further concerns as the inflammatory burden increases include consumptive coagulopathy, worsening hepatic synthetic function, ARDS, and poor glycemic control [38].

The choice of vasopressor agent has been as controversial as the choice of resuscitative fluid. Norepinephrine is a potent vasoconstrictor, and is the first choice of agent for its ability to increase MAP with little change in heart rate [39,40]. If additional agents are required, epinephrine is the second choice for achievement of MAP goals, and may be substituted for norepinephrine [41,42]. Vasopressin in low doses (up to 0.03 U/min) may be added as well, reserving higher doses for salvage therapy [43,44]. Vasopressin has the interesting property of affecting only the SVR, with no effect on pulmonary vascular resistance, and so deserves special consideration in patients with pulmonary hypertension or evidence of right ventricular failure [45]. Dopamine is reserved as an alternative only for patients who have a low risk of tachyarrhythmia, because the incidence is much higher with dopamine than norepinephrine [40]. Phenylephrine, a pure vasoconstrictor (alpha agonist), causes a reflex bradycardia and decrease in cardiac output, which can be deleterious for septic patients. As a vasopressor for septic patients, it is reserved for circumstances in which other agents have caused unacceptable tachyarrhythmia, known high cardiac output states, or as salvage therapy in addition to other agents [30,46].

Inotropic support should be added when there is evidence of systemic hypoperfusion despite adequate filling pressures and MAP. A mixed agent, such as epinephrine, is the first choice in most situations, particularly when the patient's cardiac output is unknown [42]. Dobutamine is the first choice in patients with measured or suspected low cardiac output. A dobutamine infusion challenge of up to 20 μg/kg/min may be added to vasopressor therapy or initiated in situations of known myocardial dysfunction [42,47].

Along with changes in preload, contractility, and SVR, changes in pulmonary function, particularly the onset of ARDS, can occur quickly in septic patients. ARDS may present in several ways in the operative theater. Changes in lung compliance, increases in airway pressures, and worsening oxygenation may be early signs of ARDS. If an arterial line is in place, and arterial blood gases are being checked, a decrease in the PaO_2 relative to the inspired O_2 (P/F ratio) to less than 150 mm Hg necessitates changes in ventilator and NMB strategies. In patients with ARDS, the evidence is clear that low tidal volume (6–8 mL/kg of ideal body weight) and high positive end-expiratory pressure (PEEP) (5–15 cm H_2O) improve outcomes [48]. It is also becoming increasingly clear that the low tidal volume, higher PEEP mechanical ventilation strategy is a reasonable approach in patients other than those with ARDS [49]. In addition, septic patients who develop ARDS may benefit from a 48-hour course of neuromuscular blockade with cisatracurium early in the disease process [29].

Following arterial blood gases at regular intervals during the maintenance phase of anesthesia allows the clinician to closely monitor pH, bicarbonate, base deficit, and $PaCO_2$. When the pH decreases to less than 7.15, myocardial dysfunction and vasoplegia are exacerbated, resulting in hypoperfusion and hypotension [50]. It is reasonable to treat the acidemia with sodium bicarbonate if the patient is without ventilation defects, as indicated by an end-tidal CO_2 to $PaCO_2$ gradient less than 20 [30]. If the patient has a significant ventilation defect, then a different buffer should be chosen, such as tris(hydroxymethyl) aminomethane [51].

Other issues that are likely to require attention during the maintenance phase of anesthesia include blood glucose control, confirmation of adequate antibiotic coverage, venous thrombosis (VTE) prophylaxis, and enteral (gastric or small bowel) feeding. Blood glucose should be maintained at less than 180 mg/dL [52,53]. VTE prophylaxis should be stopped before arrival in the operating theater. However, source control is the prime directive, and a recent dose of a VTE prophylactic agent should not delay definitive therapy. Nil-by-mouth guidelines for gastric and postpyloric feeds are controversial. In general, gastric bolus or continuous feeds should be held 2 hours before a procedure. Postpyloric feeds should be held for 1 hour before a procedure. However, similar to VTE prophylaxis guidelines, definitive therapy should not be delayed on this basis [54].

No specific recommendations exist for the optimal agent during maintenance of anesthesia in septic patients. There are no absolute contraindications to any volatile agents or intravenous anesthetics in the septic population. However, most anesthetic agents have deleterious effects on myocardial performance, contractility, and SVR, and they may exacerbate the hypotension, hypoperfusion, and myocardial dysfunction of sepsis. As such, clinicians should be prepared to support patients with fluid, vasopressors, and inotropes as indicated by monitored parameters.

EMERGENCE

Extubation of septic patients is subject to the same goals as for nonseptic patients:

- Adequate pain control
- Adequate but not excessive minute ventilation
- Tidal volume greater than 4 mL/kg
- Respiratory rate less than 30 per minute
- PEEP less than or equal to 10 cm H_2O
- Pressure support less than or equal to 10 cm H_2O
- Tolerable secretion burden
- Evidence of full reversal of NMB: sustained head lift longer than 5 seconds, forced inspiratory pressure more than 30 cm H_2O
- Vasopressors and inotropes either stable or decreasing [55]

These goals require strict adherence in septic patients. Septic patients frequently require large-volume fluid resuscitation, often with large volumes of blood products. Consideration of the patient's trajectory is paramount. Is the patient stable from a pulmonary and hemodynamic standpoint? Is the patient improving or getting worse? It is common (and often prudent) to forego extubation in the operating room in this challenging patient population.

SUMMARY

Septic patients present many challenges to the anesthesiologist. They are frequently brought to the operating room emergently with the hope of achieving source control, which is the definitive therapy for septic shock. Safe induction can be achieved in several ways, most of which require catecholamine supplementation. Adequate hemodynamic monitoring, often with an arterial line and a CVC, can aid clinical decision making. Central venous access also provides a safe, reliable route for vasoactive infusions. Goal-directed therapy includes maintenance of MAP greater than 65 mm Hg, volume resuscitation to a CVP of 8 to 12 mm Hg, and $Scvo_2$ greater than 70 mm Hg. Norepinephrine is the first-line agent after adequate fluid resuscitation. Epinephrine is an appropriate second-line agent. It is important for the clinician to be constantly vigilant for changes in the patient's hemodynamic and pulmonary function. Maintain or institute lung protective ventilation (low tidal volume ventilation and higher PEEP) early. Avoid NMBs when possible, unless ARDS develops. Continue appropriate and timely dosing of antibiotics throughout the procedure. Strict adherence to extubation criteria helps to decrease the incidence of urgent reintubation.

References

[1] Dellinger RP, Carlet JM, Masur H, et al. Surviving sepsis campaign guidelines for management of severe sepsis and septic shock. Crit Care Med 2004;32:858–73.

[2] Rivers E, Nguyen B, Havstad S, et al. Early goal-directed therapy in the treatment of severe sepsis and septic shock. N Engl J Med 2001;345:1368–77.
[3] Evaluation for severe sepsis screening tool. 2014. Available at: http://www.survivingsepsis.org/files/tools/evaluationforseveresepsisscreeningtool.pdf. Accessed July 10, 2014.
[4] Ventilation with lower tidal volume as compared with traditional tidal volumes for acute lung injury and the acute respiratory distress syndrome. N Engl J Med 2000;342:1301–8.
[5] Weinstein MP, Reller LB, Murphy JR, et al. The clinical significance of positive blood cultures: a comprehensive analysis of 500 episodes of bacteremia and fungemia in adults. I. Laboratory and epidemiologic observations. Rev Infect Dis 1983;5:35–53.
[6] Ananthakrishnan AN. *Clostridium difficile* infection: epidemiology, risk factors and management. Nat Rev Gastroenterol Hepatol 2011;8:17–26.
[7] Mermel LA, Maki DG. Detection of bacteremia in adults; consequences of culturing an inadequate volume of blood. Ann Intern Med 1993;119:270–2.
[8] Turner KL, Moore LJ, Todd SR, et al. Identification of cardiac dysfunction in sepsis with B-type natriuretic peptide. J Am Coll Surg 2011;213(1):139–46.
[9] Cowie B, Kluger R, Kalpikas M. Left ventricular volume and ejection fraction assessment with transoesophageal echocardiography: 2D vs 3D imaging. Br J Anaesth 2012;110(2):201–6.
[10] Ogundele O, Bose E, Pinsky MR. Pulmonary artery catheterization. In: Ehrenfeld JM, Cannesson M, editors. Monitoring technologies in acute care environments. New York: Springer New York; 2014. p. 53–64.
[11] Harvey S, Harrison DA, Singer M, et al. Assessment of the clinical effectiveness of pulmonary artery catheters in management of patients in intensive care (PAC-Man): a randomised controlled trial. Lancet 2005;366:472–7.
[12] Marik PE, Cavallazzi R. Does the central venous pressure predict fluid responsiveness? An updated meta-analysis and a plea for some common sense. Crit Care Med 2013;41(7):1774–81.
[13] Marik PE, Baram M, Vahid B. Does central venous pressure predict fluid responsiveness? A systematic review of the literature and the tale of seven mares. Chest 2008;134(1):172–8.
[14] Richter HP, Petersen C, Goetz AE, et al. Detection of right ventricular insufficiency and guidance of volume therapy are facilitated by simultaneous monitoring of static and functional preload parameters. J Cardiothorac Vasc Anesth 2011;25(6):1051–5.
[15] Marik PE. Noninvasive cardiac output monitors: a state-of-the-art review. J Cardiothorac Vasc Anesth 2013;27:121–34.
[16] Varpula M, Tallgren M, Saukkonen K, et al. Hemodynamic variables related to outcome in septic shock. Intensive Care Med 2005;31:1066–71.
[17] Radtke FM, Franck M, Hagemann L, et al. Risk factors for inadequate emergence after anesthesia: emergence delirium and hypoactive emergence. Minerva Anestesiol 2010;76(6):394–403.
[18] Riker RR, Shehai Y, Bokesch PM, et al. Dexmedetomidine vs. midazolam for sedation of critically ill patients. JAMA 2009;301(5):489–99.
[19] Ely EW, Shintani A, Truman B, et al. Delirium as a predictor of mortality in mechanically ventilated patients in the intensive care unit. JAMA 2004;291(14):1753–62.
[20] Allolio B, Dorr H, Stuttmann R, et al. Effect of a single bolus of etomidate upon eight major corticosteroid hormones and plasma ACTH. Clin Endocrinol (Oxf) 1985;22:281–6.
[21] Chan CM, Mitchell AL, Shorr AF. Etomidate is associated with mortality and adrenal insufficiency in sepsis: a meta-analysis. Crit Care Med 2012;40:2945–53.
[22] McPhee LC, Badawi O, Fraser GL, et al. Single-dose etomidate is not associated with increased mortality in ICU patients with sepsis: analysis of a large electronic database. Crit Care Med 2013;41:774–83.
[23] Cuthbertson BH, Sprung CL, Annane D, et al. The effects of etomidate on adrenal responsiveness and mortality in patients with septic shock. Intensive Care Med 2009;35:1868–76.

[24] Jacobi J, Fraser GL, Coursin DB, et al. Clinical practice guidelines or the sustained use of sedatives and analgesics in the critically ill adult. Crit Care Med 2002;30(1): 119–41.
[25] Jabre P, Combes X, Lapostolle F, et al. Etomidate versus ketamine for rapid sequence intubation in acutely ill patients: a multicentre randomised controlled trial. Lancet 2009;374: 293–300.
[26] Freebairn RC, Derrick J, Gomersall CD, et al. Oxygen delivery, oxygen consumption, and gastric intramucosal pH are not improved by a computer-controlled, closed-loop, vecuronium infusion in severe sepsis and septic shock. Crit Care Med 1997;25:72–7.
[27] Lacomis D, Petrella JT, Giuliani MJ. Causes of neuromuscular weakness in the intensive care unit: a study of ninety-two patients. Muscle Nerve 1998;21:610–7.
[28] De Jonghe B, Cook D, Sharshar T, et al. Groupe de réflexion et d'étude sur les neuromyopathies en réanimation: acquired neuromuscular disorders in critically ill patients: a systematic review. Intensive Care Med 1998;24:1242–50.
[29] Papazian L, Forel JM, Gacouin A, et al. Neuromuscular blockers in early acute respiratory distress syndrome. N Engl J Med 2006;363:1107–16.
[30] Dellinger RP, Levy MM, Rhodes A, et al. Surviving sepsis campaign: International guidelines for management of severe sepsis and septic shock, 2012. Intensive Care Med 2013;39:165–228.
[31] Gann M, Sardi A. Improved results using ultrasound guidance for central venous access. Am Surg 2003;69:1104–7.
[32] Guidet B, Martinet O, Boulain T, et al. Assessment of hemodynamic efficacy and safety of 6% hydroxyethylstarch 130/0.4 vs 0.9% NaCl fluid replacement in patients with severe sepsis: the CRYSTMAS study. Crit Care 2012;16:R94.
[33] Perner A, Haase N, Guttormsen AB, et al. Hydroxyethyl starch 130/0.42 versus Ringer's acetate in severe sepsis. N Engl J Med 2012;367:124–34.
[34] Schortgen F, Lacherade JC, Bruneel F, et al. Effects of hydroxyethyl starch and gelatin on renal function in severe sepsis: a multicentre randomised study. Lancet 2001;357:911–6.
[35] Hendrickson JE, Hillyer CD. Noninfectious serious hazards of transfusion. Anesth Analg 2009;108(3):759–69.
[36] Hebert PC, Wells G, Blajchman MA, et al. A multicenter, randomized, controlled clinical trial of transfusion requirements in critical care. N Engl J Med 1999;340:409–17.
[37] Villanueva C, Colomo A, Bosch A, et al. Transfusion strategies for acute upper gastrointestinal bleeding. N Engl J Med 2013;368:11–21.
[38] Hotchkiss RS, Karl IE. The pathophysiology and treatment of sepsis. N Engl J Med 2003;348:138–50.
[39] Martin C, Papazian L, Perrin G, et al. Norepinephrine or dopamine for the treatment of hyperdynamic septic shock? Chest 1993;103:1826–31.
[40] De Backer D, Creteur J, Silva E, et al. Effects of dopamine, norepinephrine, and epinephrine on the splanchnic circulation in septic shock: which is best? Crit Care Med 2003;31: 1659–67.
[41] Myburgh JA, Higgins A, Jovanovska A, et al. A comparison of epinephrine and norepinephrine in critically ill patients. Intensive Care Med 2008;34:2226–34.
[42] Annane D, Vignon P, Renault A, et al, For the CATS Study Group. Norepinephrine plus dobutamine versus epinephrine alone for management of septic shock: a randomized trial. Lancet 2007;370:676–84.
[43] Russell JA, Walley KR, Singer J, et al. Vasopressin versus norepinephrine infusion in patients with septic shock. N Engl J Med 2008;358:877–87.
[44] Dünser MW, Mayr AJ, Ulmer H, et al. Arginine vasopressin in advanced vasodilatory shock: a prospective, randomized, controlled study. Circulation 2003;107:2313–9.
[45] Tayama E, Ueda T, Shojima T, et al. Arginine vasopressin is an ideal drug after cardiac surgery for the management of low systemic vascular resistant hypotension concomitant with pulmonary hypertension. Interact Cardiovasc Thorac Surg 2007;6(6):715–9.

[46] Morella A, Ether C, Rothberg S, et al. Phenylephrine versus norepinephrine for initial hemodynamic support of patients with septic shock: a randomized, controlled trial. Crit Care 2008;12:R143.
[47] Seguin P, Bellissant E, Le-Tulzo Y, et al. Effects of epinephrine compared with the combination of dobutamine and norepinephrine on gastric perfusion in septic shock. Clin Pharmacol Ther 2002;71:381–8.
[48] Sevransky JE, Levy MM, Marini JJ. Mechanical ventilation in sepsis-induced acute lung injury/acute respiratory distress syndrome: An evidence based review. Crit Care Med 2004;32(11):S548–53.
[49] Futier E, Constantin JM, Paugam-Burtz C, et al. A trial of intraoperative low-tidal-volume ventilation in abdominal surgery. N Engl J Med 2013;369:428–37.
[50] Hunter JD, Doddi M. Sepsis and the heart. Br J Anaesth 2010;104(1):3–11.
[51] Diaz JV, Brower R, Calfee CS, et al. Therapeutic strategies for severe acute lung injury. Crit Care Med 2010;38(8):1644–50.
[52] van den Berghe G, Wilmer A, Hermans G, et al. Intensive insulin therapy in the medical ICU. N Engl J Med 2006;354:449–61.
[53] The NICE-SUGAR Study Investigators, Finfer S, Chittock DR, et al. Intensive versus conventional glucose control in critically ill patients. N Engl J Med 2009;360:1283–97.
[54] McElroy LM, Codner PA, Brasel KJ. A pilot study to explore the safety of perioperative postpyloric enteral nutrition. Nutr Clin Pract 2012;27(6):777–80.
[55] MacIntyre NR, Cook DJ, Ely EW Jr, et al. Evidence-based guidelines for weaning and discontinuing ventilatory support: a collective task force facilitated by the American College of Chest Physicians; the American Association for Respiratory Care; and the American College of Critical Care Medicine. Chest 2001;120(Suppl 6):375S–95S.

Advances in Anesthesia 32 (2014) 205–235

ADVANCES IN ANESTHESIA

Advances in Spinal Cord Protection from Perioperative Ischemic Injury

Philip E.F. Roman, MD, MPH[a,*], Ashanpreet S. Grewal, MD[b], Bradley S. Taylor, MD, MPH[c], Alina M. Grigore, MD, MHS[b]

[a]Division of Cardiothoracic Anesthesia, Department of Anesthesiology, University of Maryland School of Medicine, 22 South Greene Street, S11C07, Baltimore, MD 21201, USA; [b]Division of Cardiothoracic Anesthesia, Department of Anesthesiology, University of Maryland School of Medicine, 22 South Greene Street, S8D12, Baltimore, MD 21201, USA; [c]Division of Cardiac Surgery, Department of Surgery, University of Maryland School of Medicine, 110 South Paca Street, 7S164, Baltimore, MD 21201, USA

Keywords

• Thoracic aorta • Thoracoabdominal aorta • Type B dissection • Aneurysm • Spinal cord injury • Spinal cord ischemia • Paraplegia • Thoracic endovascular aortic repair

Key points

- Thoracic aortic dissections and thoracoabdominal aortic repairs may be complicated by spinal cord injury leading to paraplegia or paraparesis.
- The anterior spinal cord is particularly vulnerable during periods of decreased blood flow, as happens during both open and endovascular repairs.
- Strategies to reduce the risk of spinal cord injury are based on augmenting blood flow during periods of ischemia.
- A multimodal approach, with augmented circulation and aggressive intercostal artery reimplantation, lumbar drainage of cerebrospinal fluid, and intraoperative neuromonitoring of motor evoked potentials, reduces the risk of spinal cord injury.
- This review summarizes the recent advances in our understanding of techniques to protect the spinal cord during major descending aortic surgery.

Disclosure: No author has funding sources or conflicts of interest.

*Corresponding author. *E-mail address:* proman@anes.umm.edu

0737-6146/14/$ – see front matter
http://dx.doi.org/10.1016/j.aan.2014.08.010

INTRODUCTION

Operative management of descending thoracic and thoracoabdominal aortic disease continues to be associated with significant mortality and morbidity. Paraplegia and paraparesis persist as the leading and most feared morbidities, despite advancements in surgical and anesthetic techniques. The goal of this article is to summarize important understandings in spinal cord protection and to review more recent advancements.

ANATOMY AND PHYSIOLOGY OF THE SPINAL CORD

The arterial circulation of the spinal cord is provided by internal and external sources (Fig. 1) [1]. The internal blood supply comes from a single anterior spinal artery (ASA), which courses along the ventral aspect of the cord and ultimately distributes blood to the bulk of the cord substance through penetrating arteries, and paired posterior spinal arteries (PSA). The principal

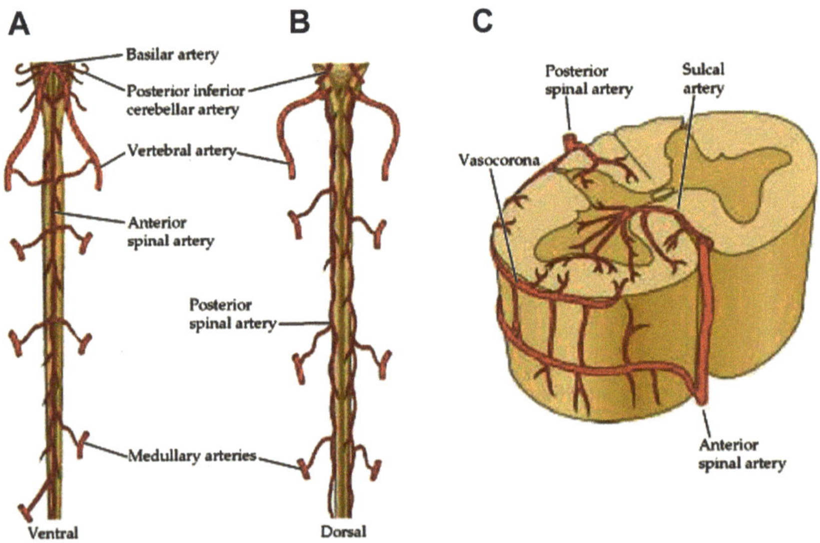

Fig. 1. Blood supply of the spinal cord. (*A*) View of the ventral (anterior) surface of the spinal cord. At the level of the medulla, the vertebral arteries give off branches that merge to form the anterior spinal artery. Approximately 10 to 12 segmental arteries (which arise from various branches of the aorta) join the anterior spinal artery along its course. These segmental arteries are known as medullary arteries. (*B*) The vertebral arteries (or the posterior inferior cerebellar artery) give rise to paired posterior spinal arteries that run along the dorsal (posterior) surface of the spinal cord. (*C*) Cross section through the spinal cord, illustrating the distribution of the anterior and posterior spinal arteries. The anterior spinal arteries give rise to numerous sulcal branches that supply the anterior two-thirds of the spinal cord. The posterior spinal arteries supply much of the dorsal horn and the dorsal columns. A network of vessels known as the vaso corona connects these 2 sources of supply and sends branches into the white matter around the margin of the spinal cord. (*From* Purves D, Augustine GJ, Fitzpatrick D, et al. Neuroscience. 2nd edition. Sunderland (MA): Sinauer Associates; 2001; with permission.)

extrinsic blood sources in the thoracolumbar cord are the intercostal and lumbar arteries. The conus is supplied by the lateral sacral branches of the hypogastric vessels. Radiculomedullary arteries irregularly distribute to the spinal cord. The thoracolumbar region is at the most risk for ischemic injury because in this region the blood is typically provided by a single radiculomedullary artery, better known as the artery of Adamkiewicz or arteria radicularis magna. This artery has been shown to arise from T9-T12 in about 75% of individuals. Because this area falls within the segment of the aorta that is clamped during reconstruction, clamping can compromise the blood supply to the cord.

Over the past several decades it was thought that the best strategy for protecting the spinal cord postoperatively was to preserve flow via the artery of Adamkiewicz, considered a critical segmental artery (SA). The concept of a uniquely important SA has been challenged recently by several clinical observations and laboratory studies, which introduced a novel idea of spinal cord circulation as being part of a continuous network that includes the subclavian artery, hypogastric arteries, and the blood supply to the paravertebral muscles (Fig. 2) [2–5]. Physiologic and anatomic studies have now documented the existence of this network, and have provided insight into its response to deprivation of SA input. The ASA, as the predominant intraspinal vessel, is connected to a series of pentagonal epidural arterial arcades, which are connected to the SAs, and also anastomose with the extraspinal network, which feeds the paravertebral muscles (Fig. 3). This extensive collateral network communicates cranially to the subclavian artery and caudally to the hypogastric artery, both of which have been shown, in physiologic experiments, to play an important role in spinal cord protection following SA sacrifice.

The central nervous system (CNS) is a converter, consumer, and conserver of energy. The metabolic substrate for the CNS is glucose produced by glycogenolysis of stored glycogen in the liver, muscle, and other organs. Through glycolysis, glucose undergoes complete oxidation, resulting in the production of adenosine triphosphate (ATP) and the formation of carbon dioxide and water. ATP is consumed in the maintenance of neuronal transmembrane electrical and ionic gradients during both resting state and depolarization. ATP is also used for synthesis, packaging, release, and reuptake of neurotransmitters. A coupling process between the production and delivery of energy substrates and demand enables the CNS to conserve and maintain a proper balance between ATP utilization and production.

Spinal cord perfusion pressure (SCPP) is the difference between distal mean aortic pressure and cerebrospinal fluid (CSF) pressure or central venous pressure (CVP), whichever is higher. Autoregulation of spinal cord blood flow (SCBF) is similar to cerebral autoregulation, and usually SCBF is maintained constant over the range of 50 to 125 mm Hg SCPP. The capillary network of the gray matter is more extensive than that of the white matter, reflecting a higher metabolic demand. Accordingly, there are various regional differences in SCBF between the gray and white matter, and also between different regions of the spinal cord. The cervical and lumbar regions are known to have 40% higher metabolic

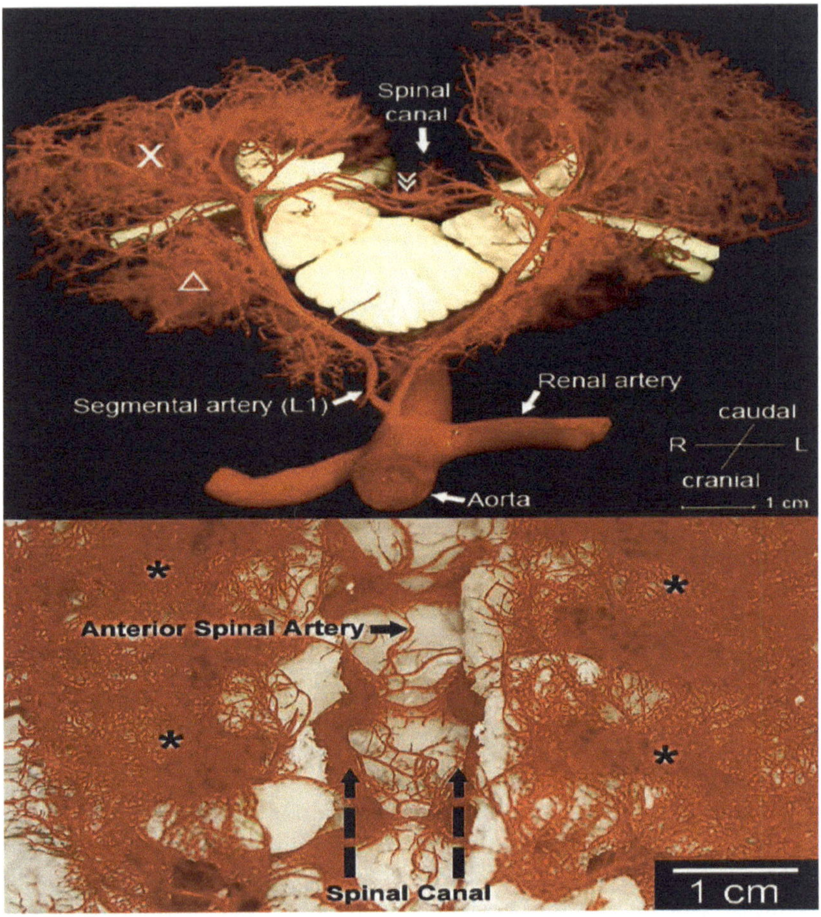

Fig. 2. Methylmethacrylate casts of juvenile pig lumbar vasculature, demonstrating the extensive collateralization between spinal cord and muscle, and cranially caudally within the paraspinous muscles. ASA, anterior spinal artery; asterisks, paraspinous muscles; triangle, erector spinae muscles; X, iliopsoas muscle. (*From* Etz CD, Kari FA, Mueller CS, et al. The collateral network concept: a reassessment of the anatomy of spinal cord perfusion. J Thorac Cardiovasc Surg 2011;141:1023; with permission.)

requirements compared with thoracic regions [6]. Aortic cross-clamping results in a decrease in distal mean aortic pressure and a significant increase in CSF pressure, which leads to a dramatic decrease in SCPP. The increase in CSF pressure with cross-clamping is primarily due to proximal arterial hypertension and venous congestion. During hypoxia and hypercarbia, autoregulation of SCBF is impaired, and flow becomes linearly related to perfusion pressure. For this reason, adjuncts that decrease CSF pressure will increase SCPP. The rationale for using a CSF drain is based on experimental data showing that (1) CSF pressure increases during aortic clamping, and (2) reducing CSF pressure improves spinal cord perfusion.

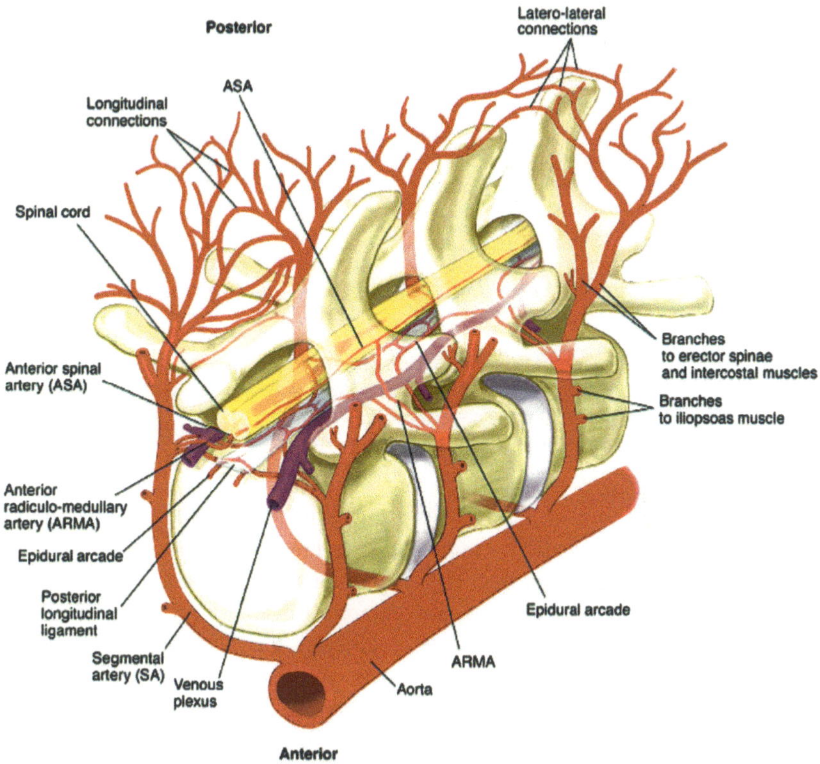

Fig. 3. Blood supply to the spinal cord: relationships, relative sizes, and interconnections among segmental arteries (SAs), anterior radicomedullary arteries (ARMAs), epidural arcades, and the anterior spinal artery (ASA). Longitudinal anastomoses along the dorsal processes of the spine, in addition to dorsal communications between the right and left branches of the SAs, are also shown. (*From* Etz CD, Kari FA, Mueller CS, et al. The collateral network concept: a reassessment of the anatomy of spinal cord perfusion. J Thorac Cardiovasc Surg 2011;141:1024; with permission.)

MOLECULAR MECHANISM OF SPINAL NEURONAL INJURY

Ischemia is the major cause of metabolic injury to the CNS, and represents an imbalance between the metabolic demand and supply. The biochemical disturbances that occur during both ischemia and reperfusion processes contribute to ultimate neuronal damage. The functional state and recovery of neurons depend on the upper and lower ischemic threshold (Fig. 4) [7]. Upper ischemic threshold defines the flow at which neuronal function ceases while neuronal structural integrity is maintained. Full recovery occurs with restoration of blood flow. By contrast, lower ischemic threshold is associated with ATP depletion, membrane failure, loss of neuronal structural integrity, and neuronal death. Postischemic reperfusion is also associated with decreased

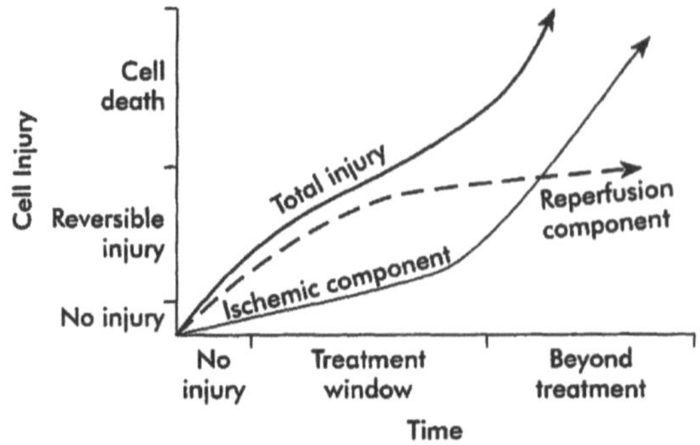

Fig. 4. Relationship between ischemic and reperfusion cellular changes leading to irreversible cell death. (*From* Cottrell J, Smith D. Anesthesia and neurosurgery. 3rd edition. Philadelphia: Mosby; 1994; with permission.)

blood flow as the result of edema and vasospasm, which leads to intracellular acidosis, release of excitatory amino acids, increased catecholamine release, hypermetabolism, secondary decrease in previously recovered metabolic activity, intracellular calcium overload, and neuronal death (Fig. 5) [8].

Complete neuronal ischemia depletes glucose and glycogen stores within 4 minutes and ATP stores in 5 to 7 minutes. As a result, neuronal membrane sodium pump failure allows intracellular influx of Na^+ and Cl^-, extracellular efflux of K^+ leading to membrane depolarization, and irreversible neuronal injury [9]. Ischemia predisposes to formation of free radicals and free fatty acids, which further induce biochemical alterations and cellular damage [10].

OPERATIVE TECHNIQUES FOR SPINAL CORD PRESERVATION

The most important factors in protecting the spinal cord during and after thoracic and thoracoabdominal aortic surgery are perfusion, metabolism, and oxygen delivery to the spinal cord during the vulnerable period of aortic occlusion, when SCBF is significantly reduced, as well as after aortic replacement while the coaxial collateral network is recruited to return resting blood flow to near-normal levels [11–13]. Assisted circulation and intercostal reimplantation by themselves have failed to reduce paraplegia risk both experimentally and clinically. This failure seems counterintuitive to the anatomic paradigm for spinal cord preservation [2,14–16]. However, reducing the vulnerability of the spinal cord during aortic surgery has always centered on collateral circulation, increasing ischemic tolerance, and protecting the spinal cord while collateral blood flow accommodates.

There continues to be controversy regarding paraplegia risk and prevention in the surgical treatment of the descending thoracic and thoracoabdominal aorta. There are 2 paradigms of causation: the purely anatomic paradigm, which postulates that paraplegia can only be prevented by reattaching specific intercostal arteries, and a more complex paradigm of collateral blood flow and

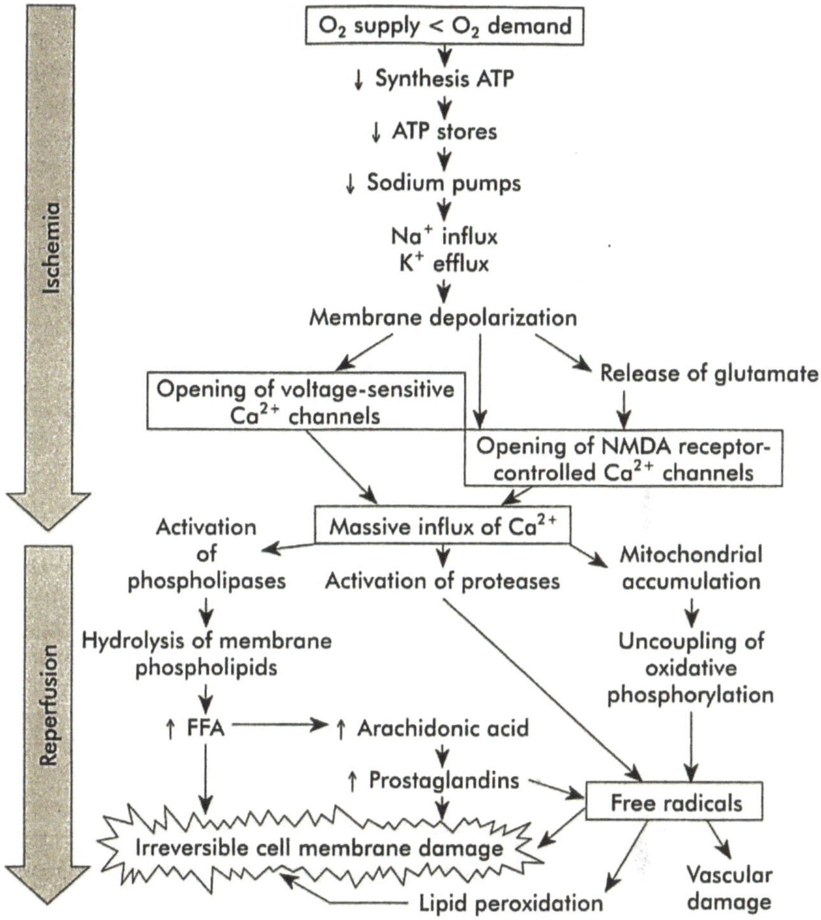

Fig. 5. Ischemic/reperfusion injury. Two components of tissue injury contribute to the ultimate neurologic damage. The ischemic component includes the processes of tissue damage occurring during ischemia. Cell death caused by the ischemic component alone depends on the severity and duration of ischemia. The secondary consequences of ischemia include the biochemical changes that take place at the time of reperfusion and reoxygenation after ischemia. The duration of these secondary processes and the extent to which they contribute to ultimate neurologic damage determine the therapeutic window during which treatment administered after ischemia may be effective. ATP, adenosine triphosphate; FFA, free fatty acids; NMDA, *N*-methyl-D-aspartic acid. (*From* Cottrell J, Smith D. Anesthesia and neurosurgery. 3rd edition. Philadelphia: Mosby; 1994; with permission.)

physiologic factors such as perfusion pressure, temperature, neurotransmitters, CSF pressure, and cardiac function, which is supported in the literature. Regardless of the surgical technique, there are equally good outcomes with the application of physiologic principles of assisted circulation with full cardiopulmonary bypass or partial left heart bypass, deep hypothermic circulatory arrest, or cross-clamping without assisted circulation. Thoracic endovascular aortic repair (TEVAR) has been shown to reduce early mortality, paraplegia (when adjunctive measures are used), and blood transfusion requirements. The fact that TEVAR alone without adjunctive measures carries the same risk of paraplegia as open procedures supports the observation that spinal cord ischemia (SCI) is primarily a matter of collateral blood flow and ischemic tolerance, rather than assisted circulation and selective intercostal reattachment. Nonselective intercostal reimplantation (IRP) in high-risk patients has added an additional 7% to 10% decrease, bringing about a 90% reduction in paralysis risk overall [17].

Indications

All patients with thoracic aortic aneurysm (TAA) or thoracoabdominal aortic aneurysm (TAAA), dissections, penetrating ulcer, and intramural hematoma should be evaluated by an aortic specialist. Asymptomatic patients with an aneurysm diameter that is twice the size of a normal aorta, aneurysm diameter greater than 6 cm in patients with familial disorders such as Marfan syndrome or 6.5 cm in patients without familial disorders, or patients with evidence of progressive aneurysm enlargement of 0.5 cm per year should be evaluated for surgery. Patients with symptomatic aneurysms should undergo urgent surgical repair, even if smaller in size. Patients with multiple or significant comorbidities that prohibitively increase operative risk or those with a limited life expectancy should not undergo surgery. Surveillance of smaller asymptomatic TAAs or TAAAs typically involves serial computed tomography (CT) or magnetic resonance imaging (MRI) scans performed at 6-month intervals.

Repair of descending thoracic aortic aneurysm

Outcomes of patients requiring thoracic and thoracoabdominal aortic surgery have improved significantly because of advances in perioperative management. The patient undergoing descending thoracic aortic repair is placed in the right lateral decubitus position for a left posterolateral thoracotomy, which provides optimal exposure of the proximal and distal necks of most such aneurysms. For more extensive descending TAAs, a rib resection and/or access via an additional intercostal space may be necessary. In patients with TAA with an adequate proximal neck, partial cardiopulmonary bypass (femoral artery and femoral vein cannulation) with full systemic heparinization and an oxygenator is often used. Alternatively, left atrial-femoral artery cardiopulmonary bypass can be used for distal perfusion. When the aneurysm involves the origin of the left subclavian artery, the optimal approach is to avoid aortic clamping and the risk of cerebral embolization by utilizing femoral-femoral or femoral-axillary cardiopulmonary bypass and profound hypothermic circulatory arrest. The proximal aortic anastomosis is performed to an open graft in a bloodless field during circulatory arrest. Using this technique, the patient is gradually rewarmed while performing the distal anastomosis.

In patients undergoing conventional repair, once partial cardiopulmonary bypass is instituted and the aorta clamped, adjustments in the rate of venous return and infusion of vasodilators minimize left ventricular strain and hemodynamic fluctuations. A longitudinal aortotomy is made over the aneurysm, and any thrombus is evacuated. The intercostal branches in the proximal aorta are controlled with suture ligatures. When patent intercostal arteries in the region of T8 to L1 are encountered, reimplantation of these arteries into the graft is performed. One option is to anastomose a smaller-caliber Dacron graft to the island of lower intercostal vessels and perfuse selectively via a side limb of the cardiopulmonary bypass circuit (this graft is later anastomosed to the main aortic graft after completion of the proximal and distal aortic anastomoses). Proximal and distal aortic full-thickness cuffs are defined, and a woven Dacron graft is anastomosed to the cuffs. Before securing the distal anastomosis, the native aorta and graft are flushed both antegrade and retrograde, thereby removing air and debris. Cardiopulmonary bypass is gradually weaned and the heparin neutralized with protamine. After decannulation, the femoral artery and femoral vein are repaired. After assuring hemostasis, the residual aneurysm sac is closed over the graft and the chest incision is closed.

Thoracoabdominal aortic aneurysm

Surgical treatments of TAAAs require extensive thoracic and abdominal exposure, with particular attention directed to reimplantation of the renal and visceral arteries. The patient's abdomen and pelvis are positioned supine with a slight rotation, and the thorax is rotated to a right lateral decubitus position. A left thoracoabdominal incision is made dividing the costal margin and extending down the abdominal midline. The exposure of the thoracic aorta is achieved in the pleural cavity, whereas exposure of the abdominal aorta is via the retroperitoneal plane after division of the diaphragm circumferentially. The proximal neck of the TAA is exposed and the abdominal portion of the aorta, the left renal artery, and the origin of the celiac and superior mesenteric arteries are identified. After systemic heparinization and cannulation of femoral artery and vein (or left atrium and femoral artery), cardiopulmonary bypass is instituted. Normothermia or mild hypothermia is maintained during the procedure to permit continued cardiac contraction. The proximal thoracic aorta and abdominal aorta are clamped, and the aortic pressure proximal to the clamp is maintained by increasing or decreasing the venous drainage into the cardiopulmonary bypass circuit. The TAA is incised and the proximal neck of the aneurysm defined. A woven Dacron graft is sewn to the proximal neck. Intercostal arteries are selectively reimplanted into the graft. The proximal clamp is then replaced distal to the site of reimplanted intercostal arteries. The distal aorta (ie, abdominal aorta) is prepared depending on the extent of the abdominal involvement. If the aneurysm extends to the celiac artery and visceral arteries but not beyond (as in type I), the abdominal aorta can be partially divided tangentially and the distal anastomosis performed without separate reimplantation of the visceral vessels (Fig. 6). If the abdominal component of the aneurysm is more extensive (as in types II, III, and IV), the visceral and right renal arteries may be reimplanted using the graft inclusion method as

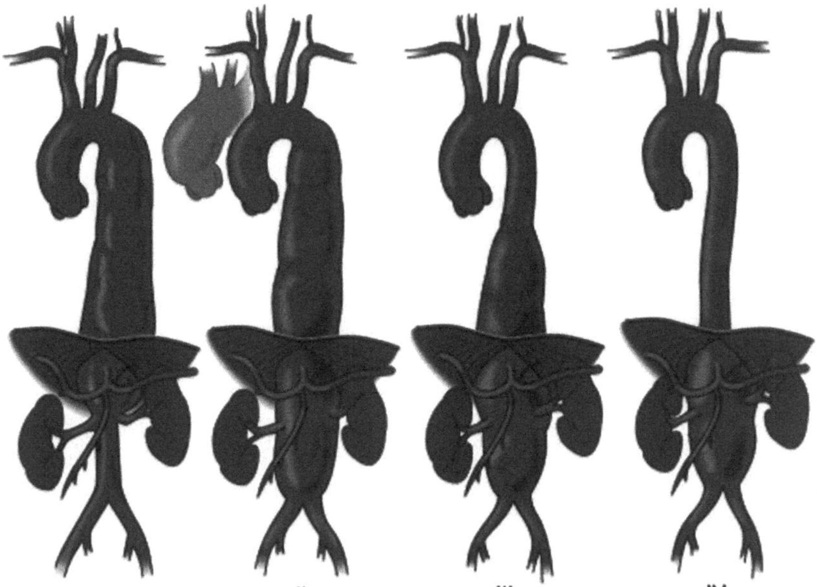

Fig. 6. The Crawford classification of thoracoabdominal aneurysms defined by anatomic location. (*From* Norris EJ. Anesthesia for vascular surgery. In: Miller RD, Eriksson LI, Fleisher LA, et al, editors. Miller's anesthesia. 7th edition. Maryland Heights (MO): Churchill Livingstone; 2009; with permission.)

one large island with the left renal artery reimplanted as a separate button. The distal neck of the aneurysm is defined and the graft sewn to it in an end-to-end fashion. After sequential flushing of air and debris from the graft and aorta, the aortic clamps are released and the patient is weaned from cardiopulmonary bypass.

Thoracic endovascular aortic repair

Indications for endovascular repair of a TAA are the same as for open repair. However, the patient should have proximal and distal "landing zones" of at least 2 cm without significant calcification or thrombus. Access vessels of at least 7 mm luminal diameter, without extreme tortuosity, are necessary and must be assessed by preoperative imaging.

The patient is placed in a supine position. Both groins and the entire abdomen are prepped and draped. If the right radial/brachial artery needs to be accessed, the right arm is prepped and draped. TEVAR may be performed under general, regional, or local anesthesia. CSF drainage is recommended for patients with previous abdominal aortic aneurysm repair in whom iliac conduit or intentional occlusion of the subclavian artery is planned. Furthermore, the patients with underlying TAA requiring extensive stent-graft coverage will require a prophylactic placement of the CSF drainage catheter, owing to the increased risk of neurologic deficits. The most common access site is the femoral artery (80%), conduit access to the common iliac artery is used sometimes (15%), and rarely access is obtained via the ascending aorta or distal abdominal aorta (5%). The right brachial/radial artery is also accessed when planning on excluding any brachiocephalic vessels with the covered stent graft (Zone 0–2 deployment in the aortic arch). Options for management of intraoperative changes seen on neuromonitoring during TEVAR include CSF drainage and alteration of hemodynamics to optimize SCPP and blood flow (see the section Treatment of spinal cord ischemia).

NONOPERATIVE TECHNIQUES FOR SPINAL CORD PROTECTION

Risk of injury

The primary mechanism of SCI in thoracic aortic operations is temporary or permanent interruption of blood supply. In a prospective database study from 2001 to 2009, Drinkwater and colleagues [18] evaluated outcomes for 235 patients undergoing thoracic aortic stent grafting. SCI in all forms (permanent or transient, early or delayed, partial or complete) and paraplegia were 9.8% and 5.5%, respectively. TEVAR was associated with the lowest risk of SCI (1.8%) or paraplegia (0.9%). Hybrid procedures including the abdominal viscera had the greatest risk of SCI (20%) and paraplegia (11.3%). Logistic regression modeling showed the percentage of aorta stented to be the greatest risk factor, with an adjusted odds ratio (OR) per 10% increased coverage of 1.78 (95% confidence interval [CI] 1.18-2.71). Drinkwater and colleagues enrolled both elective and emergency procedures, whereas Chiesa and colleagues [19] prospectively studied elective TEVARs. The incidence of delayed neurologic deficit was 4%, without permanent paraplegia. Only perioperative hypotension (mean arterial pressure [MAP] <70 mm Hg) was a significant risk factor for SCI on univariate analysis.

Transient and permanent spinal cord injury has been a long recognized complication from open descending aortic operations. In a recent review of 224 elective and emergent surgeries performed at the University of Pennsylvania, 75 (33%) patients developed intraoperative or postoperative SCI [20]. Twenty of 58 patients (34%) undergoing intraoperative somatosensory evoked potential (SSEP) monitoring demonstrated ischemia, with 9 having persistent changes. Of 75 patients, 72 (96%) had clinical evidence of postoperative SCI. Risk factors by univariate analysis included absence of a lumbar drain, surgical repair crossing the diaphragm, intraoperative permanent SSEP changes, renal failure, preoperative paraplegia, and stroke. Multivariate analysis showed that only surgical repair crossing the diaphragm (OR 4.8, 95% CI 1.4–16.7), near to complete paraplegia at diagnosis (OR 4.5, 95% CI 1.4–14), and renal failure (OR 6.1, 95% CI 1.7–21.2) were independently associated with poor outcome.

In a prospectively enrolled study of 571 patients undergoing open TAAA repair from 1981 to 2008, Schepens and colleagues [21] found a 4.4% incidence of paraplegia from surgical procedures that included left heart bypass.

Protective factors for postoperative SCI were age greater than 75 years (OR 0.14, 95% CI 0.19–1.09), presence of postdissection aneurysm (OR 0.4, 95% CI 0.17–0.94), and combined use of CSF drainage and motor evoked potentials (MEPs) (OR 0.28, 95% CI 0.14–0.56). A retrospective review of 858 TAA repairs from 1990 to 2006 showed a similarly low rate of paraplegia at 2.7% [22]. Ten cases of delayed SCI (within 48 hours) occurred despite normal SSEPs at the end of the operation. When compared with 10 matched controls who did not have SCI, postoperative mean CVP (hours 1–5) was greater in those patients with SCI ($P = .03$). Although absolute MAP was not significantly different, the relative MAP was lower than the patients' preoperative MAP ($P = .027$). This result supports the hypothesis that spinal cord hypoperfusion is the central mechanism of SCI during and immediately after extensive aortic surgery.

Hemodynamic monitoring

The unique surgical techniques used during descending aortic and thoracoabdominal aortic repairs frequently dictate the hemodynamic monitors used. The goal of monitoring is to optimize end-organ function, including the heart, brain, spinal cord, and visceral organs.

Arterial blood pressure monitoring

Invasive arterial pressure monitoring is mandatory given the sudden fluctuations seen, and the frequent use of some form of pump-based perfusion (full or partial cardiopulmonary bypass, left heart bypass) leading to nonpulsatile flow. Upper extremity blood pressure is needed to monitor perfusion pressure above the proximal aortic cross-clamp. This goal is frequently accomplished with a right radial artery catheter. Right upper extremity pressure monitoring is preferred, as the left subclavian artery may be temporarily clamped during proximal aortic dissection and clamping. Left radial artery pressure monitoring may also be needed if left subclavian perfusion via cannula or graft is performed. When distal aortic perfusion is provided, typically via the femoral artery but also with direct descending aortic cannulation, a femoral artery pressure transduced from the contralateral leg is needed. During aortic cross-clamping, the distal perfusion pressure represents the spinal cord MAP. The most prudent approach is to monitor all 3 locations, which provides the surgeon with the greatest flexibility should the operative finding mandate an unanticipated change in technique.

Central venous pressure

CVP, along with its trend, has traditionally been viewed as a proxy for blood volume or a predictor of fluid responsiveness. In a systematic review of 24 studies encompassing 803 patients, the pooled correlation coefficient between CVP and blood volume was 0.16 (95% CI 0.03–0.28), indicating very poor correlation. The trend in CVP/ΔCPV demonstrated equally poor correlation [23]. The effect of the lateral open chest position on CVP is unknown and renders the intraoperative CVP unreliable [24].

Pulmonary artery catheter

The use of pulmonary artery catheters (PACs) in critically ill patients is controversial, yet frequent. PACs continue to be used routinely in cardiac anesthesia despite evidence demonstrating lack of clinical efficacy. Critical appraisal of the literature is beyond the scope of this review, but the use of a PAC may be indicated in select patients (such as those with pulmonary hypertension or ventricular dysfunction). During partial cardiopulmonary bypass or left heart bypass, the cardiac output derived by PAC may not be accurate. Thermodilution calculations may be skewed by temperature variations during venous drainage and rapid transfusion. In addition, mixed venous saturations (Svo_2) may be accurate during left heart bypass but not partial cardiopulmonary bypass, as an oxygenator is used during partial cardiopulmonary bypass. Although there are limitations to the use of intraoperative PACs, their data may be useful in optimizing spinal cord oxygen delivery (assessed by Svo_2 and cardiac output) in the immediate postoperative period.

Spinal cord perfusion pressure

SCPP equals MAP minus the greater of either CVP or CSF pressure. As shown earlier, intraoperative CVP measurements are unreliable, and CSF pressure should be preferentially used.

A preoperative lumbar intrathecal catheter can directly measure CSF pressure. This catheter may also be used for drainage of CSF (see later discussion). The CSF pressure should be continuously monitored except during drainage of CSF. Modern anesthesia and intensive care unit monitors are capable of calculating SCPP when provided with MAP and CSF pressure. During aortic cross-clamping, one must be aware that the distal aortic MAP, not upper extremity MAP, is the forward pressure feeding most spinal cord arteries, and should be used when calculating SCPP.

Intraoperative neuromonitoring

Evoked potentials

Real-time monitoring of the neurophysiologic status of the spinal cord has proved useful in both open and endovascular aortic repairs. Changes in evoked potentials (EPs) correlate with ischemia, and EP monitoring has been associated with a reduction in spinal cord infarction. Several modalities are available, with SSEPs and MEPs being the most common. Understanding of the principles and limitations of electrophysiologic monitoring allows the operative team to tailor both the anesthetic and surgical approach to reduce the risk of paraplegia.

Monitoring SSEPs and MEPs provides information on the integrity of the dorsal and anterior horns of the spinal cord, respectively. Both SSEPs and MEPs monitor the central gray matter of the spinal cord. Somatosensory monitoring is performed with stimulation of a peripheral nerve and recording of the electrical potential at multiple sites including the peripheral nerve, spinal cord, cervical spinal cord, and sensory cortex. SSEPs are sensitive to ischemia in the peripheral nerve, spinal cord, brainstem, and sensory cortex. SSEPs are also sensitive to changes in perfusion pressure without ischemia, which limits their utility in aortic surgery.

Intraoperative MEPs are most commonly produced by transcranial electrical stimulation. The stimulating electrodes may be standard spiral needles, straight needles, or electroencephalography cup electrodes, and are placed overlying the motor cortex. Risks of stimulating electrodes include seizures, cardiac dysrhythmia or hemodynamic instability, and thermal, electrochemical, movement-induced, or bite injury. Relative contraindications are epilepsy, cortical lesions, convex skull defects, elevated intracranial pressure, and intracranial electrodes, clips, or shunts.

MEP monitoring is typically performed after the induction of anesthesia, owing to the painful transcranial electrical stimulation required. Repetitive stimulation produces a compound muscle action potential from the tibialis anterior muscle in the leg and abductor pollicis brevis muscle in the hand. The amplitude and latency of the MEP is recorded via limb-surface electrodes, with the amplitude being most important for detection of ischemic changes. The MEP amplitude reflects function of the spinal cord α motor neurons [25].

The ascending pathways assessed by SSEP monitoring contain few, if any, spinal cord synaptic connections. The white matter pathways of the dorsal column are more resistant to ischemia in comparison with the synaptic-rich anterior motor pathways.

Acute anterior horn ischemia produces attenuation or loss of lower extremity MEPs within 2 minutes (Fig. 7). Infarction may begin after 10 minutes of normothermic ischemia [26]. The contribution of pairing MEP with SSEP monitoring was evaluated in a prospective study of 56 patients undergoing descending TAA or TAAA procedures. Sixteen patients (28.6%) had significant MEP changes, but only 4 of these patients had deterioration of SSEPs. The addition of SSEP monitoring, though not solely predictive of paraplegia, may control for confounding conditions, such as isolated leg ischemia from femoral artery cannulation [27].

Influence of anesthetic technique

Both SSEP and MEP neurophysiologic monitoring are sensitive to the effects of anesthetic drugs and temperature. EPs may be successfully obtained in the presence of both volatile and intravenous anesthetics. A total intravenous anesthetic (TIVA) with propofol plus and an opiate infusion approach seems to be the most successful at preserving the full integrity of elicited EPs. When compared with isoflurane, MEP monitoring during a propofol-based TIVA technique was successful in 97% versus 67% of the patients undergoing corrective spine surgery [28]. In a comparison of equipotent anesthetic levels, Chen [29] demonstrated 100% success with MEP monitoring with propofol up to 25 mg/kg/h, 58.8% success with 0.6 vol% end-tidal isoflurane, and 17.8% success with 0.8 vol% end-tidal isoflurane.

Neuromuscular blocking agents, or paralytics, are commonly used during cardiac and vascular surgery, but profound muscle relaxation is incompatible

A

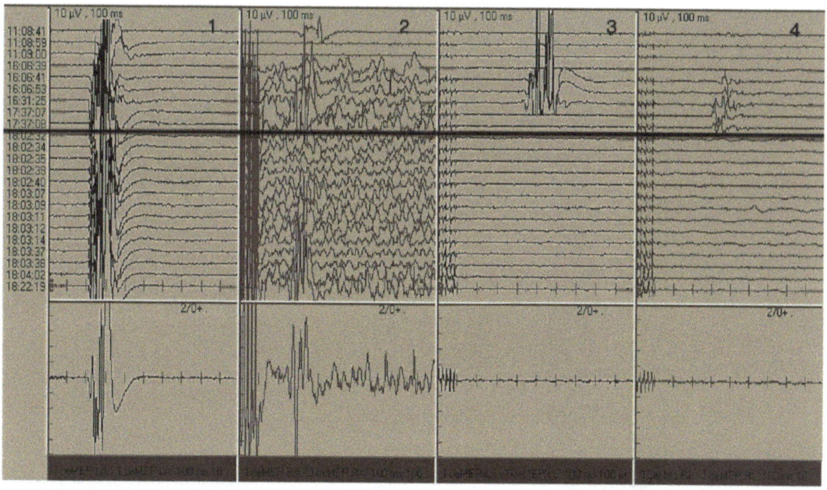

B

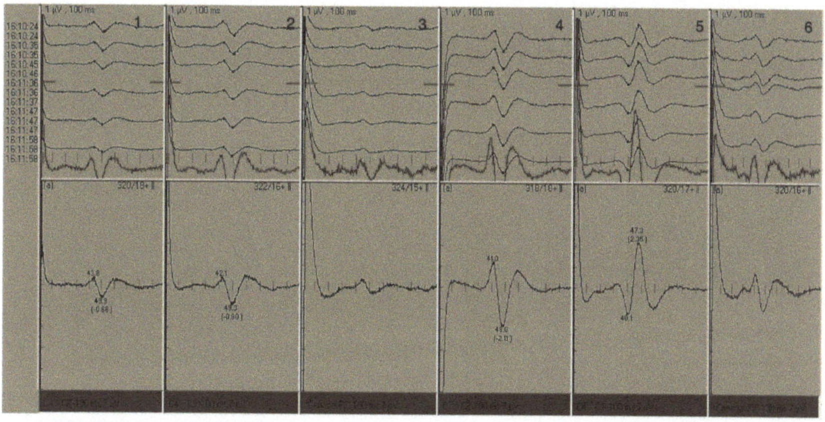

Fig. 7. Evoked potentials during a thoracic endovascular aortic repair in an 85 year-old woman. (*A*) Motor evoked potentials (MEPs) over time. Boxes 1 and 2 are left and right arms, respectively. Boxes 3 and 4 are left and right legs, respectively. Left leg demonstrates attenuation before stent deployment, likely from occlusion of left femoral artery from intravascular device. Black line demonstrates deployment of stent with rapid attenuation of right-leg MEPs despite increased stimulation. (*B*) Somatosensory evoked potentials (SSEPs) at posterior tibial nerve baseline demonstrating bilateral response. Boxes 1 to 3, left leg; boxes 4 to 6, right leg. (*C*) SSEPs now demonstrate attenuation in left leg (boxes 1–3), likely due to femoral artery occlusion. Right leg waveforms are slightly diminished but still present (boxes 4–6). (*D*) SSEPs at posterior tibial nerve now demonstrate complete bilateral attenuation 30 minutes after stent deployment (boxes 1–6).

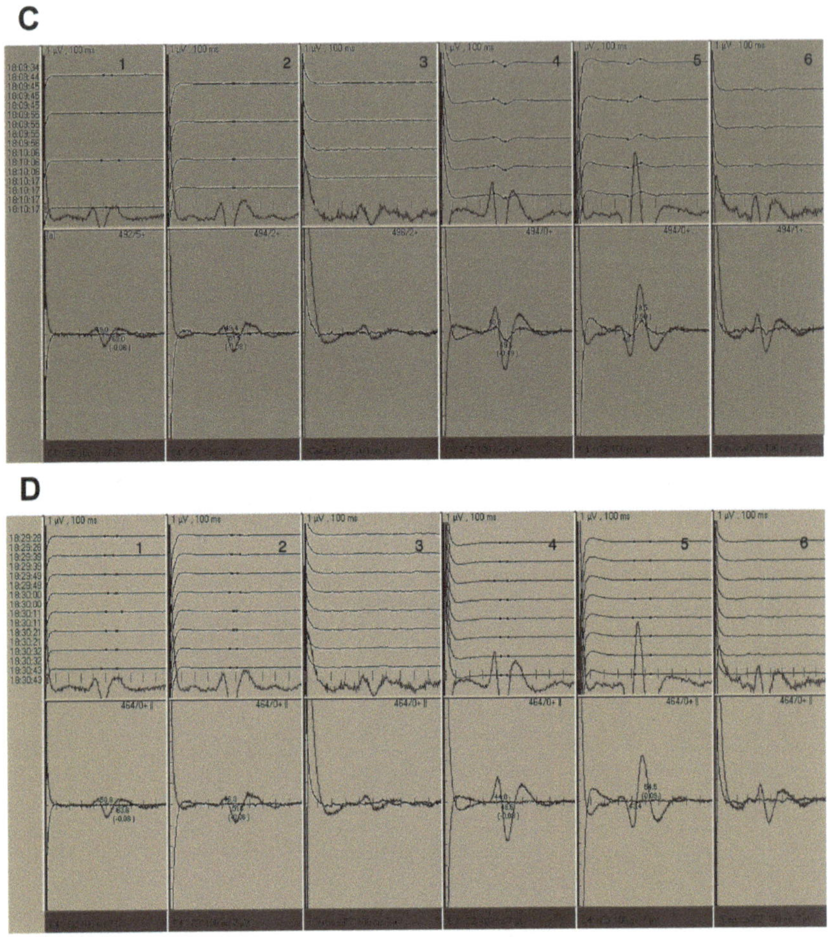

Fig. 7. *(continued).*

with successful MEP monitoring. The MEP depends on a functioning neuromuscular junction, the site of action of paralytics. Deep muscle paralysis facilitates endotracheal intubation and the initial dissection phase of aortic procedures, but should be incomplete during intraoperative MEP monitoring. Repeated doses of paralytics risk abolishing the MEP response, and may frequently be omitted. Should intraoperative muscle relaxation be needed, good communication between the anesthesiologist and neuromonitoring personnel is essential.

Hypothermia

MEPs are affected by changes in temperature and may not be a reliable predictor of paraplegia during deep hypothermia. Mild hypothermia, defined as 32°C to 34°C, is compatible with successful MEP monitoring. In a study of 15 consecutive patients undergoing descending and thoracoabdominal aortic operations with deep hypothermic circulatory arrest (DHCA), MEP amplitude decreased linearly in a temperature-dependent fashion in both hands and legs [30]. Both upper and lower extremity MEP amplitude was greatly diminished compared with baseline, even after rewarming. These limitations should be considered when interpreting MEPs during DHCA.

Cerebrospinal fluid drainage

Optimization of the SCPP requires measurement of MAP and intraspinal pressure. MAP is easily measured with noninvasive or invasive blood pressure monitors. Intrathecal pressure monitoring requires direct invasive measurement via a percutaneously placed catheter, most commonly in the lumbar spine.

The technique and rationale for lumbar cerebrospinal drainage was recently reviewed in detail by Federow and colleagues [31]. The institution of multimodal spinal cord protection, including routine CSF drainage, has been associated with a decrease in spinal cord injury [32]. In a large, unblinded, randomized controlled trial of 156 patients, Coselli and colleagues [33] demonstrated a reduction in paraplegia or paraparesis from 12.2% in the control group to 2.7% in the CSF drainage group ($P = .03$). Both groups underwent standardized operative technique including left heart bypass, mild hypothermia, and reattachment of intercostal and lumbar arteries. In a retrospective review of 402 consecutive patients from 1981 to 1994, the addition of CSF and EPs were associated with decreased morbidity. Protective factors for spinal cord injury included if the operation was performed after 1995 (OR 0.31, 95% CI 0.15–0.65) and a history of previous aortic dissection (OR 0.38, 95% CI 0.15–0.9) [34].

Patients undergoing endovascular repair of thoracic aortic disease with stent grafting still appear to be at risk of spinal cord injury. In a review of 36 stent-graft procedures in 31 patients, 11 of 31 demonstrated evoked potential changes during graft deployment, and 12 of 31 had an increase in CSF pressure. After initiation of CSF drainage, 10 of 11 patients had recovery of EP changes. There was 1 documented case of neurologic deficit, occurring 25 days after the procedure [35].

A recent update to the Cochrane Peripheral Vascular Diseases Group 2004 review failed to identify any new randomized controlled trials [36]. The evidence supporting the use of CSF drainage is equivocal, as there are only 3 main randomized controlled trials. The inclusion of case reports and retrospective studies does increase the strength of evidence for routine CSF drainage, in conjunction with an operative technique that optimizes distal aortic perfusion.

Hypothermia

Hypothermia has long been recognized as the primary neuroprotective technique in operations requiring DHCA. Hypothermia remains the sole intervention that reduces both functional and structural components of neuronal oxygen consumption [37]. Deeply hypothermic temperatures (<26°C) may not be necessary, as mild to moderate hypothermia (35–26°C) may provide beneficial effects during periods of inadequate cerebral blood flow or oxygenation [38]. Although the effects of temperature on spinal cord neurons are less well known than for cerebral neurons, clinical studies do support the use of both systemic and regional cooling during aortic operations.

Cooley and Jones [39] long realized the neuroprotective value of mild to moderate hypothermia on spinal cord injury. A recent retrospective review of 151 descending thoracic aortic repairs under DHCA, from 1989 to 2008, demonstrated a 1.3% incidence of SCI [40]. A variety of methods have been attempted to achieve regional spinal cord cooling, but the simplest and most easily reproducible seems to be cooling via an epidural catheter. In conjunction with distal aortic perfusion and CSF drainage, the addition of cold saline infusion through a T11 to T12 epidural catheter resulted in a very low incidence of spinal cord injury (3.9%) [41]. It should be noted that the highest mean CSF pressure seen in one patient was 36.8 mm Hg (range 10–70). The clinical significance of this elevated pressure is uncertain. In an experimental pig model of aortic cross-clamping, epidural cooling appears to prevent delayed spinal cord hypoperfusion and to stimulate inducible nitric oxide synthase expression during reperfusion [42]. Thus, the addition of regional epidural cooling, when available, seems to be beneficial in high-risk patients who do not undergo DHCA.

Pharmacologic interventions

There are few human clinical trials evaluating the ability of pharmacologic interventions to ameliorate the sequelae of SCI. Potential targets for the impact of drug treatments include the preischemic, ischemic, and postischemic/reperfusion periods.

As with the heart and brain, ischemic preconditioning (brief nonlethal ischemia that acts to protect against irreversible injury during subsequent ischemia) may be demonstrated with the spinal cord. Volatile anesthetics seem to confer “preconditioning” effects in the spinal cord, as have been observed in myocardial ischemic preconditioning. Preconditioning with isoflurane may decrease the neurotoxicity of SCI [43]. This effect appears to be mediated via the transcription factor nuclear factor κB, which, among many effects, regulates expression of inducible nitric oxide synthase [44].

The opioid antagonist naloxone may be beneficial in reducing the excitotoxic response to ischemia. In one small study of 27 patients undergoing thoracoabdominal aortic operations, the addition of intravenous naloxone (1 μg/kg/h) to conventional CSF drainage, distal aortic perfusion, and mild hypothermia was associated with lower levels of CSF excitatory amino acids [45]. An older study demonstrated a decrease in paraplegia from 21% to 3.4% when both CSF drainage and intravenous naloxone were used [46].

Traditional strategies to augment SCBF during periods of aortic cross-clamping have relied on modifying operative techniques (reimplantation of intercostal arteries or distal aortic perfusion). SCBF may also be manipulated pharmacologically. In a nonrandomized prospective study, the addition of intrathecal papaverine to a protocol including CSF drainage and moderate hypothermic distal aortic perfusion demonstrated a significant reduction in spinal cord injury. Permanent paraplegia decreased from 7.5% to 3.6% ($P = .01$) and paraparesis decreased from 6.3% to 1.6% ($P = .01$) in the treated group [47]. The exact mechanism of intrathecal papaverine is unknown, but may be related to phosphodiesterase inhibition [48]. Similarly, in an experimental rat model, magnesium administration was associated with greater blood flow during ischemia, probably through enhanced vasodilation [49]. The vasodilator sodium nitroprusside may be associated with increased intraspinal pressure and decreased distal perfusion pressure, which may result in decreased SCBF and increased risk of ischemia, and for these reasons is best avoided [50].

It is unlikely that a single agent will be found that protects against SCI during aortic cross-clamping. There is, however, the potential to use common medications to lessen the severity of injury and expand tolerance to SCI when used in conjunction with other modalities.

PERIOPERATIVE DIAGNOSIS OF SPINAL CORD INJURY

Postoperative diagnosis of spinal cord injury primarily depends on serial neurologic examinations performed until the patient recovers from general anesthesia and is able to report symptoms of numbness or weakness. The ideal anesthetic technique permits rapid emergence to facilitate neurologic examination. Neurologic examination should evaluate lower extremity sensation, muscle strength, and reflexes. Postoperative use of SSEPs in the intensive care unit before patient recovery from general anesthesia has been described, but this practice is not widespread [51,52]. When detected on the patient awakening from anesthesia, neurologic deficits are defined as immediate, whereas if deficits develop after a period of normal neurologic examination the patient is considered to have delayed neurologic deficits. Delayed neurologic deficits can occur as late as 10 days postoperatively. Several investigators have recently reported a 50% to 80 % incidence of delayed neurologic deficits [53,54].

Other than intraoperative SCI, causes of neurologic deficit in patients who have undergone descending aortic repair include stroke, localized nerve injury, and perfusion defects secondary to operative injury or intra-arterial thrombus. In cases of an indeterminate or nonspecific neurologic examination, further evaluation using imaging and consultation with neurologists is warranted. Stroke is a common adverse event, with an incidence as high as 8% [55–57]. A detailed neurologic examination evaluating cortical and brainstem function, in addition to a noncontrast CT scan of the brain, should help differentiate stroke from perioperative SCI as the cause for new neurologic deficits.

Distinguishing between a nerve injury and SCI will depend on a focused neurologic examination assessing a particular nerve distribution complemented by an electromyogram or nerve conduction study, with the latter being the gold standard for detection of peripheral nerve injuries. The absence of distal pulses along with a possible neurologic deficit should alert the health care team to the possibility of a perfusion defect as the causative or contributing factor. An angiogram detailing the perfusion of the affected area would help elucidate perfusion disturbance as a possible cause.

One important caveat to consider is that not all SCI and neurologic deficits are due to the operative procedure. Spinal and cerebral epidural hematoma is a risk of CSF drainage, and should be included in the differential diagnosis of paraplegia or paraparesis [58,59]. For those patients with delayed neurologic deficits, imaging of the thoracolumbar spine, ideally with MRI (or CT if MRI is not readily available), should be considered before placement of an intrathecal catheter, particularly if one was recently removed.

TREATMENT OF SPINAL CORD ISCHEMIA

When evidence of SCI is detected, immediate action is warranted. Intraoperative measures to optimize SCBF include more aggressive reimplantation of intercostal arteries, particularly if there is a temporal association with recent aortic clamping.

As illustrated earlier, SCPP is the difference between distal MAP and spinal cord pressure. Augmenting distal MAP may require increasing distal flow during left heart bypass, transfusion or volume administration, and vasoconstrictor infusion. The ideal MAP or SCPP is not known, but case reports support a MAP goal of greater than 80 mm Hg and an SCPP goal of greater than 70 mm Hg (Fig. 8) [60]. Drainage of CSF is also likely helpful, as already discussed. The removal of CSF decreases spinal cord pressure, and helps increase SCPP and, presumably, SCBF. Delayed spinal cord injury and neurologic changes may benefit from postoperative placement of a lumbar CSF drain [61]. Aggressive drainage of CSF is not without risk, although most patients tolerate drainage to a pressure of 10 mm Hg. Should the initial increase in MAP be unsuccessful, progressively increasing the MAP to greater than 100 mm Hg may be attempted.

POSTOPERATIVE CARE

Spinal cord injury remains a risk during the immediate postoperative period. Delayed paraplegia may occur days to weeks after the operation and may respond to increased MAP [62]. A retrospective analysis of 858 TAA repairs from 1990 to 2006 reported that 10 of 20 cases of paraplegia occurred within the first 2 postoperative days. Early mean CVP was significantly greater in patients who developed paraplegia ($P = .03$), although MAP did not differ [22]. The relative postoperative MAP (percentage of preoperative MAP) may be more clinically relevant. Griepp and colleagues [2] found that the immediate

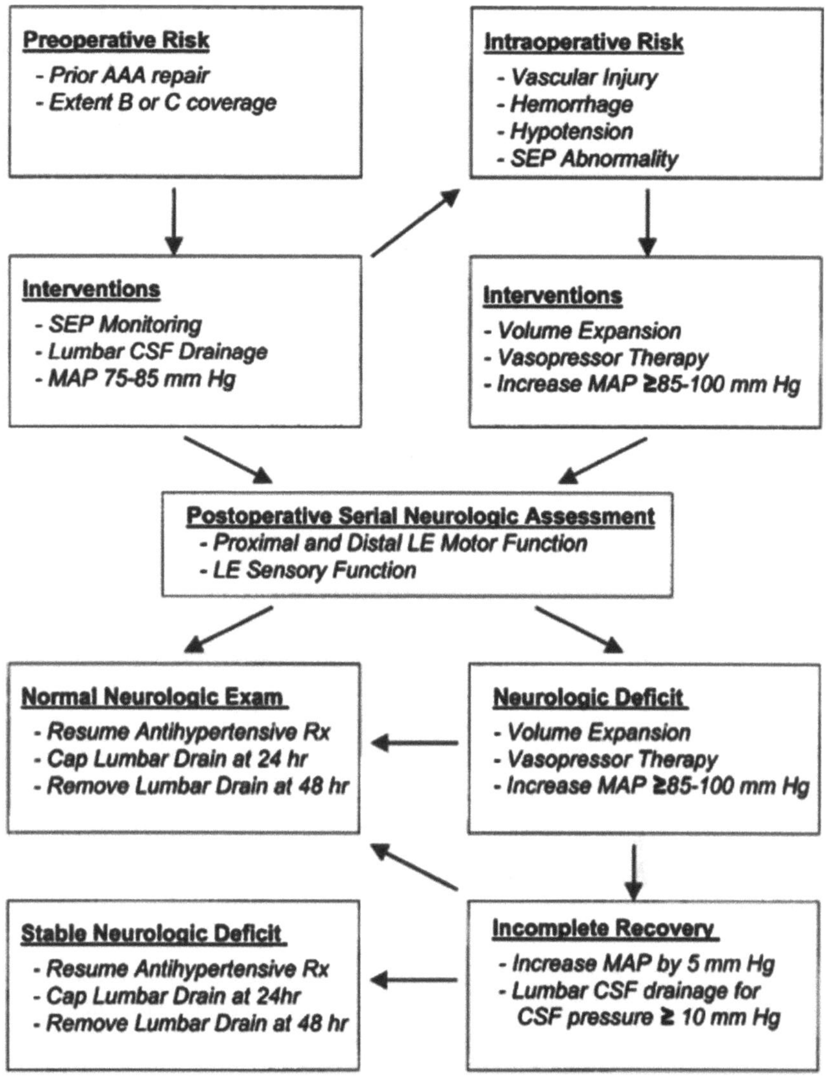

Fig. 8. Proposed algorithm for management of ischemia during endovascular repair. AAA, abdominal aortic aneurysm; CSF, cerebrospinal fluid; hr, hours; LE, lower extremity; MAP, mean arterial pressure; Rx, drug therapy; SEP, somatosensory evoked potential. (*From* Cheung AT, Pochettino A, McGarvey ML, et al. Strategies to manage paraplegia risk after endovascular stent repair of descending thoracic aortic aneurysms. Ann Thorac Surg 2005;80:1287; with permission.)

postoperative relative MAP (within the first 5 hours) was significantly lower in the paraplegic group ($P = .027$). This finding would support a postoperative hemodynamic management strategy that incorporates the preoperative MAP as a goal.

There are limited data guiding the length of time to maintain lumbar drains postoperatively. Given the risk of immediate-delayed paraplegia, it seems reasonable to gradually alter parameters for spinal cord pressure. In the first 24 hours, SCPP should be kept less than 10 mm Hg; in the second 24 hours the SCP may be kept less than 20 mm Hg, after which the drain may be clamped for an additional 24 hours [63]. The ideal coagulation parameters for discontinuation of lumbar drains are unknown but are extrapolated from the neuraxial anesthesia literature. Catheters should not be removed until normal coagulation parameters are restored. The authors' institution uses the following criteria: international normalized ratio 1.3 or less, platelet count 90,000 or more, fibrinogen 200,000 mg/dL or more. If the platelet count is between 60,000 and 90,000, thromboelastography (TEG) is performed. If TEG indicates normal coagulation, the drain is removed. If the maximum amplitude is less than 55 mm, platelets are transfused before drain removal. Platelets are empirically transfused if the count is less than 55,000. Subcutaneous heparin is held for a minimum of 1 hour after removal. As required for any patient undergoing TAA repair, frequent neurologic examinations are performed, and the patient is instructed to notify staff of any change in sensation or strength.

CSF drainage may be reinstituted in patients with delayed paraplegia occurring after 48 to 72 hours. Several case reports suggest the occurrence in some patients of spinal cord hypoperfusion days to weeks after their operation. Institution of CSF drainage may restore adequate spinal cord perfusion in these patients [62,64,65]. Imaging of the lumbar spine should be considered to exclude epidural or subdural hematoma as the cause of the new onset of neurologic changes.

OUTCOMES

Open versus endovascular

Open surgical repair was the only surgical option for the treatment of descending aorta abnormality from the 1950s to the mid-1990s. The perioperative mortality for descending thoracic aorta repair has ranged from 4% to 10%, with recent studies showing mortality in the lower range [66–71]. In addition, SCI with development of paraplegia or paraparesis has ranged from 2% to 13% [71–76]. Parodi and colleagues [77] were the first to describe endovascular repair of abdominal aortic aneurysm. Shortly thereafter, Dake and colleagues [78] published a study describing endovascular treatment of descending TAAs. Since then there have been 3 device trials and several multicenter and single-center studies investigating endovascular repair of descending thoracic aortic diseases. While some of these studies have retrospectively or prospectively selected cohorts of open repair to compare with the TEVAR results, there have been no randomized controlled trials comparing TEVAR with open repair. Comparing outcomes between open and endovascular repairs is complicated by the fact that many patients who undergo endovascular repair are not considered candidates for open repair, and that patients undergoing the 2 different procedures may not suffer comparable comorbidities.

Descending thoracic aortic aneurysms

The Gore-TAG thoracic endoprosthesis was the first commercially developed stent to be studied in a prospective, nonrandomized, phase II multicenter trial [79]. In this trial of 142 patients, the 30-day mortality rate was 2.1% and the SCI rate was 3%. The midterm results report of this trial compared the 140 study patients with 94 control open surgical repair patients, 44 of whom were prospectively enrolled during the study and 50 of whom were historical patients. TEVAR patients had a favorable 30-day mortality rate (2.1% vs 11.7%) and SCI rate (3% vs 13.8%). In addition, the average intensive care unit stay and the total length of stay in hospital were significantly shorter in the study group [80]. The 5-year results for this trial showed significantly decreased aneurysm-related mortality in the study group (2.8% vs 11.7%), but the overall mortality was similar between the 2 groups.

The VALOR trial (Vascular Talent Thoracic Stent Graft System for the Treatment of Thoracic Aortic Aneurysms) was a prospective multicenter study that enrolled 195 patients and compared the results with retrospective open surgical data of 189 patients. Although both the 30-day all-cause mortality and the 12-month all-cause mortality were lower in the study group (2.1% vs 7.9% and 16.1% vs 20.6%, respectively), only the 30-day mortality difference was statistically significant. The incidence of SCI (paraplegia and paraparesis combined) was 8.7% [81]. The recently published 5-year outcomes of this trial demonstrated 5-year all-cause mortality of 43.9% and aneurysm-related mortality of 4%.

The Cook Zenith TX1 and TX2 thoracic endograft trial was a multicenter, nonrandomized, prospective clinical trial of 100 patients with varied aortic pathology including aneurysm, chronic aortic dissections, and aortobronchial or aortoesophageal fistulas. Overall mortality and aneurysm-related mortality at 1 year were 17% and 14%, respectively. SCI was suspected in 6 patients (6%), and 2 patients developed complete and permanent paraplegia [82]. Morales and colleagues [83] reported the intermediate and 5-year results of a study of 160 patients who underwent TEVAR with the Cook Zenith devices for varied aortic pathology. The 30-day mortality was 6.9% and the 5 year survival rate was 70%.

Since approval of these devices from the Food and Drug Administration for TAA repairs, there has been a large increase in the number of endovascular repairs carried out within the United States [84]. The number of hospitals performing open thoracic repairs has decreased, whereas the number performing endovascular repairs has increased tremendously [85], despite there being limited data documenting the long-term efficacy of endovascular repair. A meta-analysis by Cheng and colleagues [86] that included 38 studies and 4 registries for a total 5888 patients, comparing endovascular aortic repair with open surgical repair for descending thoracic aortic disease, showed statistically significant reductions in 30-day mortality and paraplegia for TEVAR. A Medicare population study comparing survival in more than 30,000 patients who underwent either open or endovascular repair of descending TAAs also showed better perioperative outcomes with TEVAR, but worse long-term survival [87]. These 2 large reviews seem to concur with the long-term results of the initial device trials, in that while TEVAR may decrease perioperative mortality it does not appear to improve long-term survival. In addition to the on-label uses for TAA repairs, endovascular repair techniques and devices have been used for multiple off-label repairs, including type B dissections and ruptured aneurysms.

Type B dissections

Type B dissections may be divided into uncomplicated and complicated. Medical therapy alone has been shown to have better outcomes in uncomplicated type B aortic dissections [88]. However, because medical therapy alone does not stop blood flow into the false lumen, some patients ultimately develop dilatation of the false lumen that requires intervention. The INSTEAD (Investigation of Stent Grafts in Aortic Dissection) trial of 140 patients with chronic aortic dissection who were randomized to either medical therapy alone or medical therapy plus TEVAR failed to show a survival benefit at 2 years after treatment [89,90]. The SCI rate was also the same between the 2 groups, at 1.3%. The ADSORB (European Study of medical Management versus TAG device and Medical Management for Acute Uncomplicated Type B Dissection) trial is currently under way and should shed further light on the role of TEVAR in patients with acute uncomplicated type B aortic dissection.

Patients presenting with rupture or impending rupture (aortic dilation >55–60 mm), end-organ malperfusion, limb ischemia, unrelenting pain, and/or uncontrollable hypertension are designated as having a complicated type B aortic dissection, and require urgent surgical intervention. Historically, the open repair of complicated type B aortic dissection has had a mortality rate of 11% to 21% and an SCI rate as high as 32% [91,92]. Endovascular treatment of these patients is a relatively new technique, with no randomized controlled trials and no long-term results in comparison with open techniques available, but the short-term results have been encouraging. Sachs and colleagues [92] published an analysis of 5000 National Inpatient Sample (NIS) database patients who underwent open or endovascular repair of acute type B dissections from 2005 to 2007. Patients were selected based on International Classification of Diseases, 9th edition (ICD-9) diagnosis codes. Their analysis showed a statistically higher mortality for emergent open repair compared with endovascular repair (19% vs 10.6%). These results were consistent with a later NIS database review of patients from 2005 to 2008. However, the difference in SCI rates was not statistically significant. A recent review of 942 patients who underwent endovascular repair of acute complicated type B aortic dissection selected through a MEDLINE search showed a mortality rate of 9% and SCI rate of 1.9% [93]. A recent International Registry of Acute Aortic Dissection database analysis showed in-hospital mortality rates of 33.9% versus 10.6% in patients who underwent open versus endovascular repair. The paraplegia rates were also lower in the endovascular group (1.5% vs 5%) [94]. Just as centers of excellence with high volumes performing open repairs have better outcomes than those with low volumes, the same has been shown to be true for endovascular repairs [95]. In addition, recent reports of open repair have also shown improvement in mortality and paraplegia rates in comparison with the historical results reported earlier. Di Luozzo and colleagues [71] published excellent results of 294 patients who were treated from 2002 to 2010 with open repair. The in-hospital mortality rate was 4.7% and the paraplegia rate was 0.9%. The optimal treatment of complicated type B dissections with an endovascular versus an open approach is still controversial, and long-term data from endovascular repairs are needed before a more uniform standard can be adopted.

Ruptured aneurysms

Ruptured aneurysms, both abdominal and thoracic, have the worst overall outcomes of the indications for descending aorta diseases requiring surgical repair. Open repair of ruptured abdominal aortic aneurysms was associated with only a 64% survival at 5 years, and this number dropped further to 33% at 10 years [96]. Survival from ruptured TAA and TAAA is even more dismal. Girardi and colleagues [97] reported a 17.5% in-hospital mortality rate and a 5%

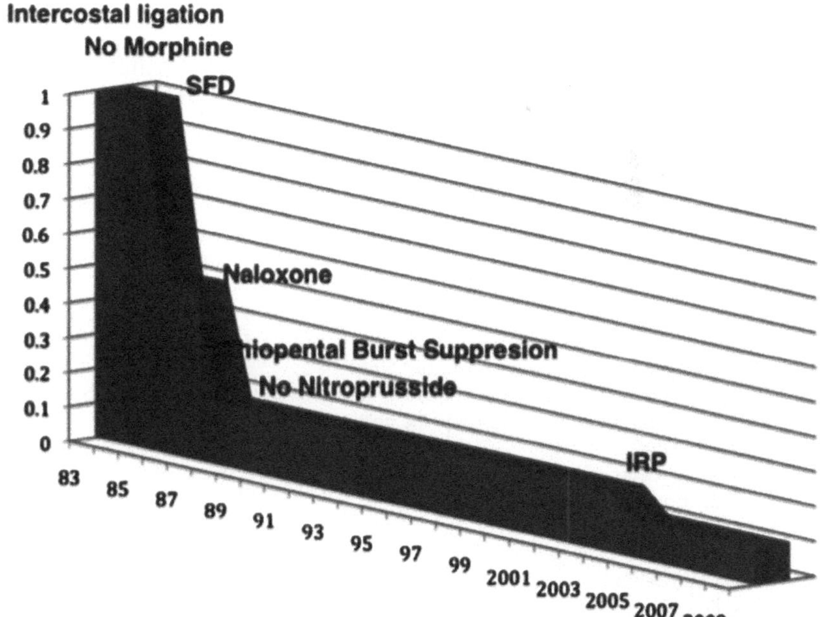

Fig. 9. Observed/expected (O/E) ratios by year for spinal cord injury. IRP, intercostal reimplantation; SFP, spinal fluid drainage. (*From* Acher C. It is not just assisted circulation, hypothermic arrest, or clamp and sew. J Thorac Cardiovasc Surg 2010;140:S137; with permission.)

paraplegia rate in patients with ruptured descending TAA and TAAA. A study comparing elective TAAA repair in 1108 patients with emergency repair in 112 patients (76% were ruptured) showed large differences in 30-day mortality (6% vs 17%) and paraplegia rates (4% vs 14%). Paraplegia was the worst in type II TAAAs (28%) [98]. A recent US Nationwide Inpatient sample data review of 364 TEVAR and 559 open repairs of ruptured descending TAAs showed no statistically significant difference in mortality. However, in smaller hospitals, TEVAR was associated with lower complication and mortality rates [55]. Jonker and colleagues [99] published a meta-analysis of all studies published after 1995 describing the outcomes of ruptured descending TAA treated with either open repair or TEVAR, showing statistically significant lower 30-day mortality in the TEVAR patients but no statistically significant difference in the incidence of paraplegia.

SUMMARY

Despite advances in the understanding of the unique pathophysiology of SCI during descending thoracic or thoracoabdominal aortic operations, spinal cord injury continues to occur with high frequency. The most promising approaches to protecting the spinal cord during these operations optimize SCBF during critical periods of ischemia. A multimodal approach centered on CSF drainage and augmenting perfusion pressure seems to be the most promising (Fig. 9) [17]. Our understanding of prevention and treatment of spinal cord injury is limited by the few randomized clinical trials that have been conducted. Further high-quality controlled trials are needed to appropriately investigate current and proposed interventions.

References

[1] The blood supply of the brain and spinal cord. In: Purves D, Augustine GJ, Fitzpatrick D, et al, editors. Neuroscience. 2nd edition. Sunderland (MA): Sinauer Associates; 2001. Available at: http://www.ncbi.nlm.nih.gov/books/NBK11042.

[2] Griepp RB, Ergin MA, Galla JD, et al. Looking for the artery of Adamkiewicz: a quest to minimize paraplegia after operations for aneurysms of the descending thoracic and thoracoabdominal aorta. J Thorac Cardiovasc Surg 1996;112:1202–13.

[3] Griepp RB, Griepp EB. Spinal cord perfusion and protection during descending thoracic and thoracoabdominal aortic surgery: the collateral network concept. Ann Thorac Surg 2007;83:865–9.

[4] Bischoff MS, Griepp RB. Spinal cord preservation in thoracoabdominal aneurysm repair. Perspect Vasc Surg Endovasc Ther 2011;23:214–22.

[5] Etz CD, Kari FA, Mueller CS, et al. The collateral network concept: a reassessment of the anatomy of spinal cord perfusion. J Thorac Cardiovasc Surg 2011;141:1020–8.

[6] Marcus ML, Heistad DD, Ehrhardt JC, et al. Regulation of the total and regional spinal cord blood flow. Circ Res 1977;41:128.

[7] Heiss WD. Flow threshold of functional and morphologic damage of brain tissue. Stroke 1983;14:329.

[8] Hossmann KA, Zimmerman V. Post-ischemic resuscitation of the brain: selective vulnerability versus global resistance. Prog Brain Res 1985;63:3.

[9] Siesjo BK. Cerebral circulation and metabolism. J Neurosurg 1984;60:883.

[10] Park E, Velumian AA, Fehlings MG. The role of excitotoxicity in secondary mechanism of spinal cord injury: a review with an emphasis on the implications of white matter degeneration. J Neurotrauma 2004;21:754–74.
[11] Gelman S, Reves JG, Fowler K, et al. Regional blood flow during cross-clamping of the thoracic aorta and infusion of sodium nitroprusside. J Thorac Cardiovasc Surg 1983;85:287–91.
[12] Svensson LG, Rickards E, Coull A, et al. Relationship of spinal cord blood flow to vascular anatomy during thoracic aortic cross-clamping and shunting. J Thorac Cardiovasc Surg 1986;91:71–8.
[13] Etz CD, Di Luozzo G, Bello R, et al. Pulmonary complications after descending thoracic and thoracoabdominal aortic aneurysm repair: predictors, prevention, and treatment. Ann Thorac Surg 2007;83:S870–6 [discussion: S890–2].
[14] Adams HD, Van Geertruyden HH. Neurologic complications of aortic surgery. Ann Surg 1956;144:574–610.
[15] Lowell RC, Gloviczki P, Bergman RT, et al. Failure of selective shunting to intercostal arteries to prevent spinal cord ischemia during experimental thoracoabdominal aortic occlusion. Int Angiol 1992;11:281–8.
[16] Svensson LG, Von Ritter CM, Groeneveld HT, et al. Cross-clamping of the thoracic aorta: influence of aortic shunts, laminectomy, papaverine, calcium channel blocker, allopurinol, and superoxide dismutase on spinal cord blood flow and paraplegia in baboons. Ann Surg 1986;204:38–47.
[17] Acher C. It is not just assisted circulation, hypothermic arrest, or clamp and sew. J Thorac Cardiovasc Surg 2010;140:S136–41.
[18] Drinkwater SL, Goebells A, Haydar A, et al. The incidence of spinal cord ischaemia following thoracic and thoracoabdominal aortic endovascular intervention. Eur J Vasc Endovasc Surg 2010;40:729–35.
[19] Chiesa R, Melissano G, Marrocco-Trischitta MM, et al. Spinal cord ischemia after elective stent-graft repair of the thoracic aorta. J Vasc Surg 2005;42:11–7.
[20] Becker DA, McGarvey ML, Rojvirat C, et al. Predictors of outcome in patients with spinal cord ischemia after open aortic repair. Neurocrit Care 2013;18:70–4.
[21] Schepens MA, Heijmen RH, Ranschaert W, et al. Thoracoabdominal aortic aneurysm repair: results of conventional open surgery. Eur J Vasc Endovasc Surg 2009;37:640–5.
[22] Etz CD, Luehr M, Kari FA, et al. Paraplegia after extensive thoracic and thoracoabdominal aortic aneurysm repair: dose critical spinal cord ischemia occur postoperatively? J Thorac Cardiovasc Surg 2008;135:324–30.
[23] Marik PE, Baram M, Vahid B. Does central venous pressure predict fluid responsiveness? A systematic review of the literature and the tale of seven mares. Chest 2008;134:172–8.
[24] Slinger P, Sullivan EA. Anesthetic management for surgery of the lungs and the mediastinum. In: Hensley FA, Martin DE, Gravlee GP, editors. A practical approach to cardiac anesthesia. Philadelphia: Lippincott Williams & Williams; 2008. p. 694–740.
[25] Jacobs MJ, Mess WH. The role of evoked potential monitoring in operative management of type I and type II thoracoabdominal aortic aneurysms. Semin Thorac Cardiovasc Surg 2003;15:353–64.
[26] MacDonald DB, Dong CC. Spinal cord monitoring of descending aortic procedures. In: Nuwer MR, editor. Monitoring neural function during surgery, Handbook of Clinical Neurophysiology. Amsterdam: Elsevier; 2008. p. 815–28.
[27] Dong CC, MacDonald DB, Janusz MT. Intraoperative spinal cord monitoring during descending thoracic and thoracoabdominal aneurysm surgery. Ann Thorac Surg 2002;74:S1873–6.
[28] Pelosi L, Stevenson M, Hobbs GJ, et al. Intraoperative motor evoked potentials to transcranial electrical stimulation during two anaesthetic regimens. Clin Neurophysiol 2001;112:1076–87.

[29] Chen Z. The effects of isoflurane and propofol on intraoperative neurophysiological monitoring during spinal surgery. J Clin Monit Comput 2004;18:303–8.
[30] Shinzawa M, Yoshitani K, Minatoya K, et al. Changes of motor evoked potentials during descending thoracic and thoracoabdominal aortic surgery with deep hypothermic circulatory arrest. J Anesth 2012;26:160–7.
[31] Fedorow CA, Moon MC, Mutch WA, et al. Lumbar cerebrospinal fluid drainage for thoracoabdominal aortic surgery: rationale and practical considerations for management. Anesth Analg 2010;111:46–58.
[32] Acher CW, Wynn MM, Hoch JR, et al. Combined use of cerebral spinal fluid drainage and naloxone reduces the risk of paraplegia in thoracoabdominal aneurysm repair. J Vasc Surg 1994;19:236–46 [discussion: 247–8].
[33] Coselli JS, LeMaire SA, Koksoy C, et al. Cerebrospinal fluid drainage reduces paraplegia after thoracoabdominal aortic aneurysm repair: results of a randomized clinical trial. J Vasc Surg 2002;35:631–9.
[34] Schepens M, Dossche K, Morshuis W, et al. Introduction of adjuncts and their influence on changing results in 402 consecutive thoracoabdominal aortic aneurysm repairs. Eur J Cardiothorac Surg 2004;25:701–7.
[35] Weigang E, Hartert M, Siegenthaler MP, et al. Perioperative management to improve neurologic outcome in thoracic or thoracoabdominal aortic stent-grafting. Ann Thorac Surg 2006;82:1679–87.
[36] Khan SN, Stansby G. Cerebrospinal fluid drainage for thoracic and thoracoabdominal aortic aneurysm surgery. Cochrane Database Syst Rev 2012;(10):CD003635.
[37] Roman PE, Grigore AM. Pro: hypothermic cardiopulmonary bypass should be used. J Cardiothorac Vasc Anesth 2012;26:945–8.
[38] Klementavicious R, Nemoto EM, Yonas H. The Q10 ratio for basal cerebral metabolic rate for oxygen in rats. J Neurosurg 1996;85:482–7.
[39] Cooley DA, Jones BA. Use of selective hypothermia to protect the spinal cord during resection of thoracoabdominal aneurysm. Tex Heart Inst J 2000;27:29–31.
[40] Kulik A, Castner CF, Kouchoukos NT. Replacement of the descending thoracic aorta: contemporary outcomes using hypothermic circulatory arrest. J Thorac Cardiovasc Surg 2010;139:249–55.
[41] Tabayashi K, Saiki Y, Kokubo H. Protection from postischemic spinal cord injury by perfusion cooling of the epidural space during most or all of a descending thoracic or thoracoabdominal aneurysm repair. Gen Thorac Cardiovasc Surg 2010;58:228–34.
[42] Ishikawa A, Mori A, Kabei N, et al. Epidural cooling minimizes spinal cord injury after cross-clamping through induction of nitric oxide synthase. Anesthesiology 2009;111:818–25.
[43] Sang H, Cao L, Qiu P, et al. Isoflurane produces delayed preconditioning against spinal cord ischemia injury via release of free radicals in rabbits. Anesthesiology 2006;105:953–60.
[44] Kim H, Jae-Woo Y, Chang-Ju K, et al. Delayed preconditioning effect of isoflurane on spinal cord ischemia in rats. Neurosci Lett 2008;440:211–6.
[45] Kunihara T, Matsuzaki K, Shiiya N, et al. Naloxone lowers cerebrospinal fluid levels of excitatory amino acids after thoracoabdominal aortic surgery. J Vasc Surg 2004;40:681–90.
[46] Tefera G, Acher CW, Wynn MM. Clamp and sew techniques in thoracoabdominal aortic surgery using naloxone and CSF drainage. Semin Vasc Surg 2000;13:325–30.
[47] Lima B, Nowicki E, Blackstone E, et al. Spinal cord protective strategies during descending and thoracoabdominal aortic aneurysm repair in the modern era: the role of intrathecal papaverine. J Thorac Cardiovasc Surg 2012;143:945–52.
[48] Rudzinkski P, Wegrzyn P, Lis GJ, et al. Vasodilatory effect and endothelial integrity in papaverine- and milrinone-treated human radial arteries. J Physiol Pharmacol 2013;64:41–5.

[49] Kohno H, Ishida A, Imamake M, et al. Efficacy and vasodilatory benefit of magnesium for protection against spinal cord ischemia. Ann Vasc Surg 2007;21:352–9.
[50] Shine T, Nugent M. Sodium nitroprusside decreases spinal cord perfusion pressure during descending thoracic aortic cross-clamping in the dog. J Cardiothorac Anesth 1990;4: 185–93.
[51] Zoli S, Roder F, Etz CD, et al. Predicting the risk of paraplegia after thoracic and thoracoabdominal aneurysm repair. Ann Thorac Surg 2010;90:1237–45.
[52] Di Luozzo G. Visceral and spinal cord protection during thoracoabdominal aortic aneurysm repair: clinical and laboratory update. J Thorac Cardiovasc Surg 2013;145(Suppl 3):S135–8.
[53] Conrad MF, Ye JY, Chung TK, et al. Spinal cord complications after thoracic aortic surgery: long-term survival and functional status varies with deficit severity. J Vasc Surg 2008;48: 47–53.
[54] Ullery BW, Cheung AT, Fairman RM, et al. Risk factors, outcomes, and clinical manifestations of spinal cord ischemia following thoracic endovascular aortic repair. J Vasc Surg 2011;54:677–84.
[55] Gopaldas RR, Dao TK, LeMaire SA, et al. Endovascular versus open repair of ruptured descending thoracic aortic aneurysms: a nationwide risk-adjusted study of 923 patients. J Thorac Cardiovasc Surg 2011;142:1010–8.
[56] Scali ST, Feezor RJ, Chang CK, et al. Efficacy of thoracic endovascular stent repair for chronic type B aortic dissection with aneurysmal degeneration. J Vasc Surg 2013;58:10–7.e1.
[57] Desai ND, Pochettino A, Szeto WY, et al. Thoracic endovascular aortic repair: evolution of therapy, patterns of use, and results in a 10-year experience. J Thorac Cardiovasc Surg 2011;142:587–94.
[58] Jeong YB, Choi WJ, Han SH, et al. Cerebral epidural hematoma following fluid drainage during thoracoabdominal aortic repair. Acta Anaesthesiol Scand 2009;53:1221–2.
[59] Yamauchi T, Takano H, Miyamoto Y, et al. Subdural hematoma induced by cerebrospinal fluid drainage: potentially catastrophic complication of spinal cord protection after thoracoabdominal aneurysm repair. Jpn J Thorac Cardiovasc Surg 2004;52:466–8.
[60] Cheung AT, Pochettino A, McGarvey ML, et al. Strategies to manage paraplegia risk after endovascular stent repair of descending thoracic aortic aneurysms. Ann Thorac Surg 2005;80:1280–8.
[61] Azizzadeh A, Huynh TT, Miller CC, et al. Reversal of twice-delayed neurologic deficits with cerebrospinal fluid drainage after thoracoabdominal aneurysm repair: a case report and plea for a national database collection. J Vasc Surg 2000;31:592–8.
[62] Wong DR, Coselli JS, Amerman K, et al. Delayed spinal cord deficits after thoracoabdominal aortic aneurysm repair. Ann Thorac Surg 2007;83:1345–55.
[63] Lam CH, Vatakencherry G. Spinal cord protection with a cerebrospinal fluid drain in a patient undergoing thoracic endovascular aortic repair. J Vasc Interv Radiol 2010;21: 1343–6.
[64] Appoo JJ, Gregory AJ, Toeg HD, et al. Successful reversal of recurrent spinal cord ischemia following endovascular repair of a descending thoracic aortic aneurysm. HSR Proc Intensive Care Cardiovasc Anesth 2012;4:182–6.
[65] Weiss SJ, Hogan MS, McGarvey ML, et al. Successful treatment of delayed onset paraplegia after suprarenal abdominal aortic aneurysm repair. Anesthesiology 2002;97: 504–6.
[66] Svensson LG, Kouchoukos NT, Miller DC, et al. Expert consensus document on the treatment of descending thoracic aortic disease using endovascular stent-grafts. Ann Thorac Surg 2008;85:S1–41.
[67] Coselli JS, LeMaire SA, Miller CC, et al. Mortality and paraplegia after thoracoabdominal aortic aneurysm repair: a risk factor analysis. Ann Thorac Surg 2000;69:409–14.
[68] Coselli JS, Conklin LD, LeMaire SA. Thoracoabdominal aortic aneurysm repair: review and update of current strategies. Ann Thorac Surg 2002;74:S1881–4.

[69] Black JH 3rd, Cambria RP. Contemporary results of open surgical repair of descending thoracic aortic aneurysms. Semin Vasc Surg 2006;19:11–7.
[70] Davies MG, Younes HK, Harris PW, et al. Outcomes before and after initiation of an acute aortic treatment center. J Vasc Surg 2010;52:1478–85.
[71] Di Luozzo G, Geisbusch S, Lin HM, et al. Open repair of descending and thoracoabdominal aortic aneurysms and dissections in patients aged younger than 60 years: superior to endovascular repair? Ann Thorac Surg 2013;95:12–9.
[72] Conrad MF, Ergul EA, Patel VI, et al. Evolution of operative strategies in open thoracoabdominal aneurysm repair. J Vasc Surg 2011;53:1195–201.
[73] Conrad MF, Crawford RS, Davison JK, et al. Thoracoabdominal aneurysm repair: a 20-year perspective. Ann Thorac Surg 2007;83:S856–61.
[74] Coselli JS, LeMaire SA, Conklin LD, et al. Morbidity and mortality after extent II thoracoabdominal aortic aneurysm repair. Ann Thorac Surg 2002;73:1107–15.
[75] LeMaire SA, Miller CC, Conklin LD, et al. Estimating group mortality and paraplegia rates after thoracoabdominal aortic aneurysm repair. Ann Thorac Surg 2003;75: 508–13.
[76] Coselli JS, LeMaire SA, Conklin LD, et al. Left heart bypass during descending thoracic aortic aneurysm repair does not reduce the incidence of paraplegia. Ann Thorac Surg 2004;77:1298–303.
[77] Parodi JC, Palmaz JC, Barone HD. Transfemoral intraluminal graft implantation for abdominal aortic aneurysms. Ann Vasc Surg 1991;5:491–9.
[78] Dake MD, Miller DC, Semba CP, et al. Transluminal placement of endovascular stent-grafts for the treatment of descending thoracic aortic aneurysms. N Engl J Med 1994;331: 1729–34.
[79] Makaroun MS, Dillavou ED, Kee ST, et al. Endovascular treatment of thoracic aortic aneurysms: results of the phase II multicenter trial of the Gore TAG thoracic endoprosthesis. J Vasc Surg 2005;41:1–9.
[80] Go MR, Cho JS, Makaroun MS. Mid-term results of a multicenter study of thoracic endovascular aneurysm repair versus open repair. Perspect Vasc Surg Endovasc Ther 2007;19: 124–30.
[81] Fairman RM, Criado F, Farber M, et al. Pivotal results of the Medtronic Vascular Talent Thoracic Stent Graft System: the VALOR trial. J Vasc Surg 2008;48:546–54.
[82] Greenberg RK, O'Neill S, Walker E, et al. Endovascular repair of thoracic aortic lesions with the Zenith TX1 and TX2 thoracic grafts: intermediate-term results. J Vasc Surg 2005;41:589–96.
[83] Morales JP, Greenberg RK, Morales CA, et al. Thoracic aortic lesions treated with the Zenith TX1 and TX2 thoracic devices: intermediate- and long-term outcomes. J Vasc Surg 2008;48:54–63.
[84] Scali ST, Goodney PP, Walsh DB, et al. National trends and regional variation of open and endovascular repair of thoracic and thoracoabdominal aneurysms in contemporary practice. J Vasc Surg 2011;53:1499–505.
[85] Patel VI, Mukhopadhyay S, Ergul E, et al. Impact of hospital volume and type on outcomes of open and endovascular repair of descending thoracic aneurysms in the United States Medicare population. J Vasc Surg 2013;58:346–54.
[86] Cheng D, Martin J, Shennib H, et al. Endovascular aortic repair versus open surgical repair for descending thoracic aortic disease a systematic review and meta-analysis of comparative studies. J Am Coll Cardiol 2010;55:986–1001.
[87] Goodney PP, Travis L, Lucas FL, et al. Survival after open versus endovascular thoracic aortic aneurysm repair in an observational study of the Medicare population. Circulation 2011;124:2661–9.
[88] Hiratzka LF, Bakris GL, Beckman JA, et al. 2010 ACCF/AHA/AATS/ACR/ASA/SCA/SCAI/SIR/STS/SVM guidelines for the diagnosis and management of patients with thoracic aortic disease. Circulation 2010;121:e266–369.

[89] Nienaber CA, Rousseau H, Eggebrecht H, et al. Randomized comparison of strategies for type B aortic dissection: the Investigation of STEnt grafts in Aortic Dissection (INSTEAD) trial. Circulation 2009;120:2519–28.
[90] Trimarchi S, Nienaber CA, Rampoldi V, et al. Role and results of surgery in acute type B aortic dissection: insights from the International Registry of Acute Aortic Dissection (IRAD). Circulation 2006;114:1357–64.
[91] Safi HJ, Miller CC, Reardon MJ, et al. Operation for acute and chronic aortic dissection: recent outcome with regard to neurologic deficit and early death. Ann Thorac Surg 1998;66:402–11.
[92] Sachs T, Ponposelli F, Hagberg R, et al. Open and endovascular repair of type B aortic dissection in the Nationwide Inpatient Sample. J Vasc Surg 2010;52:860–6.
[93] Parker JD, Golledge J. Outcome of endovascular treatment of acute type B aortic dissection. Ann Thorac Surg 2008;85:1707–12.
[94] Fattori R, Tsai TT, Myrmel T, et al. Complicated acute type B dissection: is surgery still the best option? A report from the International Registry of Acute Aortic Dissection. JACC Cardiovasc Interv 2008;1:395–402.
[95] Eggebrecht H, Nienaber CA, Neuhauser M, et al. Endovascular stent-graft placement in aortic dissection: a meta-analysis. Eur Heart J 2006;27:489–98.
[96] Cho JS, Gloviczki P, Martelli E, et al. Long-term survival and late complications after repair of ruptured abdominal aortic aneurysms. J Vasc Surg 1998;27:813–9.
[97] Girardi LN, Krieger KH, Altorki NK, et al. Ruptured descending and thoracoabdominal aortic aneurysms. Ann Thorac Surg 2002;74:1066–70.
[98] LeMaire SA, Rice DC, Schmittling ZC, et al. Emergency surgery for thoracoabdominal aortic aneurysms with acute presentation. J Vasc Surg 2002;35:1171–8.
[99] Jonker FH, Trimarchi S, Verhagen JM, et al. Meta-analysis of open versus endovascular repair for ruptured descending thoracic aortic aneurysm. J Vasc Surg 2010;51:1026–32.

Advances in Anesthesia 32 (2014) 237–243

INDEX

Note: Page numbers of article titles are in **boldface** type.

0737-6146/14/$ – see front matter
http://dx.doi.org/10.1016/S0737-6146(14)00023-9

T

FSC
www.fsc.org
MIX
Papier | Fördert gute Waldnutzung
FSC® C083411

Kolibri 360 GmbH
Ferdinand-Jühlke-Straße 7
99095 Erfurt, Deutschland
produktsicherheit@kolibri360.de